The
Fertility
Sourcebook

Other books by M. Sara Rosenthal

The Thyroid Sourcebook
The Gynecological Sourcebook
The Pregnancy Sourcebook
The Breastfeeding Sourcebook
The Breast Sourcebook
The Gastrointestinal Sourcebook
The Type 2 Diabetic Woman
The Thyroid Sourcebook for Women
Women and Depression
Women of the '60s Turning 50
Women and Passion
Managing PMS Naturally
The Canadian Type 2 Diabetes Sourcebook
The Hypothyroid Sourcebook
Women Managing Stress
50 Ways to Prevent Colon Cancer
50 Ways Women Can Prevent Heart Disease
50 Ways to Relieve Heartburn, Reflux, and Ulcers
50 Ways to Manage Type 2 Diabetes
50 Ways to Prevent and Manage Stress
50 Ways to Fight Depression Without Drugs

SarahealthGuides™

These are M. Sara Rosenthal's own line of health books dedicated to rare, controversial, or stigmatizing health topics you won't find in regular bookstores. They are written by Sara Rosenthal and other health authors. SarahealthGuides™ are available only at online bookstores such as amazon.com. Visit sarahealth.com for upcoming titles.

Stopping Cancer at the Source
Women and Unwanted Hair
Living Well With Celiac Disease by Claudine Crangle

The
Fertility
Sourcebook

Third Edition

M. Sara Rosenthal, Ph.D.

Foreword by **Masood A. Khatamee, M.D., F.A.C.O.G.**

Executive Director, Fertility Research Foundation

Contemporary Books

*Chicago   New York   San Francisco   Lisbon   London   Madrid   Mexico City
Milan   New Delhi   San Juan   Seoul   Singapore   Sydney   Toronto*

Library of Congress Cataloging-in-Publication Data

Rosenthal, M. Sara.
    The fertility sourcebook / M. Sara Rosenthal ; foreword by Masood A. Khatamee.—3rd ed.
       p. cm.
    Includes bibliographical references and index.
    ISBN 0-7373-0380-8 (alk. paper)
    1. Infertility—Popular works.   I. Title.

RC889 .R84 2001
616.6'92—dc21   2001032390

Contemporary Books

*A Division of The **McGraw-Hill** Companies*

1 2 3 4 5 6 7 8 9 DOC/DOC 1 0 9 8 7 6 5 4 3 2

ISBN 0-7373-0380-8

This book was set in Sabon by Rattray Design
Printed and bound by R. R. Donnelley—Crawfordsville
Cover design by Jeanette Wojtyla

McGraw-Hill books are available at special discounts to use as premiums and sales promotions, or for use in corporate training programs. For more information, please write to the Director of Special Sales, Professional Publishing, McGraw-Hill, Two Penn Plaza, New York, NY 10121-2298. Or contact your local bookstore.

The purpose of this book is to educate. It is sold with the understanding that the publisher and author shall have neither liability nor responsibility for any injury caused or alleged to be caused directly or indirectly by the information contained in this book. While every effort has been made to ensure its accuracy, the book's contents should not be construed as medical advice. Each person's health needs are unique. To obtain recommendations appropriate to your particular situation, please consult a qualified health care provider.

This book is printed on acid-free paper.

Contents

Foreword to the First Edition

IN THE TWENTY years I've devoted to infertility patients in New York City, it can be safely said that the couples with the most tangible success were those who sought accurate information and thoroughly educated themselves about their conditions and treatment needs. *The Fertility Sourcebook* gives you the proper tools you need to accomplish this goal. The crucial element in achieving successful fertility treatment is carefully choosing the right doctor. The commitment couples make to their skilled clinician, regardless of the treatment's outcome, affects their treatment options. Staying the course with a single practitioner as opposed to "physician hopping" avoids the possibility of gaps in treatment that may lead to important clinical signs being overlooked.

The standard of quality care dictates that a fertility investigation should not exceed a duration of two months, nor should an investigation be halted and treatment commenced as soon as a single factor, such as a cervical factor, is discovered. Couples should be aware of the possibility of "iatrogenic infertility" arising. This occurs when the origin of infertility goes undiscovered as a result of lack of knowledge or interest on the part of the physician, causing procrastination of treatment if not permanent or irreversible infertility related to the physician's mismanagement of the problem.

Infertility specialists are usually devoted to that sole issue and do not generally diverge into the areas of obstetrics to avoid the obvious distractions that are inherent to these practices. For example, if your physician canceled your postcoital test due to a delivery, it is time to search for another doctor. The time and attention devoted to your individual case is as important as the timing of various clinical tests.

For example, in my own practice, we strongly believe in the consultation, done in the initial visit. Regarded as the most important step in the fertility investigation, this allows the physician the opportunity to take a couple's thorough medical and reproductive histories, as well as allowing time to get to know them and assess their personal needs regarding effective treatment that is right for them as *individuals*. Treatment will take into account their current needs as well as past treatments. It is always important that both partners be present for this crucial visit, preferably at the beginning of the female partner's menstrual cycle. An uninterrupted session lasting from sixty to ninety minutes should be devoted to this initial interview, while instructions and educational material will lead to more effective treatment.

Generally, no testing is performed at this initial visit unless time constraints and scheduling concerns (as in the case of a patient traveling out of state) make it difficult for the patient to return for a subsequent visit. When scheduling an appointment, it is important that the male patient be advised to abstain from intercourse for at least two days, as the semen analysis would most likely be performed on the first visit. The premise of bringing male patients into the office for testing is, in itself, difficult to achieve, as the majority of male partners encountered hesitate to come with their female partners for evaluation. However, it is an important component of the educational phase of their treatment. Male partners need to have their semen analyzed, discuss the results based on what is visible under the microscope, and, if possible, be allowed to view their own specimens under the microscope to enhance their awareness.

For females, a pelvic exam is performed at the first consultation. This usually involves a Pap smear, urine tests, some hormonal testing, as well as screenings for various sexually transmitted diseases and other conditions (such as rubella), which could pose a danger to a potential pregnancy. Although patient compliance is less than optimal in our less-motivated patients, it is also advised that patients take their basal body temperature and bring these charts to each visit. On the day of the initial visit, they are shown how to use the basal temperature thermometer (if they are not acquainted with one), while all of their questions are answered.

The first cycle should be devoted to noninvasive testing, including a postcoital test (PCT), discussed in chapter 6 of this book. Once the clinical data has been compiled from these preliminary tests, a detailed consultation should then be scheduled with the couple to discuss the results and further treatment options. The second cycle is usually devoted to more invasive diagnostic measures, and condom use is recommended to our patients to avoid possible ill effects of certain tests on undiagnosed early pregnancy.

It is abundantly clear that a fertility investigation—even in the event of endoscopic surgery—should not have a duration of more than two or three months. On the other hand, when a single factor is isolated, and the investigation is halted to begin treatment, precious months may be sacrificed if another factor is overlooked due to an *incomplete* investigation.

Fertility treatment can be lengthy and frustrating. It would seem, at times, that the necessary collaboration between specialists prolongs the procurement of the end result. Nevertheless, keep in mind that all treatment must adhere to a reasonable timetable, and the parameters for all modes of therapy must be made clear by your physicians. For instance, if a physician tells you to "take clomiphene citrate for six months and come back if you are not pregnant," it would indicate to the well-informed patients that this practitioner is either less than interested in helping you achieve pregnancy, or unschooled in the monitoring and administration of clomiphene citrate. It could also indicate that he or she is less than interested in treating infertility. Such an instance is cause for concern.

Take care that your testing and analyses, including ultrasound, are *directly* monitored by your physician. It is not in the best interest of the patient to be juggled between various practitioners to obtain testing. For example, in our practice, many tests are performed by our office using an outside facility. This affords us the opportunity to establish that all-important continuity with the patient, as well as to monitor the safety and accuracy of imaging equipment. We also ensure that a certified radiologist is in attendance.

Regarding the issue of assisted reproductive technology (ART), it has sparked a virtual revolution for practitioners, opening up a wellspring of hope for both infertile and sterile couples. New procedures surface almost every month as this new science is advancing exponentially. In many cases, our moral and legal evolution lags behind our scientific evolution. One is hard-pressed to give answers to the many questions that arise concerning inheritance of the offspring and disclosure issues.

This book provides you with guidelines that will aid you in choosing a reputable ART clinic. Valuable information to consider and questions to ask your health care provider when you are an ART candidate are also provided. Of primary concern is the distinction between the rate of live births and the rate of pregnancies. The latter will always be higher. Always be more concerned with the "take-home baby" percentage.

Be certain that before considering ART, complete and thorough treatment for infertility conditions has been attempted. Some centers will try to coerce patients into rushing directly into ART treatment before other, less costly options have been explored. Stringent medical guidelines governing proper medical and surgical treatment must be adhered to, and patients should beware of centers that want hasty decisions regarding ART, as this would be an obvious scheme for monetary gain.

Finally, an issue close to my heart, and held by many physicians as being of paramount importance, is that of *infertility prevention*—also discussed in this book. Twenty percent of North American couples to date are infertile, and the numbers are increasing according to the American College of Obstetrics and Gynecology. This figure accounts for roughly twelve million couples in the United States alone and more than fifty-eight million couples worldwide. Infertility prevention, as a component of sex education, is not widely addressed.

Infertility is caused mostly by sexually transmitted diseases (STDs), and even in well-educated, industrialized countries, such as the United States and Canada, the medical community is failing to stem the tide of STDs, which lead to infertility. Other causes of infertility are ovarian dysfunction, abnormal sperm physiology, and endometriosis. Unfortunately, information about their origins and prevention is grossly lacking. In 1985, I proposed to the medical community that we should endeavor to prevent infertility at all costs. The commonsense modalities we encourage physicians to implement with their patients have received approval from leading health authorities such as the World Health Organization, the American Medical Association, the American Fertility Society, the American College of Physicians and Surgeons, and the Surgeon General of the United States.

By focusing on infertility prevention, we will be able to help eliminate some of the common but completely preventable causes of infertility: STDs. Second, the success rate for pregnancy in infertility intervention is dismal: a mere 13 percent. Logically, it is more cost-effective for the medical community to concentrate on prevention rather than treating resulting conditions. Unfortunately, it appears from the low success rates inherent in infertility treatment that this is the only medical discipline that permits a failure rate of no less than 87 percent! Prevention must be addressed to ward off further tragedy.

The ramifications of infertility treatment are the tremendous costs involved with investigation and treatment. *Only 1 percent of infertile couples can afford the expense of ART.* At this rate, couples in the United States alone invest over seventy million dollars in procedures that offer only a 13 percent success rate, according to the United States Congress Office of Technology Assessment 1989 estimate. In addition to the financial burdens this presents, infertility leaves emotional and psychological scars. Relationships erode under the strain, families flounder, and the very fabric of society, the family unit, is undermined.

Currently, while the World Health Organization acknowledges that infertility prevention lags behind treatment, there are some practical suggestions I give my patients regarding prevention. Even if you, personally, cannot practice these measures, pass them on to your friends, relatives, and—hopefully—your children:

1. Women aged eighteen to twenty-eight are optimally fertile. Fertility decreases with passing time, sharply declining at age thirty-five, and by age forty, becoming the exception rather than the rule. ART is substantially less effective after age thirty-eight.

2. STDs pose the greatest threat to the reproductive tract in both men and women. Oral contraceptives will prevent pregnancy but not STDs. Condoms should be used at all times.

3. If you've never had children, and would like to, do *not* use an intrauterine device (IUD). IUDs are associated with pelvic infections and subsequent infertility.

4. If you have symptoms of endometriosis (discussed in chapter 7 of this book), you *must* have a diagnostic laparoscopy to investigate. Women with mothers or sisters afflicted with endometriosis are at high risk. This condition worsens with age and can lead to infertility.

5. Ovarian dysfunction is being associated with industrial contaminants and may be aggravated by smoking, drug abuse, and pollution. Avoid all "avoidable" toxins! (See chapter 3.)

6. Male subfertility is increasing at alarming rates. In 1960, it was estimated that 6 to 10 percent of adult males were subfertile. By 1990, estimates rose to 35 to 40 percent. Environmental factors are undoubtedly responsible, but more research needs to be done. Be aware and watch the headlines (see chapter 1).

This book will help an infertile couple seek proper advice and treatment. It will also help to educate you about quality fertility treatment and tell you how to maximize your own fertility. Ultimately, the combination of sound prevention and early treatment will preserve the ability of individuals to procreate in the future and allow loving couples to raise the dear families they so strongly desire.

MASOOD A. KHATAMEE, M.D., F.A.C.O.G.
Associate Clinical Professor, Department of
Obstetrics/Gynecology
New York University School of Medicine
New York, New York

Executive Director
Fertility Research Foundation
New York, New York

Acknowledgments

I WISH TO thank the following people, whose expertise and dedication helped to lay so much of the groundwork for this edition of the book: Masood Kahthamee, M.D., F.A.C.O.G., Executive Director of the Fertility Research Foundation, who served as medical advisor on the first edition of this book. Keith Jarvi, M.D., F.R.C.S., and Jerald Bain, F.R.C.S., who served as content advisors on the male-factor infertility sections for the first edition of this book.

A number of past medical advisors on previous works helped me to shape the content for this work. And so I wish to thank the following people (listed alphabetically): Gillian Arsenault, M.D., C.C.F.P., IB.L.C., F.R.C.P; Kelly MacDonald, M.D., F.R.C.P., Micheal Policar, M.D., F.A.C.O.G., Suzanne Pratt, M.D., F.A.C.O.G., and Robert Volpe, M.D., F.R.C.P., F.A.C.P.

William Harvey, Ph.D., L.L.B., University of Toronto Joint Centre for Bioethics, whose devotion to bioethics has inspired me, continues to support my work, and makes it possible for me to have the courage to question and challenge issues in health care and medical ethics. Irving Rootman, Ph.D., Director, University of Toronto Centre for Health Promotion, continues to encourage my interest in primary prevention and health promotion issues. Irving Rootman, Ph.D., Director, University of Toronto Centre for Health Promotion, continues to encourage my interest in primary prevention and health promotion issues. Helen Lenskyj, Ph.D., Department of Sociology and Equity Studies, Ontario Institute for Studies in Education/University of Toronto, and Laura M. Purdy, Professor or Philosophy and Ethics, Wells College, have been central figures in my understanding the complexities of women's health issues and feminist bioethics.

I'd also like to thank Meredith Schwartz, Editorial Assistant on the this edition, and Larissa Kostoff, Editorial Consultant on this edition and past editions.

Introduction

THE MORE THINGS CHANGE, THE MORE THEY STAY THE SAME

WELCOME TO THE third edition of *The Fertility Sourcebook*! Since the first edition of this book came out, much has changed in some areas, but unfortunately, too many things have *not* changed. When I first wrote this book in 1995, I had envisioned most of my words to become obsolete by the 21st century. This has not happened. Costly treatments (financially and psychologically) with low success rates is still the norm when looking at Western-style, conventional fertility treatment offered by most fertility clinics. I was alarmed, when revising this book, to learn, too, that many questionable treatments that were being done in the mid-to-late 1990s are still being done. It's important for you to note, too, that male doctors still dominate the fertility industry, and some feminist critics argue that what have become standard issue treatments at the best teaching hospitals are nothing less than unethical experimentation on women's bodies. Indeed, many male doctors were after "stardom" in their field at the expense of their patients' health. For example, throughout the 1990s, shocking tales of implanting more than half a dozen embryos at once abounded; today this is frowned upon, but the fact that there is still no law against this is noteworthy. In fact, fertility treatment remains largely unregulated. What *has* changed are the questions surrounding fertility treatments. There are more than ever before, and now there are many questions surrounding the disposal or usage of the unused embryos that have piled up since fertility treatment became a "norm" in the Western world. Questions regarding stem-cell research and cloning, for example, abound. Another thing that has changed between editions of this book is me. In 1995, I was married and unable to get pregnant. I thought one of the best ways to research my infertility was to write this book. After I learned more, it became clear to me that I would not be able to submit myself to the kind of workups and treatments that were the norm at the time, and I remained childfree. Shortly after the first edition of this book was published (and hailed), I was invited to be a keynote speaker for an infertility organization in my home city of Toronto. Some women, I was told, were so offended by my criticism of treatments, and my choice to live childfree, they complained to the organizer of the talk. The organizer told me that my talk would have been more accepted if I had "cried" when giving my story of infertility. Apparently I seemed too composed about my circumstances, and therefore, must not have "really" wanted a child. People who paid to see me speak were refunded their money by this organization, which was embarrassed to have presented a speaker with an alternate approach to her infertility. I argued with the organizer of this talk at the time, that surely, seeing someone who had taken a "different road" might contribute to a more informed perspective, but she felt that I had harmed the audience by suggesting that what they were doing might be unhealthy. It became clear to me then (circa 1996) that I was alone in my questioning of the fertility industry. My life took a different direction. I became interested in the field of bioethics and attended a lecture at the University of Toronto's Joint Centre for Bioethics on the ethics of fertility treatment. To my surprise, I was approached by a woman who told me that she saw me speak at that infamous lecture. She was doing her Ph.D. thesis on infertility organizations, and she told me: "You were the only speaker they had who said something new and different, and I really appreciated it." When I told her about the outcome of that talk, she said: "I'm not surprised. These organizations get their funding from fertility drug companies." That explained a lot. Today, I have completed my doctorate in sociology and bioethics, and much of what I do is to look at reproductive health in a more critical fashion.

This edition of *The Fertility Sourcebook* presents you with all the information you need if you are seeking answers to infertility in the conventional, Western medical framework. Let's face it: this is the medical model we're stuck with, and much as I'd like to, I can't "reinvent" our fertility industry. So . . .

I'll tell you what's done, what's not, what ought to be, and questions you should raise each step of the way. This book also has a lot of information about possible causes of your infertility—causes that you may have some control over, and causes that may be beyond your control. Without exception, every chapter has been revised, particularly chapter 9 entitled "Out-of-Body Experiences" which discusses the reproductive technologies in detail, including ethical issues surrounding their use. As a result of the popularity of reproductive technologies in the gay and lesbian community, I've also devoted a separate chapter to the unique issues surrounding fertility and parenting for same sex couples.

Finally, I call your attention to chapter 1, "Infertile Ground" which discusses the social and environmental causes of infertility. Many of you may also find the section on alternative systems of healing a good place to start.

I sincerely hope that this book puts you on the right path, regardless of the outcome. Many readers of *The Fertility Sourcebook* have taken the time to contact me and tell me about their progress. I'm eager to hear from all of you. In fact, much of the information in this edition comes from past readers of *The Fertility Sourcebook* who have made suggestions for content. I'm thrilled that so many couples have come to embrace *The Fertility Sourcebook* as their conception health resource.

For those of you who are successful in getting pregnant and having a child, you may benefit, too, from *The Pregnancy Sourcebook* and *The Breastfeeding Sourcebook*. For more information, visit me online at www.sarahealth.com.

The
Fertility
Sourcebook

1

Infertile Ground:
Social and Environmental
Causes of Infertility

In 2002, ONE-THIRD of women who reach forty have not yet had a baby. Regardless of the hype and hope surrounding the infertility treatment market, the "Age Bomb" is the largest contributing factor to infertility. If you've never had a child, you're probably curious about the state of your reproductive organs. That's only natural in light of the fact that we are in the midst of an infertility epidemic. The funny thing about this infertility epidemic, though, is that we really can't prove that it exists. Interpreting the statistics regarding fertility rates (production of children) and fecundity rates (the capacity to reproduce) can be tricky.

Approximately 5.3 million couples experience infertility each year, according to the American Society for Reproductive Medicine. Surveys indicate about 15 percent of all couples will experience infertility at some time during their reproductive lives.

This chapter helps you to make sense of what's going on "out there," that is, what is affecting your own fertility and contributing to a very real infertility crisis. Sweeping changes in social attitudes about sexuality and marriage combined with economic realities have forced women into a position of delaying childbirth. Women more than men are also paying a high price for "un-condomed" sexual encounters they had in their teens and twenties: Asymptomatic sexually transmitted diseases such as chlamydia can travel up the reproductive tract, scarring fallopian tubes and rendering women in their thirties and forties infertile as a result.

And then there is the environmental toxin story. Sperm counts are down all over the world. Estrogen-related conditions affecting women, such as endometriosis and fibroids, are also on the rise. Environmental toxins are believed to be the cause, discussed in detail beginning on page 8. The focus of this chapter is not lifestyle factors affecting fertility, but social and environmental factors you cannot easily control, if at all.

A Sign of the Times

If we simply look at birthrate statistics, there's no doubt that they've declined since the late 1950s and early 1960s. But that's because there has been a major upheaval in the size of families and the nature of "family." Couples are marrying later in life, fewer people are marrying, fewer married women are having children, women are having fewer children, and more planned first pregnancies are occurring in women over thirty-five—which, not so long ago, used to be the "cutoff" date for childbearing. In 1994, 13 percent of all live births were to mothers aged thirty-five or older; in 1987, only 5 percent of all live births were to mothers in this age group, which represents a 9 percent increase in less than a decade. This is considered to be a significant increase.

Beginning around the mid-1980s, we began to experience a second-wave baby boom (called the Echo Boom) that brought about a significant rise in fertility rates—a rise not seen since the 1950s. Obviously the children of the first baby boom had grown up and were having children themselves. But they were having fewer children than were the couples of the 1950s and early 1960s, and fewer of these first-wave boomers were even having children in the first place. There are so many first-wave boomers that any reproductive activity on their part profoundly affected the almost stagnant birthrate of the time. We also have no way of knowing how many of the newborns included in this second wave were conceived through assisted conception techniques, the aid of fertility drugs, spontaneous lovemaking, or carefully planned lovemaking. Furthermore, how many of these births were to teenage mothers? How many births were wanted? Remember, in today's social trends, more teenagers are sexually active, resulting in more teenage pregnancies and unplanned births (discussed further on).

What can we prove about fertility by examining the rate of "nonbirths"? For example, in the late 1980s, a study in Sweden by Princeton University and Lunds University revealed that the rate of childless white women was no higher in 1981 than it was in 1941. (Remember, the attack on Pearl Harbor didn't happen until December. In the United States, there were plenty of white men around until about January 1942.) The same study revealed that the rate of childless non-white women over the age of thirty has dropped since the 1950s. Again, the social trends of the times greatly affect this statistic. The real translation: Fewer white women got pregnant during the Great Depression (which really wasn't over in the United States until 1941, when the Americans entered the war). And since the 1950s, more non-white women have joined the poverty line, gotten pregnant as teenagers, or gotten pregnant as a way to get more money through government assistance. (Single mothers in North America with no higher education can make more money on welfare with two or more children than they can working to support one child!)

As for fecundity, here's what the statisticians have to say: If you compare women of the same age from the 1960s and the 1980s, their capacity to reproduce remains at exactly the same rate. Because women in the 1980s are choosing to have children at an older age, however, the overall infertility rate has risen. A nineteen-year-old woman today is just as fertile as a nineteen-year-old woman in 1960; a forty-year-old woman today is just as fertile (and probably in better shape) as a forty-year-old woman in 1960. But more forty-year-olds in the 1980s (and even more today) desire pregnancy than did the forty-year-olds of 1960 or the nineteen-year-olds of today. Therefore, more women are having difficulty conceiving today than in the 1960s.

There's another wrinkle we need to add to the fecundity statistic: More nineteen-year-old men and women were having unprotected sex with multiple partners in the 1970s and 1980s than they were in the 1950s and 1960s. As a result, more people in their thirties and forties today have sexually transmitted diseases (STDs), which can or did wreak havoc on their fecundity. (See further on.)

Many sociologists argue that the so-called infertility crisis is created to feed the infertility industry, which boasts annual revenues exceeding two billion dollars. For example, some statistics quote that in 1965 the U.S. infertility rate was 13.3 percent compared to 13.7 percent in 1988. According to the U.S. Office of Technology Assessment, infertility rates for married women have even dropped from 11.2 percent in 1965 to 8 percent in 1988. The problem with these statistics, however, is that criteria has changed between 1965 and 1988. The age of the average infertile couple in 1965 was considerably younger than the 1988 couple. The median age for first-time mothers (planned children, that is) was twenty-four in the 1960s and twenty-nine in the 1980s and early-to-mid 1990s. And as we've entered the new millennium, that median age is increasing. In addition, as infertility often goes unreported, statistics are usually lower than the actual rate anyway. As for the "married women" statistic, it is more likely that fewer women were married in 1988, compared to 1965. Additionally, none of these statistics factor in same-sex couples who require assistance through new reproductive technologies (NRTs) to get pregnant.

A more interesting statistic is the increase in physician consults over infertility. In the United States, 600,000 women visited physicians for this problem in 1968; by 1982, the number increased to 1.6 million.

But since 1988, infertility rates have increased because there are more women in the population between the ages of thirty-five and forty-four who desire children. In fact, there were four million more women in that age group in 1988 than there were in 1982. So statistically, the number of childless women increased by 37 percent in just six years. And, since at least 40 percent of all infertile couples will seek help, the problem of infertility becomes far more prevalent in our society.

We're also living much longer these days. Life expectancy has increased to seventy-eight in the 1990s from forty-five in the 1900s. Better standards of living (for example, wealth, education, better sanitation, better nutrition, and a safer food supply) are all contributing factors. As a result, more women are experiencing menopause than ever before, while more women who reach menopause are feeling robbed of their reproductive capacity too early. Therefore the baby boomers are in their peak "envelope pushing years," which has led to an explosion in fertility treatments all over the developed world. When the first edition of this book was published, women were "pushing" the limits of fertility at forty-five. Today, postmenopausal pregnancies are not uncommon, while as of this writing, women have made headlines by having babies in their sixties, discussed more in the section "Pregnancy after fifty," on page 221.

Pregnant Teenagers . . . and You

What has teenage pregnancy got to do with you and this current infertility crisis? Quite a lot! The answer to the question "When are you most likely to get pregnant?" is: When you're in high school! Fertility actually begins to decline after twenty-five, and considerably more so after thirty. Ninety-seven percent of all twenty-year-old women are fertile; by forty-five, that number dwindles to 5 percent (see Table 1.1). As women age, there is also an increase in conditions such as endometriosis, discussed in chapter 7.

Your grandmothers or mothers were likely pregnant teens—who got married. Or they were when they got married, and then got pregnant. The United States has more than double the teenage pregnancy rate of any Western industrialized country, with more than a million teenagers becoming pregnant each year. In a 1953 study, it was estimated that a large percentage of all marriages were to pregnant teenage girls. By 1978, the number of pregnant teenagers who married dwindled to 31 percent. Today, 70 percent of all pregnant teenagers remain single. As attitudes about sexuality and women's roles in society have shifted over the last forty years, the marriage rates have declined while sexual activity has increased. So that means a few things:

- Fewer people are willing to commit themselves to a life partner earlier in life, thereby making it more difficult for women in their twenties and thirties to find suitable life partners and resulting in a further delay in childbearing.
- More casual, unprotected sexual encounters earlier in life have led to an explosion in STDs, which can damage reproductive organs (particularly in women), causing infertility in their thirties and forties.

Table 1.1 Fertility Through the Ages*

Age	Likelihood of Getting Pregnant*	Likelihood of Infertility
20–24	100%	3%
25–29	94%	5%
30–34	86%	8%
35–39	70%	15%
40–44	36%	32%
45–49	5%	69%
50+	0%	100%

Source: Adapted from Khatamee, Masood, M.D. "Infertility: A Preventable Epidemic?" *International Journal of Fertility*, vol. 33, no. 4 (1988): 246–51.

*Presuming optimum health

More choices equals fewer choices

At one time, women could choose between a career or having a baby. The choice for most women today is whether they will have a baby *and* work, or not have a baby *and* work. In other words, few women have the luxury to choose between staying home or working. How did this happen?

The declining rate of teenage marriage in North America since the 1960s is directly related to more educational opportunities and career choices for women, as well as a general acceptance of common law living versus marriage. But a decline in blue collar jobs has led to poor job prospects for young adults without higher education, meaning that more women have had no choice but to enter the blue or pink collar workforce. Younger women are also competing for jobs with older, divorced women, who must work in order to make ends meet. The high cost of living has also made it virtually impossible for most young adults to afford a family until they're in their mid-to-late twenties. Therefore, while marriage or family plans are often delayed, intercourse is not. The prospect of "waiting until marriage" becomes more and more unrealistic as marriage seems unaffordable until relatively late in life, or even unlikely to teens growing up in dysfunctional or broken homes (I'll get to this).

Consequences of Sex Before Marriage

As a society, we all pay for unplanned or unwanted pregnancy, as well as a teenage mother's unpreparedness for raising children. For example, 80 percent of teenage mothers drop out of school and raise their children in poverty. We also know that 83 percent of the teenagers who become pregnant are already poor. Meanwhile, one-third of those mothers will become pregnant again with a second child within two years, usually to boost welfare incomes. And those baby girls who are born in poverty are more likely to grow up in abusive or violent homes; pregnancy is often used as a form of escaping an abusive home or circumstance. So what happens is that the circumstances leading to teenage pregnancy in the first place feed off each other, perpetuating the problem.

Furthermore, students are becoming sexually active at younger ages compared to just one decade ago. Seventy percent of teenagers are sexually active prior to their high school graduation. Most surveys show that the average age of sexual intercourse is sixteen years. In fact, it is not unusual for a twelve-year-old student to have had at least one sexual encounter. Meanwhile, roughly 63 percent of students aged fourteen to twenty-one are sexually active; 40 percent of all teenage girls become pregnant; and 20 percent go to term. Add to all this the increase in sexually explicit media, and you get an explosion in sexual activity among teenagers. The most haunting statistic is that the sisters of teenagers who become pregnant are four times more likely to get pregnant themselves.

The consequences of all this sex at younger ages is that the likelihood of casual sexual encounters without appropriate protection from STDs has increased. Women who were having casual sex in the early-to-mid 1980s may have been using birth control, but may not have been using condoms to protect themselves from STDs. At least three million cases of chlamydia and one million cases of gonorrhea are diagnosed annually in the United States alone. Right now, 80 percent of all female-factor infertility is believed to be caused by untreated sexually transmitted diseases that have scarred the fallopian tubes or caused damage to the reproducive tract. This is discussed more in chapter 2.

The impact of safe sex

It's estimated that at least half of all infertility is 100 percent preventable through safe sex. A 1987 article pointed out that well over sixty-five billion dollars annually was spent in the United States on infertility workups and treatments; but by supplying free condoms to all for the bargain price of roughly $350,000, the savings could be enormous, while 50 percent of infertility could be prevented.

The impact of abortion

As a staunch prochoice advocate, delivering this news to you is all the more difficult: When abortion was illegal, older, infertile women had more choices in terms of adoption. But because so many unwanted pregnancies end in abortion, the pool of available newborns in developed countries has dried up, making it cheaper in some respects to go for more exotic fertility treatments than to adopt. Fewer babies has also created a market for exotic fertility treatments. Adoption is discussed in more detail in chapter 12.

There is another problem. Since women are not being educated properly about how their fertility can decline beginning at age twenty-five, some women may have made a different choice about having an abortion if they were given all the facts. In fact, one-third of all infertile women have had an abortion at some point in their lives. Perhaps women should be lobbying for informed choice, not just prochoice.

The Impact of Sexism in the Workplace

The term *paternalism* means, in layterms, "old boys club." What has this got to do with your fertility? Again, quite a lot. As of this writing, only 3 percent of all top level managers in corporate North America is composed of women. That's just terrible. Some female executives refer to the "glass ceiling" as a "plastic ceiling" because at least you can break glass! As any feminist will tell you, women haven't come all that far; the strides women have made in the workforce have been on male terms. The proof? Women are routinely discriminated against in the business world for wanting to bear children. Instead of being told they're terminated upon announcement of, or return from, maternity leave, other excuses such as "downsizing" or "restructuring" are used. If you look at all the money women pay to get pregnant and have children (see chapter 8), and all the money spent on childcare programs and supporting public health initiatives such as breast-feeding, you're looking at a very lopsided scale.

Companies that support women for having children are virtually nonexistent. This forces many women to delay childbearing until they're in a more secure job, or until they can afford to leave their jobs. Otherwise, most women find that they are backpeddling: Making just about enough money to pay someone else to raise their children.

Paternalistic medicine

This is entirely another book (and I'd love to write it), but there is an important link you need to understand about infertility treatment and paternalistic practices in medicine. The term paternalistic literally means "parental." A paternalistic doctor presents selected information in the hopes that you will consent to the intervention that he or she feels is in your best interests. In some cases, the doctor will not seek your consent at all and will inform you about what will be taking place. Paternalistic medicine refers, in general, to male-dominated, Western medicine in a world where women are patients 25 percent more frequently than men. It is treatment-based rather than prevention-based and tends to be focused on the disease rather than the person. It is a style of medicine that is heavy on jargon and clinical research, light on patient education. It is also deeply funded, if not controlled, by pharmaceutical companies. When you look at the cost of fertility treatments (see chapter 8), compared to the odds they offer of taking home a healthy baby at the end of the treatment, ask yourself who stands to profit? And at whose expense? Right now, most fertility programs or clinics are male-led.

Environmental Links to Infertility

In 1962, environmentalist Rachel Carson wrote a book called *Silent Spring*, which essentially said: Wake up and smell the chemicals; wildlife and humans are dying from pesticides and pollutants. Today, many renowned scientists in both the environmental and medical research communities are concluding that Rachel Carson was right all along, including Dr. Theo Colborne, senior scientist at the World Wildlife Fund and coauthor of *Our Stolen Future* (1996).

Environmental Estrogens and Male Infertility

One out of every twenty-five males is infertile. In about 30 to 40 percent of infertile men, the results of semen analysis are abnormal—including low or absent sperm count, dead sperm, abnormally shaped sperm, slow- or nonmoving sperm. Environmental scientists may provide some answers.

There is mounting evidence that male factor infertility is on the rise as a result of environmental toxins. A 1995 study published in *The New England Journal of Medicine* concluded that there has been a true decline in the quality of human semen since 1973. The characteristics of semen from a fertile man in 1973 were significantly superior to his 1995 counterpart's. This decline is attributed to a decrease in the number of Sertoli cells produced by men today. And what's causing this? Well, apparently, life on planet Earth is being threatened by a group of substances known as "environmental estrogens." A very long grocery list of organic chemicals, found in various pesticides and plastics, are transforming in the natural environment into a substance identical to the female hormone estrogen. And the results are absolutely disastrous, threatening not only human fertility, but contributing to an epidemic of reproductive cancers, such as breast and testicular cancer.

For quite some time, environmental scientists had begun to notice that several wildlife species were experiencing "hermaphroditic" traits. In the Florida swamplands, for example, alligators are simply not breeding. A concerned research team from the University of Florida went into the swamps to find out why. These researchers pulled male alligators out of the water to examine their genitals. The majority of the male alligators they found were sterile as a result of their either nondeveloped or abnormally shaped penises. A chemical spill in nearby waters was found to be the culprit, which was having an "estrogenic effect" on the alligators' natural habitat.

Twenty-three hundred kilometers north, in a Canadian creek on Lake Superior, scientists found that fish living in waters close to a pulp mill that contained certain chemicals with "estrogenic effects" were now complete hermaphrodites. The male fish in these waters had developed ovaries and were sterile; the female fish had exaggerated ovaries.

Meanwhile, Swedish and U.K. researchers have been concerned since the late 1980s over a dramatic increase in male infertility, while an increasing number of male infants are being born with a condition known as *cryptorchidism*, where the testicles do not descend into the scrotum, but remain undescended inside the abdomen. One study found that there has indeed been a huge decrease over the last fifty years in the quality of human semen. There has also been a huge increase in the incidence of testicular and prostate cancers. In Britain, testicular cancer incidence has tripled over the last fifty years; it is now the most common cancer in young men under age thirty. In Denmark alone, there has been a 400 percent increase in testicular cancer. As for prostate cancer, its incidence has doubled over the last decade.

Those troubling pesticides

Pesticides are major contributors to this environmental estrogen problem, one of the most notorious of which is DDT. DDT stands for "dichlorodiphenyl-trichloroethane" and was formally banned in most industrialized countries by the mid-1970s. It was discovered in the late nineteenth century by a German chemist, but wasn't considered an insecticide until 1939, when Switzerland's Paul Muller won a Nobel Prize for the newfound usage. DDT was considered a godsend to the agricultural world and, in fact, was thought to be an effective combatant against lice. During the second world war, soldiers, refugees, and prisoners were dusted with DDT to kill lice.

DDT was banned in North America because it was essentially wreaking havoc on several wildlife species. But its effects on the human population should be looked at. Not only is DDT considered to be an estrogen pollutant when it breaks down into its by-product, dichlorodiphenylethane (DDE), but it's a known carcinogen (cancer-causing agent) as well as a substance that lowers human sperm count. Until very recently, no one really understood why DDT seemed to target reproductive systems. However, with the discovery of environmental estrogens, the mystery is apparently solved. Unfortunately, even though DDT is banned in North America, it is still in use in other parts of the world. That's because we make it and market it to less-developed countries. Dibromochloropropane (DBCP), which was also banned in 1977 because it was known to cause sterility, was used in the banana belt (Ecuador and other countries) to fumigate bananas. Currently about twenty-five-thousand workers from twelve developing countries are working with this known hazard.

But even though DDT has been pretty much banned in most countries since 1972, it remains active in the environment for twenty-five to thirty years.

Organochlorines

Pesticides aren't the only problem. A variety of exotic chemical concoctions are in our air in abundance. Organochlorines are particularly nasty; they're nondegradable in the environment and are fat soluble in the bodies of wildlife and humans. An organochlorine is what you get when you take natural chlorine, which is found in ordinary salt, and split the salt molecule to make chlorine gas. When that chlorine gas comes into contact with any organic (that is, carbon-based) matter, you wind up with an organochlorine. So organochlorines such as DDT, DDE, dioxins, and polychlorinated biphenyls (PCBs) have accumulated and concentrated in the food chain.

It's estimated that billions of gallons of these toxic substances have been released into an unsuspecting environment. Since these chemicals are resistant to breaking down, they're spread around the world through the air and water, exposing us to these poisons in our food, groundwater, surface water, and air. A 1987 study identified 177 organochlorines in the fat, breast milk, blood, semen, and breath of the general North American population. According to a 1992 Greenpeace report on chlorine and human health, no industrial organochlorines are known to be nontoxic.

A brief history of manmade chemicals

Although PCBs were first introduced into the environment in 1929, large scale production of man-made chemicals didn't really take place until just after World War II. By 1947, the United States was producing 259,000 pounds of pesticides annually; by 1960, 636.7 million pounds of pesticides were being produced. In terms of synthetic fibers, between 1945 and 1970, the production increased by almost 6,000 percent; plastics production increased by almost 2,000 percent; nitrogen fertilizers and synthetic organic chemicals increased by about 1,000 percent; and organic solvents increased by 746 percent. Industry now produces roughly forty million tons of chlorine per year. That chlorine is then combined with petrochemicals to make organochlorine products, such as PVC plastic, solvents, pesticides, and refrigerants. After that, thousands of organochlorines occur as by-products—particularly in the pulp and paper industry. These chemicals are spread by wind and water, sprayed on plants, or ingested by animals we eat, settling in our fat and tissues.

Sperm Wars

There are many people who stand to lose a great deal of money if, in fact, sperm counts are down as a result of environmental toxins. If this news is confirmed beyond a reasonable doubt in the medical journals, then, of course, more stringent restrictions on industry would have to be imposed in the interests of environment and public health. The first news about declining sperm counts hit the media in the early 1990s when researchers from Copenhagen University reported sperm counts were falling around the world (based on an analysis of sixty-one different studies). Since then, several studies have been published about sperm counts that either contradict or at least criticize earlier studies on sperm counts.

The latest results

According to U.S. researchers, who actually set out to disprove the "falling sperm" stories, sperm counts are falling faster than anyone thought. The original sixty-one studies used by the first group of Danish researchers were reanalyzed. And guess what? The original Danish study was correct after all. In Europe and the United States, there is a "strong and significant decline" in sperm count. Regional variations in temperature were attributed to the contradictory results.

This latest study has the support of the National Institutes of Health (NIH). In a November 1997 statement, the NIH declared that sperm densities have decreased 1.5 million sperm per milliliter (1.5 percent per year) between 1938 and 1990. And in Europe, sperm counts are falling at twice that rate (about 3.1 percent per year).

This time, researchers accounted for known factors affecting sperm quality, such as age, smoking, climate/temperature, and ethnicity. The only thing left is environmental toxins with estrogenic effects, such as persistent organic pollutants (POPs), which range from pesticides such as DDT to industrial chemicals such as PCBs.

Men living in the Ukraine are experiencing record high numbers of infertility as a result of the Chernobyl disaster. In fact, The New England Cryogenic Center has a contract with the Ukraine to supply them with U.S. sperm.

Environmental Estrogens and Women

Environmental estrogens are linked to a steady rise in estrogen-dependent cancers, such as breast, ovarian, and uterine cancers, as well as estrogen-dependent conditions, such as endometriosis and fibroids, both discussed in chapter 7. For example, nobody knows for certain what causes endometriosis, but currently environmental factors are identified as the chief cause. These "environmental estrogens," as they're called, are being linked to an alarming increase in estrogen-dependent conditions such as endometriosis, fibroids, and a variety of reproductive cancers. Dioxins, in particular, have been linked to endometriosis. In a University of South Florida study, female monkeys fed very small amounts of dioxins went on to develop moderate to severe endometriosis within four years.

Obviously, a woman's fertility is threatened by reproductive cancer, too. For more information on breast cancer and environmental toxins, consult my book, *The Breast Sourcebook*.

Limiting your exposure

Right now, the only hope you and I have of eliminating these toxins is through consumer lobbying. The best place to start the environmental "clean up" is in your kitchen. Your weekly groceries probably contain residues from pesticides and other organochlorines (on store-bought fruits and vegetables); hormones in meat products, as well as a number of "extras" you may not have bargained for, which were fed to your meat when it was still alive. This includes feed additives, antibiotics, and tranquilizers. Meanwhile, anything packaged will most likely contain dyes and flavors from a variety of chemical concoctions.

Airborne contaminants, waste, and spills affect the water and soil, which affects virtually everything we ingest. In addition, when one species becomes unable to reproduce, the food chain is interrupted, and eventually trickles down to our kitchen tables. Cleaning up the food chain is all part of creating a healthy, contaminant-free diet for ourselves. So make the following grocery list before your next shopping trip:

- You can find out what your produce has eaten, and whether it was injected with anything, by calling the USDA information line at (202) 720-2791. In Canada, call Agriculture and Agrafood Canada at (613) 952-8000.
- You can find out what waters your fish has swum in by calling the above numbers.
- You can find "safe food" that is organically grown through a number of natural produce supermarkets, such as Bread and Circus, for example.
- You can find out what your grown produce was sprayed with by calling the numbers listed above.
- You can find out more about your supermarket's buying habits when it comes to produce by contacting your supermarket's head office.

Since the origin of the word *consumer* comes from the word *consume*—to eat—becoming vigilant about our groceries is the only way to help change the produce and foodstuff industry. Customers are incredibly powerful to any company. In the 1980s, it was the "vigilante consumer" who helped to make manufacturers more green friendly and value-conscious. In many instances, the sheer volume of customer complaints and customer letters has completely changed not only individual companies' habits and policies, but an entire industry's. If enough customers ban products, protest manufacturing or agricultural practices, and so on, the companies will change. Bring new meaning to the adage "The customer is always right!"

Read any good labels, lately?

Worried about the plastic that lines certain canned goods? Demand labeling that identifies the organic chemicals used to make that plastic. Worried about the plastics used in various cosmetics, detergents, and spermicides? Then write letters to manufacturers; call toll-free numbers; start a news group on the Internet; lobby; protest; ban products to help change standards. Don't be afraid to write letters to the editors of daily newspapers or call for press conferences on various labeling, packaging, or ingredient issues that concern you. What exactly is plastic wrap made out of anyway? You have a right to know! What was this spinach sprayed with? You have a right to a label that reads: "This produce sprayed with endosulfan." To date, the chemical ingredients that make up plastic products are kept from the consumer because they're considered "trade secrets." This is unacceptable. As consumers, we must use our collective voice to help get labeling details on the containers that house our produce, as well as the farmers that grew our produce.

What Your Government Is Doing

In 1958, the U.S. government passed an amendment to the federal Food, Drug and Cosmetic Act designed to protect the public from residues of carcinogenic pesticides in processed foods. It was called The Delaney Clause, which called for an absolute ban on these chemicals. But in 1965, the National Academy of Sciences (NAS) concluded that an absolute ban wasn't scientifically realistic and the clause was abandoned. Ever since, the Food and Drug Administration (FDA) and the Department of Agriculture began to set "allowable" levels of chemicals in our food.

The Environmental Protection Agency (EPA) in the United States in the late 1980s established "negligible risk tolerances" for all carcinogenic pesticides on all foods. But this particular risk assessment doesn't consider the cumulative effects of possible cancer-causing pesticides in our diet, drinking water, and air. In other words, how many "hits" can our cells take with these pesticides before turning cancerous?

By 1992, the EPA was ordered to remove food with pesticide residues from supermarket shelves. This helped get the National Cancer Institute to at least begin to study the effects of environmental contaminants.

To date, The International Joint Commission, which is an advisory body on environmental issues, has recommended to the U.S. and Canadian governments that organochlorines should be phased out as a class, not simply on a chemical-by-chemical basis. For more information about environmental contamination, see my book *Stopping Cancer at the Source*.

Now that you've covered the infertile ground, it's time to start laying the groundwork and doing your homework. The next chapter will walk you through the "preconception" steps of weeding out any STDs that might impair your fertility and finding the right doctor to put you on the path to conception.

2

Who Is a Fertility Doctor
and When Do You Need One?

IN THE SAME way that one is assumed innocent until proven guilty, one is assumed to be fertile until proven otherwise. That means that before you can start investigating why you may not be able to conceive, you must have solid, concrete proof to support your suspicions of infertility in the *first* place. (Again, infertility, as stressed in this book's introduction, can mean anything from delayed conception to temporary or permanent barriers to conception.) In other words, you shouldn't graduate to a "fertility doctor" until you do the groundwork. The first part of this chapter explains what this groundwork really involves when it comes to conception—because unless you've done *yours*, a fertility doctor cannot do *his* or *hers*.

The second part of this chapter focuses on who the appropriate fertility specialist is (which depends on who has the problem), what the appropriate diagnostic steps are, and when you need to see various specialists in the conception planning process. Finally, we discuss how to "use" a fertility specialist, which is a must if our fertility workups are to be successful.

The Groundwork

I liken the conception process to yardwork. There are several things you need to weed out before your yard is pronounced "healthy." Similarly, there are several physical problems *you* need to weed out before you can really begin "trying." Unless you're prepared to do this yardwork, a proper fertility workup cannot be done.

Preconception Weeding

Although many couples think the first step in conception planning is to take a crash course in menstrual cycle mechanics (discussed further below and in chapter 3), this actually is a later step. The absolute first step in conception planning is pulling out the weeds that may interfere with or make you question conception. In short, *pull the weeds before you conceive*!

To do the necessary weeding, you'll need a "weed doctor." Who is this person? It depends on where you live. Anywhere in Canada, or in smaller communities in the United States that are far from large medical centers, a primary care physician can do the "weeding." In larger urban centers in the United States, the task of weeding is best performed by either a genetic counselor (who any primary care physician can refer you to) or a gynecologist. A *primary care physician* can be an internist, general practitioner, or family practitioner.

You and your partner should see the weed doctor together. That way, one doctor will be managing all the necessary screenings and histories for both of you. At all times, if a woman is seeing a gynecologist with whom she's comfortable, the gynecologist may do the "weeding" for both partners as well. It is a *mistake* to seek out *any* kind of fertility specialist until this weeding process is completed.

Weeding consists of being screened for a number of problems at the outset of your conception journey rather than at the middle or at the end. The time you take to be screened now could save you months or years of frustration. If a problem is discovered now, you'll have more time to correct it. If no problem is found and if you don't conceive within a reasonable amount of time, you'll be able to cross off a number of possible problems from the list. You can then get to the bottom of your conception delay much sooner. Finally, if you do get pregnant soon after the weeding, you'll have taken every precaution to prevent or prepare for a high-risk pregnancy.

Depending on the results of the screenings, however, one or both of you may be referred to a specialist. In the case of a primary care doctor, his or her role is to manage your *overall* health. In other words, primary care doctors specialize in being *generalists*. When the time comes, they will refer you to the appropriate specialist—be it a "fertility" specialist, a gynecologist, an obstetrician, or even a perinatalogist (specializing in high-risk pregnancies).

You probably will be screened for the following:

Several genetic disorders

Don't even *think* about having children until you've been checked for genetic disorders. You can be a carrier of a disorder even if you are not personally affected by it. Some examples of these disorders are Tay-Sachs disease (if you're Jewish or French Canadian);

sickle cell anemia (if you're of Mediterranean or African descent); certain diseases linked to the X chromosome (in other words, diseases carried by the female and passed on to her male child, such as various forms of muscular dystrophy including leukodystrophies and hemophilia). When you present yourself to your doctor and tell him or her that you'd like to be screened for any possible genetic or chromosomal disorders, he or she will take it from there. Your race and family history will determine which diseases you need to be screened for. If you happen to be a carrier of a disease linked to the X chromosome, you'll need to go for genetic counseling and weigh the risks of even having a child, as well as prepare for various prenatal tests during a pregnancy. If you carry any genetic diseases that requires *both* you and your partner to be carriers before the genes can be passed on (such as Tay-Sachs), then your partner *must* be screened as well. If you're both carriers, you'll also need genetic counseling before you venture into the "trying" phase.

Rh incompatibility

Your blood type is either Rh positive (meaning you have an Rh factor in your blood, as 85 percent of us do) or Rh negative (meaning you don't have an Rh factor). Either is fine, *but* if the male partner is Rh positive and the female partner is Rh negative, the blood type of your offspring may not match *the mother's*. If not diagnosed, this can be a big problem during delivery or even in the event of a pregnancy loss or therapeutic abortion. However, once diagnosed, medications such as Rhogam can fix the problem.

German measles (rubella)

When you're planning a pregnancy, it's important to screen out rubella. In early pregnancy, this disease can damage the fetus. Most women (one in seven) were vaccinated long ago for rubella but may not remember the vaccine. Women can be screened for a rubella *titer*, a test that detects whether antibodies to rubella are present in the bloodstream. If you have the antibodies, you're immune; if you don't, you'll need to consult with your doctor about the next step, which usually involves a vaccine.

Human immunodeficiency virus (HIV)

If you have reason to suspect that you've been exposed to HIV, you must take an HIV antibody test if you're planning pregnancy. Review the risk groups and risk factors with your doctor, or call your local AIDS hotline.

Chlamydia

If you have chlamydia, you'll need to make sure it is treated before you try to conceive. (Even so, 10 percent of the time, people who have chlamydia will test negative for it.)

Chlamydia is one of the most common STDs in North America right now, and in the sexually active eighteen to thirty crowd, as many as *50 percent have chlamydia*. Chlamydia is particularly nasty because it is usually *asymptomatic* (meaning it has no symptoms). In one year, about 4.5 million women in North America will be infected with chlamydia, and 60 percent of them will not have any symptoms. But the disease can do a lot of damage and lead to *pelvic inflammatory disease* (PID), discussed in chapter 7, which is a primary cause of female infertility. Some experts estimate that chlamydia causes 50 percent of all pelvic infections and 25 percent of all tubal pregnancies (ectopic pregnancies) due to scarring and/or inflammation of the fallopian tubes. (Inflammation of the tubes is called *salpingitis*.) Chlamydia can also cause urethral infections in both men and women and cervicitis (inflammation of the cervix) in women.

The screening is simple. Your doctor takes a culture swab of cervical mucus. It can be done in conjunction with a Pap test. Chlamydia is *extremely* easy to treat: Tetracycline will cure it. The drug usually prescribed is *doxycycline* (Vibramycin), which is a derivative of *tetracycline* (Tetracyn and many other brands). Two doxycycline capsules per day for ten days will do the trick. Tetracycline, which is cheaper, must be taken four times a day, but many people forget to take that many pills; that's why doxycycline is better. If you're already pregnant or cannot be on tetracycline, you'll be given *erythromycin* (Eryc, PCE, Erythromid, and many others). Incidentally, as many as 10 percent of all pregnant women are found to have chlamydia, which can cause a host of problems during pregnancy and delivery.

Gonorrhea

Gonorrhea is another STD that's fairly common and does more damage to women than to men. If left untreated, gonorrhea can cause PID as well, and subsequent female infertility. *It is believed that gonorrhea and chlamydia account for 80 percent of all PID*. However, gonorrhea is *less* common than chlamydia. If a woman is diagnosed with gonorrhea, she'll also be treated for chlamydia. The reasoning: "If she managed to catch gonorrhea, she's got an enormous chance of already having chlamydia. Better treat her for both just in case!" In fact, women can often be simultaneously infected with both chlamydia and gonorrhea if the partner is a carrier for both infections. After one sexual contact with an infected partner, women have a 30 percent chance of contracting gonorrhea and almost a 100 percent chance if they are on hormonal contraception. Like chlamydia, early-stage gonorrhea is asymptomatic about 80 percent of the time. Symptoms depend on where the gonococcal bacteria are "living."

During an annual pelvic exam, the doctor will check the cervix for any unusual discharge and often take a culture as a routine screening. Gonorrhea tests usually are 90 percent accurate if a culture test is done; if only a "gram stain" is performed, in which the discharge is smeared onto a slide and stained, the test is only 50 percent accurate for women, but very accurate for *men with symptoms*. In men, gonorrhea can lead to sterility as their bodies may develop sperm antibodies after they've been infected. When this happens, sperm motility is reduced, which affects male fertility.

The best thing to do if you suspect gonorrhea is to request two culture tests one week apart. If you *do* have gonorrhea, you will be either screened for chlamydia or simply treated for it. Gonorrhea is easily treated with antibiotics. One dose of *ceftriaxone* (Rocephin) and a follow-up prescription of doxycycline cures the probable chlamydia.

Mycoplasma

Mycoplasma (*Ureaplasma urealyticum*) is an asymptomatic bacterial infection that is, more often than not, an STD. (In other words, virgins don't usually get mycoplasma!) Your doctor can detect mycoplasma by culturing cervical mucus during a routine Pap smear. It's important to be screened for mycoplasma prior to pregnancy because if left untreated, mycoplasma can travel to the endometrium, causing inflammation. This is known as *endometritis*—not to be confused with endometriosis. If you were pregnant with endometritis, the embryo may not implant in the uterus, and you would miscarry.

Herpes

Herpes is an STD caused by the herpes simplex virus. The virus enters the body through the skin and mucous membranes of the mouth and genitals and permanently sets up shop at the base of the spine.

There are two types of herpes: herpes simplex virus type I (HSV I), which is characterized by cold sores and fever blisters on the mouth and face, and herpes simplex virus type II (HSV II), the dreaded genital herpes. HSV I can be transmitted through kissing. You can also contract an HSV I and II "combo" if you have both oral sex and intercourse with an infected partner. Herpes *is* contagious whether the sores are active or not; it is most contagious when the sores are active, but has been found that most infection takes place when the sores are *inactive*. This is when herpes is known to be asymptomatic. When the sores are active, they're visible and stand as a warning to the other partner "not to touch." Indeed the sores are so potent that touching them with the fingers and then touching the skin of a healthy person will transmit the virus. Even if there are no visible sores, the virus can still be transmitted.

The herpes sores are called vesicles, and they are painful, watery blisters that occur anywhere from two to twenty days after infection. Within a few days, the vesicles rupture, leaving behind shallow blisters that may ooze or bleed. After three or four days, scabs form and the vesicles fall off, healing by themselves without treatment.

There is no cure for herpes, but there are some antiviral medications (pills) that can help alleviate the pain. The initial outbreaks also take longer to heal, lasting about two to three weeks. Then, the virus will start to taper off, and you may go from monthly initial outbreaks to annual outbreaks. The usual pattern is nasty initial outbreaks, and milder recurrent episodes within three to twelve months after the first outbreak. Recurrences then become milder and far more sporadic, like once every two years and so on. Generally, factors such as stress, poor diet, caffeine, and hormonal elements (menstruation, oral contraceptives, and so on) trigger herpes outbreaks. The presence of other infections, such as vaginitis (inflammation of the vagina), genital warts, or yeast can also trigger a recurrence. Usually, there aren't any recurrences with HSV I. About 25 percent of people with HSV II may also never experience a recurrence.

Diagnosing herpes isn't difficult. When the sores are active, it's usually obvious. A blood test can detect whether you have herpes antibodies present. The problem with this test is that it can only tell you that you've contracted herpes at some point; it does not tell you when the initial infection occurred.

More than thirty million North Americans are currently infected with herpes, but only about 25 percent know they have it. Roughly 30 percent of the general population have been exposed to HSV II. If you've been exposed to herpes and are planning a pregnancy, ask your primary care physician for advice. The risk of passing on herpes to your spouse or partner years after an initial outbreak may be quite low if you don't suffer from recurrent herpes. Many women with herpes go on to have normal, healthy pregnancies and deliveries, but it's more important to rule out a herpes infection in the cervical area.

For more information on herpes and pregnancy, call the Herpes Resource Center hotline: (919) 361-8488.

Human papillomavirus (genital warts)

Genital warts are also STDs and are sometimes referred to as venereal warts. They are caused by the human papillomavirus (HPV). This virus is very similar to the one that causes skin warts, but there are more than twenty types of HPV floating around. Warts are painless and can appear on the vulva or the cervix or on a man's penis. Unless the warts are on the cervix, your doctor can usually spot them and treat them with a solution that will burn off the wart. HPV on the cervix can take the form of raised (condyloma) or flat lesions. Both types of lesions can be detected through a Pap smear. If left untreated, HPV can cause the cells on the lining of the cervix to change, which can lead to cervical cancer. HPV is currently *the* most common STD in North America. It is rampant in sexually active couples aged eighteen to thirty-five. HPV can be treated but never technically cured. Once the warts are removed, the virus generally doesn't cause problems, but it remains in your bloodstream forever. For women, follow-up Pap smears for the first couple of years after HPV diagnosis, and annual Pap smears after that, will help nip HPV in the bud should it decide to erupt again (which is an extremely rare event). When HPV is treated, however, you are in effect "cured." For both sexes, treatment can encompass cryosurgery or laser surgery, and for women, a sloughing cream can also be applied to the cervix.

Syphilis

Perhaps the most famous STD, syphilis was once a very serious, incurable disease that often resulted in "madness." Today it's easily treated with antibiotics. Syphilis is caused by a bacterium known as a *spirochete*. There are three stages of syphilis: primary, secondary, and tertiary (late stage). It's transmitted through sexual or skin contact with someone who is already infected. While syphilis does not cause infertility, when you're pregnant, you can transmit the disease to your unborn child, which is known as *congenital syphilis*. The number of congenital syphilis cases reported in 1988 was the highest since the early 1950s, and in New York City alone, the number had increased more than 500 percent! Untreated syphilis during pregnancy can lead to fetal bone and tooth deformities, fetal nerve damage, stillbirth, and fetal brain damage. All couples planning pregnancy should request a syphilis test. Syphilis spreads through open sores called *chancres* or rashes that pass through the mucous membrane lining the mouth, genitals, anus, or broken skin.

In the 1970s, syphilis was virtually eliminated as an STD because it had been aggressively treated in previous decades. In 1985, however, the incidence of syphilis skyrocketed in the United States and continues to rise.

Diagnosing syphilis is tricky. Known as the "great masquerader," syphilis symptoms imitate other symptoms and can be misdiagnosed. Syphilis is diagnosed through a blood test that checks for antibodies to spirochetes in the bloodstream. Two tests are involved; the first one screens for it, the second confirms it. Syphilis is a miserable, damaging disease that is *curable* with simple antibiotics, either penicillin or tetracycline. After you've been treated for syphilis at any stage, you'll need to have a follow-up test to make sure you've been cured.

Hepatitis B

Hepatitis B is a virus that causes inflammation of the liver. It's most common in people aged fifteen to thirty-nine and is a serious STD that is on the rise. It is transmitted through contaminated needles or blood, but it is also transmitted through mucus-sharing activities that involve saliva, semen, or vaginal fluid, which enter the bloodstream of an uninfected person. *Mothers can also pass on this virus to newborns during childbirth.*

It can take up to 180 days after infection for any hepatitis symptoms to develop. Most people who get hepatitis B remain well, have no symptoms, and completely recover. Even if you're asymptomatic, the virus can cause damage to the liver, which can lead to serious illness and even death. Those who *do* get sick generally experience flulike symptoms, jaundice, dark urine, and light stools. Generally you will recover from hepatitis, but if you're unlucky, the illness can overwhelm you for several months. Some people will always carry the hepatitis B virus and thus remain infectious.

There is no cure for hepatitis B, but there is a vaccine! Safe sex is not considered adequate protection from hepatitis B; only a hepatitis B vaccine will protect you. Like HIV, hepatitis B can flourish in an anal sex "environment" and among drug users. However, tattooing and ear piercing are also common routes of infection. Those at highest risk for hepatitis B are intravenous drug users, gay men, health care workers, and prostitutes.

The vaccine is given by injection in three doses over a six-month time period. The second shot is given one month after the first shot; the third shot is given five months after the second. Other than a sore arm for a day or two, side effects from the vaccine are rare. If you do suffer from any side effects, you'll experience general feelings of "unwellness," fatigue, and so on. Contact the physician or clinic that administered the vaccine.

Vaginal infections: attention, ladies

All vaginal infections should be treated prior to the "trying" phase, or else you will *not* be able to observe the cervical mucus accurately, nor will sexual intercourse be comfortable.

The most common vaginal infection is caused by the overgrowth of vaginal yeast known as *candidiasis*. This is *not* an STD. *Trichomoniasis* and *bacterial vaginosis* are also common and can be passed on to a male partner during intercourse. All three infections are characterized by unusual, odorous vaginal discharge; cottage cheeselike discharge, coupled with the smell of baking bread, is often a classic symptom of a yeast infection.

Trichomoniasis is diagnosed by swabbing the vaginal discharge and examining it under the microscope. But "trich" can also cause urinary tract infections and can be passed back and forth between partners. Like both chlamydia and gonorrhea, if left untreated, "trich" can hitchhike up the fallopian tubes and cause pelvic inflammatory disease and eventual infertility. Sixty percent of women with "trich" are cured with an antifungal medication called *clotrimazole* (Canestan). Women taking medication for "trich" must make sure that their partners are treated as well.

For bacterial vaginosis, the treatment for both partners is with a drug known as *metronidazole*. (Pregnant women are given a different drug in a suppository form.) The male partner must wear a condom until cured.

Yeast and "trich" aren't dangerous to a developing fetus per se but could aggravate natural discomforts of pregnancy considerably. Bacterial vaginosis, however, can complicate a pregnancy if untreated and can trigger premature labor.

Group B streptococcal disease

Group B streptococcus (GBS) is a type of bacteria that adults can carry in the bowel, vagina, bladder, or throat. Roughly 10 to 30 percent of all women carry GBS, which is the leading cause of blood infections and meningitis in newborns, as well as a common cause of newborn pneumonia. In pregnancy, GBS can cause bladder infections and infections in the womb. Many people who carry GBS never get sick. During labor, however, GBS can be transferred from the rectum or vagina to the newborn. By being screened for GBS between the thirty-fifth and thirty-seventh weeks of pregnancy (when the screening test is most accurate), you can find out whether you carry GBS. If you do, administering antibiotics during labor and delivery can prevent GBS from transferring to your newborn. Routine screening for GBS isn't always offered, but you should discuss it with your health care provider. Screening involves taking a swab from the vagina and rectum and culturing it. Group B strep should not be confused with Group A streptococcus, which causes strep throat, scarlet fever, and some pneumonias.

Full physical

Both partners should have a full physical when planning pregnancy to make sure that their blood pressure, iron levels (for women), blood sugar, urine, cholesterol levels, heart rates, and so forth are all normal. The purpose is to establish that both partners are healthy and presumed fertile unless a problem is found. At this point, they should also discuss nutritional issues that may increase fertility, eliminating certain foods, tobacco, or alcohol while stockpiling on others. Make sure you bring along your family and personal medical history so that your doctor can keep an eye on anything unusual. (Family/personal history charts are discussed on page 24.)

Autoimmune disorders

Autoimmune means "self-attacking." Most autoimmune disorders are hereditary but can affect a couple's fertility if left untreated. Common autoimmune diseases include diabetes, thyroid disease, lupus, and rheumatoid arthritis. The symptoms of these diseases may interfere temporarily with fertility until the diseases are brought under control through medication. For example, thyroid disease can interfere with regular ovulation and can reduce sperm count. A classic symptom of diabetes in women is chronic vaginal yeast infections, which will interfere with cervical mucus observation. Know your family history as well as the early warning signs of these illnesses so you can be screened for them.

History 101

When it comes to laying the groundwork, History 101 is a prerequisite, not an option! Both you and your partner will need to write a complete family and personal medical history that can be given to your "weed doctor." Should you need to see a fertility specialist later on, this history will help speed up the fertility treatment process tremendously. Here are the questions you'll need to address:

1. *Have there been previous pregnancies and/or abortions?* Has *he* impregnated someone in the past (with or without her knowledge)? Has *she* been pregnant (with or without his knowledge)? For example, scarring may have resulted that could be affecting your fertility now. Previous miscarriages and any subsequent D & Cs (*dilatation and curettage*, in which the uterine lining is scraped out) may also have resulted in scarring. If you're a male who has impregnated another woman in the past, it's highly unlikely that you're infertile today unless you are taking certain medications known to reduce fertility or you have been exposed to certain toxins.

    And finally, any history of ectopic pregnancy may have resulted in tubal damage or even the removal of one or both tubes. This information is crucial to disclose!

2. *Do either of you have a history of pelvic surgeries or therapies?* Women who have had pelvic surgery or therapy of any kind (D & Cs, removal of ovarian cysts, treatment for cervical dysplasia, or laparoscopy procedures) need to disclose this information. Men who have had surgery in or around their genital area (for instance, removal of cysts around the testes) need to disclose this information, too. Again, scarring from previous surgeries or procedures may be affecting your fertility now.

3. *Do you have a history of pelvic infection or pelvic pain?* Any woman who suffers from chronic pelvic pain (this does not mean menstrual cramps) may be suffering from PID. Any woman suffering from menstrual cramps painful enough to keep her from participating in pleasurable activities, pelvic pain, constipation, or other pelvic discomforts during menstruation may have

endometriosis. Both PID and endometriosis can affect your pelvic organs and in some cases can interfere with ovarian function. You *must* report these symptoms if you have them.

4. *Do either of you have a history of cancer therapy?* Anticancer drugs and chemotherapy can affect future fertility for both men and women. Both testicular and ovarian function can be permanently affected. Some common cancers in younger adults that require chemotherapy treatments include Hodgkin's disease, leukemia, breast cancer, testicular cancer (relevant when one testicle remains), and non-Hodgkin's lymphoma. Of course, there are many other kinds of cancers for which either of you may have received chemotherapy treatments. External radiation therapy will not affect your fertility unless the radiation beam was directed at the ovaries or testicles.

5. *What is your hormonal contraceptive history?* Were you ever on combination oral contraceptives or the mini-pill? Norplant? Depo-Provera? In each case, how many years were you on hormonal contraception? Have your menstrual cycles returned to normal? (See chapter 4 for more details on the menstrual cycle and hormonal contraceptives.) Women with a long history of hormonal contraception may have a more difficult time getting pregnant. This has more to do with waiting for the return of normal menstrual cycles than any permanent infertility.

6. *What is your history of hormonal therapy?* Were you prescribed estrogen or progesterone for any reason? Were you ever on *Danazol* (a male hormone derivative that shuts down ovarian function—sometimes used to treat endometriosis)? Were you taking hormonal therapy as part of any cancer treatment (such as *tamoxifen*)? Hormonal therapy will most definitely interfere with normal ovulation, but this interference is temporary. Once you go off the medication, your menstrual cycle should resume, but you may need to stay on hormonal therapy to treat a more serious condition. Discuss your options with the doctor who is managing your therapy.

7. *What is your contraceptive history in general?* Have you ever used an IUD? What barrier methods have you used? IUDs are particularly suspicious because they can trigger bacterial infections that lead to PID (discussed in detail in chapter 7). Your condom history is also important because this will give your doctor an idea of your risk factor for exposure to STDs. Attention, men: Your condom history is important as well.

8. *Assuming neither of you have an STD today, have either of you ever been treated for an STD in the past?* This is more of a concern for women than for men. Even if a woman has already been treated for chlamydia or gonorrhea, she

may still have suffered tubal damage as a result. That's why it's crucial that you're both screened for STDs! Screening today will also ensure that past treatments worked.

9. *Do either of you suffer from chronic bladder or urinary tract infections?* This spells I-N-F-E-C-T-I-O-N. Men who have cloudy urine or experience a burning sensation when they urinate may have *nongonococcal urethritis* (NGU) (inflammation of the urethra that is not caused by gonorrhea, also known as nonspecific urethritis). When a man has NGU, he almost always has chlamydia, which can be passed on to his partner. She in turn may not show any symptoms, creating an STD merry-go-round of nightmarish proportions.

    On the other hand, women who suffer from symptoms of urinary tract infections (UTIs) may have cystitis (a bladder infection, which could affect the kidneys if left untreated), a vaginal infection, or an STD. Be on the lookout for painful urination, frequent urination, and either or both symptoms in conjunction with a sluggish or almost nonexistent urine stream and fever.

10. *Do either of you have a family history of only children? Did either mother have a late pregnancy or a history of troubled pregnancies?* The answers to these questions may mean nothing, or they may be clues to a family history of pregnancy or fertility *complications*. For example, diseases such as endometriosis (discussed in chapter 7) are hereditary, but women who suffer from endometriosis often have no symptoms. Some problems that cause male infertility may be hereditary, and so on. The bottom line is that knowing your parents' fertility history will help your doctor probe further and ask more direct questions, which may yield more definite answers for you!

11. *Are either of you DES children?* Anyone born in the United States between 1941 and 1971 (perhaps even a little beyond that) may be a DES daughter or DES son. During this period, five million pregnant women took the drug DES (*diethylstilbestrol*, a synthetic estrogen) to prevent miscarriage. Any daughter born to a mother who took DES runs a higher than normal risk for reproductive organ abnormalities (such as twisted fallopian tubes), cervical and vaginal cell changes, and cancer. All this can spell trouble when she tries to conceive. Men who are DES sons may also have anatomical abnormalities when it comes to their reproductive organs, although DES sons are not as commonly affected as are daughters.

    DES was administered under a host of different labels. If you can, find out the name of the drugs your mother took during her pregnancy and contact DES Action at (510) 465-4011. Ask them to check if any of the drugs you discovered match the drugs on their list. DES Action has a nationwide referral service of doctors who specialize in the treatment of DES-exposed women and men.

12. *Do either of you suffer from a chronic disease/condition such as diabetes, lupus, rheumatoid arthritis, thyroid disease, multiple sclerosis, asthma, ulcers, and so on?* Depending on your age and condition, pregnancy may not be recommended to begin with, or your condition may be affecting your fertility.

13. *Are either of you taking medications to control a chronic medical or psychiatric condition?* Many medications can interfere with fertility for both men and women, so you need to disclose all of this information to your primary care doctor. Certain antidepressants, any medications that contain steroids (used to control asthma, for example), and certain ulcer medications are classic examples.

14. *Have either of you been exposed to environmental toxins?* Exposure to radiation (also used in cancer therapy), toxic chemicals such as lead, pesticides, insecticides, polystyrene, xylene, benzene, mercury, Agent Orange, anesthetic gases, PCBs, or solvents can cause both temporary or, in extreme cases, permanent damage to your reproductive organs. (Are either of you Gulf War veterans?) Often just getting away from a toxic environment can restore fertility. This is discussed further in chapter 3.

15. *What are your lifestyle and nutritional habits and vices?* This is something you *really* need to explore and is the subject of chapter 3. As amazing as it may seem, cutting out certain foods and chemicals and changing habits can result in conception after months of delays.

A good primary care physician will most likely ask you these questions anyway, but addressing these issues yourselves beforehand will help you form a conception *partnership*. In addition, clearly reviewing your medical histories is an excellent way to prepare you for parenthood. Parents are the "health care contractors" for their children. Knowing your own histories will help you prepare or comfort your offspring should a future health problem arise.

When Do We Chart the Menstrual Cycle?

This is an excellent question, one to which many couples don't know the answer. At this point, you shouldn't be *trying* to conceive until you've done the weeding.

Even if your menstrual cycles are charted (see chapter 4) and are so regular that you can set your watch by them, *unless you've done your weeding and history lesson above, this will mean nothing and can waste months of time!* Fertility problems revolve around structural problems (his or hers) and hormonal problems (his or hers). Menstrual cycle abnor-malities will identify female hormonal problems only—*which account for just a small por-tion of fertility problems in general.* Today, roughly 80 percent of all female infertility is due to structural damage to the fallopian tubes from PID. And, women with PID can have perfectly normal menstrual cycles. So, while understanding both the female and male hor-monal cycles is crucial to conception (the female cycle is discussed in chapter 4; the male cycle is discussed in chapter 5), it is *not* the first step in conception *planning.*

If your screenings all came back negative (normal), then the next step is to read chap-ters 3 and 4. You're looking at about a year's worth of "trying" before you should even suspect there's a fertility problem.

If your screenings revealed a garden-variety weed of some sort (an STD or a suspected PID), you'll need to "treat and repeat." Treat the STD, go off the drugs that are making you infertile, and go for diagnostic tests to confirm the problem. You may need certain treatment or need to repeat certain tests before you complete your screening process. Then read chapters 3 and 4 and begin your "trying" phase.

The next section of this chapter may either be "in order" or "out of order" depend-ing on how your screening process goes. Essentially, the "Groundwork" = Weeding + 1 Year of Trying (based on information in chapters 3 and 4).

When the year is up and there's still no baby, both of you and your weed doctor may graduate to what's called a workup (discussed in chapters 5 and 6). The workup is a spe-cial series of tests that pinpoint hormonal, structural, or immunological problems that may be interfering with conception. Men and women require *different* workups. To avoid wasting time and money, both the male and female workups begin with a semen analy-sis—the easiest, cheapest, and least invasive test of all. Whoever is managing your pre-conception screening should manage the semen analysis. The results of the semen analysis will determine the next steps.

The "Fertility Doctor"

Today, no area has caused more confusion or lawsuits than fertility treatment. This is because there is no such thing as a fertility or infertility specialist per se—*yet.* In other words, a graduating M.D. cannot become a "board-certified fertility specialist" in the way that he or she can become a board-certified gynecologist or pediatrician. To date, no post-graduate board-certification course exists for this purpose.

This, understandably, creates enormous problems for the fertility consumer. Essen-tially, any M.D. or even Ph.D. can say that she or he is a fertility specialist, but this does not mean that he or she is *qualified* to treat a fertility problem.

The answer to "who is a fertility specialist?" is rather complicated. The doctor that manages your infertility workup will vary depending on who has the problem. Male infertility specialists are either *andrologists* (M.D.s or Ph.D. scientists specializing in male fertility and in assisted reproductive technology) or *urologists* (doctors who specialize in male and female urinary tract problems but are particularly knowledgeable about penis and testicle "design"). Many urologists are also andrologists.

As I stress repeatedly throughout this book, both the male and the female workup begin with a semen analysis. If your partner has an abnormal semen analysis, he'll be sent for a "male workup" (discussed in chapter 5). If the semen analysis is normal, you'll then go on as a couple to a gynecologist who specializes in *reproductive endocrinology*. This person is qualified to manage the "female workup" (discussed in chapter 6).

If you and your partner decide to undergo assisted reproductive technology (see chapter 9), the following combination of specialists is appropriate: A gynecologist who subspecializes in reproductive endocrinology; a urologist (for male infertility) who subspecializes in andrology; an *embryologist* (a Ph.D. scientist specializing in embryo transfers—this person should never manage the treatment, however).

A *radiologist* (a doctor specializing in imaging tests) can be called in as a consultant by your specialist, but you will rarely have occasion to meet him or her.

How to Find a Good Fertility Specialist

Never, I repeat, never go to a fertility specialist because he or she has been recommended by a friend. Picking the right fertility specialist greatly depends on who has the problem and what kind of treatment route you've decided to take. In the same way that real estate agents always sell you on "location, location, location," finding a good, *appropriate* fertility specialist depends on "referral, referral, referral." You *first* need a good primary care physician who can refer you to the appropriate specialist. This requires some medical diagnostic training—something that your friend's neighbor's sister *doesn't* have!

If you don't have a good primary physician but *do* have a good gynecologist, the gynecologist can serve as your "weed doctor" (as mentioned earlier) and can refer you to the appropriate specialist when the time comes. If this gynecologist subspecializes in reproductive endocrinology, then he or she can manage the female workup if need be.

You can also phone one of the infertility/fertility organizations listed at the back of this book and ask for a list of qualified reproductive endocrinologists, andrologists, urologists, and so on. Other ways of making short lists of potential specialists involve contacting former infertility patients from a patient support group, or contacting a specific hospital directly. Generally, seeking out a fertility specialist on your own should be done only if you're unhappy with the referral from your weed doctor and if you already know *who* needs the workup. Otherwise, you could be wasting time and money.

This leads to an obvious question: How do you find that weed doctor to begin with? Two ways: "friends, friends, friends" or "referral, referral, referral." Ask someone whose opinion you value. Who do *they* see? Who does their *spouse* see? Or, if you have an allergist, podiatrist, or pulmonary specialist whom you really like, who do *they* recommend as a primary care doctor? Who is *their* doctor, or their *spouse's* doctor? You get the idea. You can also call the American Medical Association or, in Canada, the College of Physicians and Surgeons (the provincial branches) for lists of primary care physicians in your area. *NOTE: If you live away from a major medical center or urban area, you may need to travel to a center for your care. Infertility specialists are few and far between since this is a relatively new area of specialty.*

Going for a Test Drive

The results from your semen analyses (you need at least two) are back. You're now proceeding with either a male or female workup. Whether you're seeing an andrologist, reproductive endocrinologist, gynecologist, or urologist, here are the questions you need to ask at your first appointment as a way of "test driving" your specialist:

1. *Are you board-certified?* This means that he or she has completed a residency training program that has met with the standards set by the American board of that particular field (obstetrics and gynecology, endocrinology, urology, and so on). For example, there's a one in two and a half chance that any gynecologist you see is not board-certified. To check a doctor's credentials in the United States, call 1-800-766-CERT during business hours.
2. *What are your subspecialties?* Does your gynecologist "do" reproductive endocrinology? Does your urologist "do" andrology?
3. *Who will manage the pregnancy if conception is achieved? (If you're seeing a gynecologist, does he or she do obstetrics?)* Because you're planning to get pregnant, you should have an obstetrician waiting in the wings. Also, if your treatment is successful, you *will* have a high-risk pregnancy and must be under the care of an obstetrician. A midwife or primary care doctor won't do!
4. *What kind of hospital privileges do you have?* Full operating privileges are best.
5. *Do you share copies of medical records and test results with your patients at their request?* If he or she doesn't, that's a bad sign.
6. *Are you available for occasional phone calls?* Find out if the doctor is accessible, or if you have to make an appointment just to ask a question.

7. (If the specialist is male, and you're undergoing a female workup) *Is a female assistant present in the room when you perform a pelvic exam or administer treatment/testing in the pelvic area? If not, do you object if I bring along a friend or my spouse?* If the male doctor performs "solo pelvics," it's not only a bad sign, it's illegal in most places. (Sorry, guys, there are no laws in place that call for a male nurse in the room while a female urologist examines your genitals. You may ask to bring your spouse, however. There are no laws covering same-sex doctor-patient exams either.)

8. *How much of your practice revolves around infertility treatment?* Does the urologist specialize in treating cystitis only but *dabbles* in male fertility? Does the reproductive endocrinologist have a waiting room filled with menopausal women and only *occasionally* handles the odd fertility workup? You'll want someone who focuses a good portion of his or her practice on fertility treatment.

9. *What are the costs involved?* Once you factor in the costs of both diagnostic procedures and treatments, you could be looking at a hefty price tag. You *must* get a rough estimate up front so you can make the necessary insurance arrangements for coverage. (In Canada, many procedures and therapies involving infertility are not covered by provincial health insurance. Find out what's covered before making your decisions.)

10. *How experienced are you in monitoring and administering fertility drugs?* Because these drugs are extrememly potent, you'll want a doctor who knows what he or she is doing when it comes to dosage monitoring, dosage adjusting, and side-effects. (See chapter 8 for more details.)

11. *Who will perform microsurgery?* If your fertility is being caused by a structural problem, such as blocked tubes in women, scrotal varicose veins in men, or reversal of vasectomy procedures, who will actually be *doing* the surgery? You may ask to meet with the surgeon at some point, too.

12. *What other services do you offer to patients?* Can you join a support group? Are counselors available? Are there videos or other reference materials? The more information you can sink your teeth into, the better.

13. *What percentage of live births have resulted from your treatments?* Be careful with the term *success rates* because many doctors or clinics won't distinguish pregnancies from actual births. Also, keep in mind that when a pregnancy is established, the rate of miscarriage is far higher under many of these specialized treatments than it is under standard treatment.

14. *What percentage of multiple pregnancies have resulted from your treatments?* This time, it's helpful to know how many past patients carried multiple fetuses. Multiple births are higher risk pregnancies and carry lower gestation periods.

This is an important piece of data if you can get it. Ask, again, how many *live* multiple births resulted.

What Are Your Rights as a Patient?

In a very general way, patients' rights in Western healthcare involve four basic umbrella principles. Since infertility workups and treatments are so complex, this is important information for you to have. You can challenge your doctor on any of these principles, and use the following information to launch a complaint to your state/provincial medical board if you feel your rights have been ignored. This section has been reviewed by experts at the University of Toronto's Joint Centre for Bioethics.

Respect for Persons (Also Known as Patient Autonomy)

This means to respect that each person is, in fact, a human being with full human rights. That means each person has a right to be fully informed about all things involving his or her care, his or her body, or things being done to his or her body (if you're pregnant, you have the right to know about everything that affects the fetus you're carrying), and to make his or her own decisions about care based on accurate information (this is known as "respect for persons" or sometimes "patient autonomy").

A health care provider has a duty to respect your personhood, wishes, bodily integrity and health care preferences. So information, counseling, and informed consent (see further on) are all crucial aspects of care, which support this principle. Here are some examples of when your health care provider is ignoring the Respect for Persons principle when you're seeking guidance about infertility:

- You are given no information about the causes of your infertility, and your doctor refuses to answer or address your questions.
- You refuse a certain treatment or procedure after being fully informed of all the risks and benefits of that procedure, but your health care provider tries to force you or coerce you into having the procedure anyway, which does not respect your choice.
- You request a referral to a specialist and your doctor ignores your request.
- You do not speak English and your doctor refuses to speak to a translator you've appointed.
- Your confidentiality is breached in some way (see further on).

What is "informed consent"?

Many of you have heard the term *informed consent*, but may not truly understand what it means. To uphold the principle of Respect for Persons, you have the right to accurate and full information about your health so you can make an informed decision about your health care. You cannot even know to refuse a procedure if you are not given this information first. This is known as informed consent. In order for informed consent to take place, three things have to happen:

1. *Disclosure*: Have you been provided with relevant and comprehensive information by your health care provider? For example, a description of the treatment; its expected effects (such as side-effects of drugs, duration of a particular procedure, expected time to recovery, restrictions on daily activities, scars); information about relevant alternative options and their expected benefits and relevant risks; and an explanation of the consequences of declining or delaying treatment. Have you been given an opportunity to ask questions, and has your health care provider been available to answer them?
2. *Capacity and competency*: Do you understand information relevant to a treatment decision and appreciate the reasonably foreseeable consequences of a decision or lack of a decision? Do you understand information and appreciate its implications? Do you understand what's being disclosed and can you decide on your treatment based on this information?
3. *Voluntariness*: Are you being allowed to make your health care choice free of any undue influence? To answer the question, we need to take into consideration factors such as pain and manipulation (when information is being deliberately distorted or omitted).

Other barriers to informed consent include:

- language barriers
- wide gaps in knowledge (when you're not a doctor, how informed can you really be unless you go to medical school?)
- health care provider bias (when your health care provider makes assumptions about your intelligence or character and tailors the information to those assumptions)

With respect to infertility treatments and procedures, informed consent is a continual problem. Several ART cases involve problems with clinic consent forms not being properly understood by infertility patients—particularly when it comes to issues surrounding frozen or unused embryos and ownership of embryos should the relationship of infertile couples change in the future. This is discussed more under Ethics in chapter 9.

What about confidentiality?

No matter how confidential you think your health care records are, or the information you disclose to your health care provider, your medical records are, in fact, not confidential. These are the questions you must ask your health care provider if you're concerned about confidential information getting into the wrong hands:

1. *Who owns this information?* For example, if during the course of your workup you test positive for HIV, does your health care provider have a duty to report this information to anyone other than yourself? If you're taking fertility drugs, or are pregnant from a donor egg, do you want this information to get out? Can you bar your physician from disclosing this information? And what about employers who demand that you have routine physicals?
2. *How will this information be used?* Can your health status information be used by employers or health insurers as tools of discrimination? If your employer knew you were going through infertility treatment, would this affect your job, for example?
3. *How will your health status affect other family members?* If you are found to have a genetic disease that interferes with your fertility, do you have to disclose this information to other family members that may be affected? Ought you? Ought they be tested? And what are the consequences involved?

Beneficence and nonmaleficence (doing some good and doing no harm)

This means that the health care provider must strive to maintain or promote the well-being of a patient and avoid harming that patient (this is known as "beneficence"—pronounced "be-ne-fi-cents"). At the same time, the health care provider must also strive not to inflict harm or evil on a patient (this is known as "nonmaleficence"). This means that a health care provider has a duty not to kill a patient and a duty not to refrain from aiding a patient.

In order to promote the well-being of patients and avoid harming them, therapies, treatment, or diagnostic tests that involve risks to your health need to be weighed against potential benefits. Since the success rates of fertility treatments are so low, and the potential risks from drug side effects high and costly, the risk/benefit ratio is very difficult. Here are some examples of when your health care provider is ignoring beneficence:

- Your doctor is recommending you try an experimental therapy that has not yet been proven to work better than a standard therapy and has unknown risks.

- You are given a drug or therapy and not provided with information on side effects or potential risks. For example, many women are not told that fertility drugs are linked to higher rates of ovarian cancer.
- You are in a drug study that involves some people taking a "dummy pill" (called a placebo) and some people taking a real pill. In this case, you may continue to suffer from an ailment needlessly if you are a taking the dummy pill and not offered a standard therapy that will help your ailment.
- Your health care provider breaches your confidentiality (see previous section).

Justice

This means that the health care provider/system has to ensure that all people have the same access to health care services (such as hospital beds, medicine, treatments, clinical trials, health care providers, preventive care, and so on) regardless of their ability to pay, gender, ethnicity or race, physical or mental ability, age, or any other factors, such as behavior or lifestyle. In the United States, the principle of distributive justice is almost never honored since all health care is based on one's ability to pay for health insurance. (Countries with universal health care, such as Canada and the U.K., fare better on the distributive justice scale but fall short in terms of being able to meet the demand.) When it comes to seeking treatment for infertility, coverage—regardless of what health care system you have—is not great. But new legislation has recently been introduced in the United States that would mandate insurers to cover a significant portion of infertility treatment in the form of procedures and drugs. (See chapter 9 for more information.)

Even without equal access to coverage, health care providers can at least treat all their patients equally. Single women using ART and lesbian couples using ART (see chapter 10) should be treated equally as heterosexual couples using ART, and so on. In order to be fair, all people should have equal access to health care services and resources. Being just or fair means all lives and interests are of equal importance and must be given equal weight. As well, a health care provider has a duty to provide the same standard of care and options to all patients, regardless of income, education, or race. Here are some examples of when the health care system—or your individual health care provider—is ignoring justice:

- When some people have more access to resources than other people due to privilege and wealth. (Again, this goes on all the time in fertility treatment.)
- When your health care provider places a greater value on some patients than on others.
- When poor women have babies with lower birth weights and more complications at birth than affluent women because they have less access to good prenatal care.

- When an HIV positive person is refused health care service by a health care provider who fears HIV.
- When certain groups of people die of curable diseases because they don't have the same access to screening for that disease than have other groups of people.
- When vulnerable populations (the elderly, mentally ill, people in developing countries, or certain ethnic groups) are selected for dangerous or risky medical experiments because they are perceived "expendable."

Problems with "Doing the Right Thing" for Patients

Ignoring one of the above principles can put you in jeopardy, which would make the health care provider negligent. But in many circumstances it isn't always clear what "the right thing" to do is, and it isn't always possible to do the right thing; for example:

- When people are unconscious, it's impossible to inform them and ask them about their wishes. (In this case, someone close to the unconscious person may make decisions on his or her behalf.)
- When people are not competent to make their own decisions, it's difficult to inform them. (Here, again, someone close to the incompetent patient makes the decision.)
- When the benefits of certain medications or therapies have to be weighed against certain risks, it's difficult to know what to do and what's in the patient's best interests.
- When the health care providers are faced with limited resources, such as funding for research, organs for transplant, or even hospital beds, it's difficult to decide who should get the funds, organ, or bed.
- When conducting drug studies, is it right to conduct a study where someone is taking a dummy pill (known as a placebo-controlled study)?

Whose life is worth saving? Whose life is worth risking? And who decides? These are all common, everyday questions and situations that health care providers face.

Legal Duties of Health Care Providers

Whether health care practitioners are considered to be trained in a conventional or unconventional manner, charging a fee for services ought to imply that there are standards of competence their patients or clients have a right to expect. Any health care professional who earns a salary is bound by tort law (which varies from country to country) to uphold standards of care. Moreover, there is a duty of all health care practitioners of "due awareness," meaning that they have a duty to stay educated, informed, and up-to-date on all aspects of legally enforceable duties of care to patients, their families, colleagues, and staff members. Health care providers have a basic duty to diagnose, treat, manage, or care for a health problem. They also have a duty to counsel you about potential harms you may be doing to yourself through medications you're taking, bad habits, or other practices, or harms from outside forces beyond your control, such as environmental factors. And finally, when medical records need to be transferred or copied to a third party, health care providers have a duty to disclose potentially sensitive or stigmatizing information to that party as well as to you.

When to Get a Second Opinion

When it comes to fertility treatment, getting a second opinion is often a necessary route, which translates into seeing two separate doctors about the same set of symptoms. The doctors can be in the same field or specialize in different areas. This can happen at either the diagnostic or treatment stage of an infertility investigation. It's difficult to know whether you're justified in getting a second opinion. Just because you don't like the sound of your diagnosis doesn't mean you require another opinion. Let's say your doctor suspects that your infertility is caused by endometriosis and wants to perform a laparoscopy procedure to confirm his or her suspicions. You might not like the sound of this and decide to see a holistic doctor or an herbalist instead, who may tell you that you're under stress and only need to rest and take various herbs in order to conceive. Of course, this is a much more soothing diagnosis, but in this case, your doctor is the one who is right.

The following guidelines should help you decide whether a second opinion is warranted. If you answer yes to even one of the questions below, you're probably justified in seeking a second opinion.

1. *Is the diagnosis uncertain?* If your doctor can't find out what's wrong or isn't sure whether he or she is correct, you have every right to go elsewhere.
2. *Is the diagnosis life-threatening?* In this case, hearing the same news from someone else may help you cope better with your illness or come to terms with the diagnosis. Diagnoses like cancer, however, usually won't change; the diagnosis is based on carefully analyzed test results, not just on the patient's symptoms.
3. *Is the treatment controversial, experimental, or risky?* You might not question the diagnosis but have problems with the recommended treatment, such as certain potent fertility drugs or microsurgical procedures. If you're not comfortable with the recommended treatment, perhaps another doctor can recommend a different approach.

4. *Is the treatment not working?* This is a real dilemma for fertility patients. If you've been in treatment for a reasonable length of time (see chapter 12) and you're not conceiving, maybe the wrong diagnosis was made, or perhaps the treatment recommended is not right for you. Seeing another doctor may help to confirm or alleviate concerns.

5. *Are risky tests or procedures being recommended?* If you don't like the sound of microsurgery, hearing it from someone else might make you accept the procedure more readily. Or, you may find out that microsurgery is premature and isn't necessary after all. Find out if there are alternate therapies or procedures that can yield the same results.

6. *Do you want another approach?* A forty-five-year-old woman who is entering menopause wants to prolong her fertility with fertility drugs so she can conceive. Her doctor refuses to treat her, saying that she's too old to have a child. The woman finds this approach unacceptable and sees a second doctor who *doesn't* have a problem with her age and is willing to put her on the drugs for a limited period of time.

7. *Is the doctor competent?* If you suspect that your doctor is incompetent, seek a second opinion either to reaffirm your faith in him or her or to confirm your original suspicions.

Heal Thyself

When you're investigating or treating infertility, there's a lot you need to know when it comes to choosing the right combination of doctors and making sure you're receiving the best care possible. There are also a number of ways you can heal yourself during the investigative or treatment phase of your fertility problem.

1. *Educate yourself.* Learn about the physical, psychological, and emotional processes involved with conception and pregnancy.

2. *Learn about all your options,* and choose the practitioners appropriate for you.

3. *Inform yourself about hospital policies and regulations* that will affect your treatment and possible pregnancy.

4. *Arrange for a companion or support person to help you through your treatment if your partner is unavailable.*

5. *Calmly and clearly make your preferences known to your doctors* regarding testing, alternative therapies, or objections to certain procedures at the beginning of your treatment.

6. *Research the costs of your treatment in advance.* (Canadians will need to find out what treatments are covered by the province.)
7. *Notify your practitioners if you intend to seek care elsewhere or intend to stop treatment.*

Much of the information you'll need to fulfill this list is provided throughout the book. Moving on to the "trying" phase of the process may happen immediately after you've been screened for various health problems or have been treated for one. Before you begin charting the rhythms of your individual menstrual cycle, it's important to be aware of how certain lifestyle habits can interfere with infertility. In other words, you and your partner should go through the exercise of evaluating whether your own habits are creating a barrier to conception.

3

The Seven Habits of
Highly Infertile People

ONE OF THE major differences between couples in the 1960s and couples today is that both partners usually need to be in the workforce in order to make ends meet. In many cases, this translates into two-car families, long commutes to and from work, poor eating habits as a result of skipped breakfasts, fast-food lunches and dinners, and intense physical workouts to stay in shape. To combat the stress and fatigue, most of us indulge in a few bad habits, such as gulping coffee, smoking, and drinking alcohol. Many of us will also take over-the-counter medications to fight off headaches, fatigue, and other side effects of stress. For women, these habits can mean interrupted ovulation cycles, skipped periods, and decreased libidos; for men, these habits can mean decreased sperm counts, decreased libidos, and, in extreme cases, bouts of impotence.

Your own lifestyle habits can have a powerful influence on your fertility. "Get more sleep, more rest, and eat right" are the usual words of advice. It's not enough. This chapter is devoted to outlining *all* the lifestyle habits that can affect a couple's fertility. Obviously, when there is a hormonal imbalance or structural problem at work, changing your lifestyle probably will not help you conceive. But when you're planning conception, and no delay is identified at the "weeding," it's crucial to assess whether your lifestyle is "fertility friendly" to begin with *before* you undergo an expensive workup or begin charting your fertility cycle. To continue the yardwork analogy from chapter 2: you've pulled the weeds, now you need to prepare the *soil*. Too much sun, too much water, or too little of each can profoundly affect your garden. You also need to assess whether your soil has any *contaminants*. This chapter serves as your lifestyle "checklist" and discusses seven common, not-so-healthy habits. Unlike chapter 2, this chapter identifies modifiable factors that influence your fertility, including occupational risks. In other words, while you may not be able to control the air outside, you can certainly control the air you breathe inside.

1. Bad Habits

Whether you smoke, drink coffee and/or alcohol, or use addictive drugs such as marijuana or other narcotics, your vice(s) could certainly affect your current or future fertility. The traditional thinking was that only *women* needed to purify their bodies, which most women do once they discover they're pregnant. But few couples realize the importance of purifying their systems *prior* to conception, and even fewer understand how important it is for *both* partners to rid themselves of these indulgences when planning a pregnancy. So here's the bad news about your bad habits . . .

Women

Much has been written about alcohol use during pregnancy and the risks of fetal alcohol syndrome. As a result, very few women who educate themselves about prenatal care will choose to drink during pregnancy. Unfortunately, very few women understand how alcohol can affect them in the "trying-to-get-pregnant" phase, which can be equally hazardous.

Even moderate drinking (one to two glasses of wine per week, for example) can increase the level of the hormone *prolactin*. Prolactin is the hormone responsible for milk production after pregnancy. It does this by suppressing the levels of estrogen and progesterone in your body, which, in turn, will suppress ovulation. This is why breast-feeding has been touted as a natural contraceptive, although it is by *no* means 100 percent effective. If, however, your prolactin levels are too *high* prior to conception, your ovulation cycle can go haywire and you will have difficulty conceiving. (See chapter 4 for more details about the ovulation cycle.) In extreme cases, a condition known as *hyperprolactinemia* (meaning "too much prolactin") can set in, which will render a woman infertile until the problem is corrected.

Alcohol isn't the only drug that can increase prolactin levels. Antidepressant medications (which may be prescribed), painkillers (for headaches, menstrual cramps, and so on), and hallucinogens such as marijuana have all been cited as substances that can cause hyperprolactinemia.

As for smoking, more women die from lung cancer than any other disease, and women who smoke greatly increase their chances of developing other kinds of cancers (breast, gynecological, colon). Furthermore, smoking significantly reduces a woman's fertility. *No one knows exactly why this is.* The current theory is that smoking "pollutes" all of your reproductive organs and reproductive system, affecting overall job performance. Different studies point to reduced levels of estrogen and poor cervical mucus, higher tendencies to develop pelvic infections, and subsequent tubal damage. Worse, high levels of nicotine, which can be found in cervical mucus, can be toxic to your partner's sperm. To date, all studies that tracked the effect of smoking on female fertility came to the same conclusion: More women who smoke are infertile than are women who *don't* smoke. As for the hazards of smoking in early pregnancy, the list includes an increased risk of ectopic pregnancy and miscarriage (both discussed in chapter 11).

Finally, women who drink coffee or other caffeinated beverages and who are trying to get pregnant may want to start eliminating caffeine altogether. A recent study by the U.S. National Institute of Environmental Health Sciences found that the more caffeine a woman consumes, the less likely she is to conceive. In fact, women who drank the equivalent of one cup of brewed coffee per day were found to be half as likely to conceive as women who had no caffeine. Don't panic, though. The study also found that the effects of caffeine on female fertility are *short-term*. If you drank six cups of coffee a day two years ago and have since given up caffeine, you will be just as likely to conceive now as you would if you had no history of caffeine consumption. (See Table 3.1.)

For women coping with infertility, cutting out their vices may be easier said than done. Here's a typical scenario: A woman has intercourse mid-cycle and suddenly "purifies" herself in anticipation of conception. Instead of her anxiously awaited feelings of nausea and morning sickness, she gets PMS and then her period—a scarlet reminder of another "failed" cycle. Feeling frustrated and angry, she "ties one on" and gets good and drunk. Or, she may decide to start smoking again in a what-does-it-matter-now rationale. All in all, a vicious cycle.

Men

Male fertility is also affected by smoking, alcohol, and recreational drugs. It's believed that nicotine reduces testosterone levels by altering the *Leydig cell*, the cell that produces testosterone. This can cause low sperm counts, poor motility, and an increase in abnormal sperm (two heads, no tail, or deformed tails). One Greek-American joint study found that men who smoked more than twenty cigarettes per day had significant defects in the tails of their sperm. Research also shows that cigarette smoke adversely affects the overall male reproductive tract, causing the tissues and tubules responsible for smooth sperm production to operate in a type of "smog" that reduces fertility. Finally, strong anecdotal evidence has found long-term infertility to be suddenly "cured" when the male partners stop smoking.

Alcohol consumption in men can lead to poor sperm quality, poor libido, and even impotence. As alcohol damages the liver, estrogen levels rise, which counteracts testosterone levels normally responsible for libido and sperm quality. High estrogen levels in men are linked only to long-term, heavy alcohol use, however. One beer or alcoholic beverage a day will most likely *not* cause high estrogen levels or interfere with male fertility. No one is sure, though, what constitutes "heavy" alcohol use in men. One British infertility expert suggests that the daily maximum limit for men should be no more than two to three pints of beer, which is equal to one-half bottle of wine, or two to three shots of hard liquor. Of course, even if a man does not go over his daily allowable "maximum," any amount of intoxication will significantly affect his ability to sustain an erection and hence father a child.

Table 3.1 The Java Chart

Worried about your caffeine intake? Check it out . . .

Coffee (5-oz. cup)	Milligrams of Caffeine
Brewed, drip method	60–180
Brewed, percolator	40–170
Instant	30–120
Decaffeinated, brewed	2–5
Decaffeinated, instant	1–5
Tea (5-oz. cup)	
Brewed, major brands	20–90
Brewed, imported brands	25–110
Instant	25–50
Iced (12-oz. glass)	67–76
Other	
Caffeine-containing soft drinks	15–30
Cocoa beverage (5 oz.)	2–20
Chocolate milk (8 oz.)	2–7
Milk chocolate (1 oz.)	1–15
Dark chocolate, semisweet (1 oz.)	5–35
Baker's chocolate (1 oz.)	26
Chocolate-flavored syrup (1 oz.)	4

Source: Adapted from *Infertility Helper*, December 1996.

Marijuana, barbiturates, and other narcotics are a different story. Sperm quality is affected by heavy and/or frequent marijuana use. Essentially, the sperm get "stoned" and are not able to swim as well or move as effectively (motility) up the female reproductive tract. Marijuana may also increase the number of abnormal sperm produced. As for other recreational drugs, they interfere more with performance than with sperm quality, causing impotence and various ejaculatory disorders.

2. Coping Habits

Coping with the stress of daily existence can have adverse effects on both female and male fertility. Most women have experienced at least one fouled-up menstrual cycle because of job or personal stress. (Ironically, for teens and younger women, missing periods because of stress is most often caused by worrying about being pregnant!) Similarly, most men have experienced at least one bout of impotence or ejaculatory problems that is stress related. When men *can* perform sexually under great stress, their sperm counts are actually reduced. Stress-related situations revolve around career changes, job loss, death in the family, moving, exams, stressful workloads, and emotional upheavals.

Under stress, the hypothalamus, which controls both the female and male hormonal cycles (see chapters 4 and 5) functions more slowly. This slows down the pituitary gland, which in turn slows down the sex hormones of either the stressed-out man or woman. This translates into either a missed period or a decreased sperm count. It's not really understood *why* this happens, but it is considered a protective mechanism, a sort of prehistoric parachute in the human body. Studies show that women exposed to high levels of stress have higher levels of *prolactin*, a hormone that can block ovulation. The body senses the stress levels and decides to stop either ovulation or sperm production for that month, preventing a "stressed" pregnancy. This protective mechanism isn't unique to humans; animals in cramped quarters in either laboratories or zoos often cannot reproduce. Progesterone receptors also don't function when exposed to adrenaline—the hormone produced under stress.

Currently, fertility experts assume that between 5 and 10 percent of all infertility is stress related. Translation: Stress is a factor in 5 to 10 percent of all persons with either irregular menstrual cycles or reduced sperm counts.

"Just Relax . . . "

We hear these frustrating words often from friends, relatives, or even doctors. *There's no such thing as trying to "relax" when your life is stressful.* In fact, under stressful circumstances, you should listen to your *body* and *not* try to force conception.

Finding a strategic method for coping with stress is an expansive topic that drives a good portion of the how-to book and seminar market. The strategy that works for you is *highly* individualized, so what you find helpful, your partner may not. Consult the resource list at the back of this book for more information on relaxation books, methods, and therapists. To indicate how powerful some of these methods can be, a clinical study published in a 1991 issue of *Fertility and Sterility* revealed some amazing statistics. The study compared conception rates of two groups of infertile women. Seventeen percent of the women who had only medical treatment conceived, whereas 35 percent of the women who underwent a specific program of meditation, exercise, and yoga, *in addition to medical treatment*, conceived. In short, adding this particular relaxation method to medical treatments doubled these women's chances of conception. It's important to realize that the underlying cause of your stress may pass with time, as is the case with a death, a job change, a move, and so on.

When your stress is clearly job related, there are a number of ways you can minimize your stress, which are discussed in the "Work Habits" section. Sometimes the only solution is to change either your job or your career if you want to lead a more stress-free life.

Guidelines for Seeking Help

Many of us cope with stress by indulging in some of the bad habits discussed above, or overdoing it in the exercise or eating department. When this happens, your fertility becomes even more threatened as your lifestyle becomes *more* unhealthy. Whether your stress is a short-term or long-term problem, there are certain situations that warrant counseling. In fact, if you recognize yourself in any of the following statements, going for counseling is a good idea.

1. I need a few drinks every day (wine, beer, liquor) just to unwind.
2. I need to take drugs (cocaine, marijuana) in order to cope.
3. I pig out when I'm under stress and then punish myself with a really intense workout.
4. I'm losing interest in activities I used to enjoy (including sexual activities).
5. I'm not sleeping well. I wake up very early and can't seem to get back to sleep.
6. I feel very sad and depressed and haven't been able to pinpoint why.
7. I have no appetite; it's a struggle just to eat.
8. I'm always sleepy. I seem to need constant sleep just to function.
9. I'm very irritable and anxious over issues that never bothered me before (partner's habits, and so on).

3. Eating Habits

When your eating habits are unhealthy, the worst hit your body may take is below the belt. Both male and female fertility is dependent on healthy diets and stable weights. Because of the culture we live in, women are more susceptible to eating disorders than men, but sperm count can also be lowered through obesity or being underweight (see the following "Men" section).

Women

When it comes to true obesity, most women do not become obese until they begin dieting! Only a tiny portion of women are obese because of truly hereditary factors. Most women who think they are overweight are actually at an *ideal* weight for their height and body size. There is a crippling fear of obesity in Western society. Sixty percent of young girls develop distorted body images between grades one and six and believe that they are "fat," and 70 percent of all women begin dieting between the ages of fourteen and twenty-one. This just isn't healthy. A 1991 documentary reported that most women, when given a choice, would rather be dead than fat!

Eating disorders are so widespread that abnormal patterns of eating are becoming accepted in the general population. Some parents are actually *starving* their young daughters in an effort to keep them thin. The two most common eating disorders involve starvation dieting (in extreme cases, this develops into *anorexia nervosa*) and bingeing followed by purging (eating copious amounts of food, and then self-inducing vomiting or abusing laxatives, known as *bulimia*). Perhaps the most accepted abnormal dieting conduct revolves around overexercising, discussed later in this chapter, which has spawned a new term: *exercise bulimics*. Generally, all women have displayed or will display some type of abnormal eating behavior. At the minimal level, women often will not eat one day prior to a fancy function in an effort to fit into their outfit or "look thinner." Other women will binge/purge by abusing laxatives and diuretics. Many women will define "bingeing" as eating three well-balanced meals in one day, instead of the usual no-breakfast/salad-for-lunch/salad-for-dinner routine.

The truth is, living in fear of obesity can be more dangerous to your health than being 25 to 30 pounds overweight, the technical definition of obesity. Most women have a desired weight goal set at roughly 10 pounds *under* their ideal weight; many women who think they are overweight are either at an ideal weight or 10 pounds *underweight*. Women need to relearn their eating habits, understand why they gain weight when they starve themselves, understand the *reproductive* hazards of eating disorders, and reprogram their body image to welcome normal, necessary body fat.

Starvation diets, purging and bingeing rituals, and yo-yo dieting affect ovulation. If you have difficulty eating regularly or normally, you need to see a nutritionist to get your diet under control. Unless you're eating balanced meals and are maintaining a *stable* weight, you won't be creating optimum conditions for conception. When the female body is malnourished, it stops ovulating because it can't sustain a pregnancy. One doctor told me about an aboriginal tribe in Australia that has developed a unique protective mechanism: Women of that particular tribe menstruate only at certain times of the year, when the food cycle is abundant. During World War II, up to 50 percent of the women who were in concentration camps stopped menstruating within two months after their capture.

When you are truly starving, the body's ability to adapt to adverse conditions is amazing. But when you're jumping back and forth between starving and eating normally, you'll most certainly gain weight. Here's why: Your body is very smart. When it doesn't get enough calories, it gets tougher and more efficient. When you starve yourself, *it learns how to function on fewer calories*. When you go back to eating normally or eating less than you ate before you started dieting, you'll gain weight! Your body will be jarred by the sudden calorie intake and store it as fat for "later" when the "famine" strikes again. As far as your body is concerned, it doesn't know that you're living in North America and can have food anytime you want. Your body is trying to save you, not do you in! So be good to it. The gynecological consequences of starvation diets and yo-yo dieting are irregular cycles or even long bouts of amenorrhea (discussed in chapter 4), which translates into infertility, bone loss during pregnancy and before menopause (which creates huge problems during and after menopause), and future ovarian problems. Starving yourself results in the cruelest of "vicious cycles": Unless you keep reducing your food intake until you *do* starve to death, you'll gain weight to the extent of becoming *overweight*.

How much food should you eat?

The average nonpregnant woman in her childbearing years requires about 1,680 calories a day to maintain the right energy balance and ideal weight. This is an appropriate amount of calories, assuming that your food absorption, gastric emptying, secretion of digestive juices, and motility of your digestive tract are all intact. Conditions that affect all these elements are

- weight changes (sudden weight loss, yo-yo dieting, or sudden weight gain);
- diarrhea (often caused by abusing laxatives);
- mild or severe anemia (often caused by heavy periods; see chapter 4);
- diuretics (nutrients are taken out of the blood and excreted in the urine);
- thyroid disorders (your metabolism may speed up or slow down depending on the disorder);
- lactose intolerance (interferes with a high-calcium diet);
- diabetes;
- HIV; and
- high cholesterol, hypertension, and heart problems.

The above is only a sample of the unique problems that can affect the dietary needs of each woman. The only way to meet dietary requirements is to tailor your food and vitamin intake to your weight, height, culture, medical history, and lifestyle. How do you do this? Request a referral to a nutritionist. All hospitals have nutritionists on staff, and all doctors have lists of nutritionists they can refer you to.

When you meet with your nutritionist, put together a realistic food plan that you can stick to. If you have gained weight, you should be able to lose it by eating sensibly and following your food plan. Stay away from quick-fix diets, and try to set practical goals such as losing 1 to 2 pounds a week instead of 5 to 10 pounds. Eating healthy will also help improve the efficiency of any medications you're taking, because your digestive system will be better able to absorb them. For many women, consulting a therapist to deal with an eating disorder is a more appropriate route. Your primary care physician can refer you to one.

A good way to gauge whether you're at an ideal weight is to take a look at the Body Mass Index (BMI) chart, available through your doctor or nutritionist (as well as on several cereal boxes!). A BMI of under 20 means that you are probably underweight and may have difficulty conceiving. A BMI in the mid-20s is a healthy weight, while a BMI over 30 is considered to be in the obesity range.

If you truly are obese

If you're overweight by at least 25 to 30 pounds (that is, 25 to 30 pounds over your medically ideal weight—*not* your desired weight), your ovulation cycle can also be affected. Estrogen is stored in fat cells, which is one reason why overweight women tend to be at risk for certain estrogen-dependent cancers such as breast, endometrial, ovarian, or colon. The fat cells convert fat into estrogen, creating a type of estrogen reserve that may interfere with ovulation. Slimming down to a more ideal weight *with the help of a qualified nutritionist* not only may put your ovulation cycles back on track but will also help you achieve a healthier lifestyle.

Finally, the weight may interfere with intercourse positions, which naturally will have a bearing on your fertility. Usually, though, weight-affected sexual performance is more of a problem for obese men than for women.

Men

Although women in Western culture are more prone to starving themselves, men are more prone to (and even encouraged to) overeat. This can spell trouble for male fertility. The fat cells store androgen (a collection of male hormones that *includes* testosterone), just as fat cells store estrogen in women. But the fat cells in males can convert androgen into estrogen, causing overweight men to develop breast tissue (we've all seen this before, thinking it's just fat) and even a more feminine complexion, with softer skin and less facial hair. All this boils down to reduced testosterone levels and a dramatically reduced sperm count.

Obese men will also have more trouble with sexual performance. For example, excess weight in the abdominal area may get in the way of inserting the penis high enough inside the vagina; unless the sperm is ejaculated well inside the vagina, the sperm cannot swim as effectively up the cervix and female reproductive tract. Other problems may involve intercourse comfort and positioning. The man's weight may interfere with his own and/or his partner's sexual comfort, causing premature ejaculation, premature or involuntary withdrawal, or inadequate stimulation to maintain an erection.

Males who are overweight should get down to a stable weight through the help of a qualified nutritionist and a primary care physician. In some cases, an underactive thyroid may be the cause of a sudden weight gain. In addition to fertility problems, men who are obese are at a higher risk of developing heart problems, strokes, and various kinds of cancers.

Underweight men may also experience decreased libido and sperm counts. Infertility has been seen among men who are 25 percent below their medically ideal body weight. In Western culture, underweight men are generally a rare commodity, seen only in conjunction with chronic illnesses such as colitis or with more life-threatening illnesses such as cancer or AIDS. Achieving underweight is never a *deliberate* goal among men the way it is among women. Persistent weight loss due to poor appetite, however, is often a symptom of biologic depression, which may require psychiatric treatment. Persistent diarrhea, perspiration, and prolonged fevers are symptoms of illnesses ranging from parasitical, bacterial, or viral infections. In some cases, sudden weight loss could also be a sign of an overactive thyroid gland. Unexplained weight loss should always be followed up with a full physical.

What's good for the heart is good for conception

Adopting a heart-smart diet can also do wonders to improve male fertility because many of the factors that interfere with blood flow to the heart also interfere with blood flow to the penis and testicles, adversely affecting erection and ejaculate. Cutting down on saturated fats, adding fish fats to the diet (which are high in omega-3 oils and are good for the heart), and eating a variety of fruits and vegetables can all be the right start to healthy sperm.

About Those Chemicals and Pesticides . . .

There are several nutritional and medical experts who have gone on record to say that chemically processed food is bad for your reproductive organs. They recommend avoiding food that is processed and treated or contains artificial hormones. Eating organic seasonal and local foods is a good rule to follow. The U.S. Department of Agriculture and Ministry of Food and Agriculture in Canada have consumer information lines that can direct you to stores that carry organic produce. Some nutritionists also recommend sticking to the outside aisles of a supermarket when food shopping to avoid buying an excessive amount of canned, bottled, or boxed goods.

Anne Marie Colbin, in her 1986 book *Food and Healing*, cautions women about food that involves the reproductive systems of animals or contains both natural and artificial hormones. Her list includes free-range and hormone-fed chicken eggs, as well as meat from animals raised on estrogens. Free-range animal *meat* is perfectly fine, however.

A Danish study, published in a June 1994 issue of *The Lancet*, looked into the effects of chemicals on human fertility and revealed that male organic farmers who eat pesticide-free food are able to produce roughly *double* the average number of sperm. The Danish research team maintains that this latest study seems to link pesticides and food additives to a worldwide decline in male fertility over the last half-century. See the "Sperm Wars" section in chapter 2 for more details.

Watch your peas

Although I've always considered peas to be a reasonably harmless vegetable, Jean Carper, in her 1989 book *Food and Pharmacy*, claims that they're the worst thing you can eat when you're trying to conceive. Apparently, peas contain an antifertility chemical called *m-xylohydroquinone*, which somehow interferes with progesterone and estrogen. In fact, one of the few studies done on peas and fertility found that peas have an "oral contraceptive" property. (Definitely something the Green Giant ought to know about!)

4. Exercise Habits

Regular exercise should always accompany a healthy lifestyle, but today, the definition of being "in shape" has come to mean an exaggerated physique for both men and women. For both sexes, the pressure to pump up has reproductive consequences.

Women

Rigorous, strenuous exercise has become one of the tenets of socially accepted feminine behavior in the 1990s. It's not enough to look like a concentration camp victim; women now must look like concentration camp victims with *biceps*! Strenuous exercise often accompanies an eating disorder, and together they can wreak havoc on the female hormonal cycle. The appropriate amount of exercise women require is a brisk fifteen-minute walk each day. Eliminating all fat from the female body and building up biceps is *not* what a healthy female body is all about; this trend has more to do with "masculinizing" the female body than "feminizing" it. While exercising and toning are certainly part of a healthy lifestyle, it's important to do it for enjoyment and not because you're obsessed with maintaining a toned appearance. Overexercising can interfere with ovulation, causing women to miss their periods altogether or to experience long bouts of no periods, called amenorrhea (see chapter 4). It's not unusual for female athletes to stop menstruating when they're in training.

Exercise versus exorcise

In an age of eating disorders, a new form of bulimia has come into vogue as women binge and then overexercise to exorcise the caloric demons from within. This common food/fitness perversion is a disturbing lifestyle reality for many women and may warrant the intervention of a therapist as well as a nutritionist. If you're exercising out of guilt because you think you've binged, please seek professional guidance. This is not a healthy way to exercise and can do more long-term damage than you think.

Men

Of course, the body-building trends for women originated in the male gymnasium. Unfortunately, few men are immune to the allure of an Arnold Schwarzenegger body type. This has led to some unique problems for men trapped in the body-building craze.

Anabolic steroids, which are on their way out of vogue for professional athletes, are still very much in use by men who want to achieve that pro-athlete look. In addition to numerous health problems, anabolic steroids can cause *long-term male infertility*. Anabolic steroids are essentially pure testosterone derivatives, which cause a *huge* increase in testosterone levels in the steroid user. Testosterone levels are controlled by both the pituitary and hypothalamus glands, located in the brain. (See chapters 4 and 5 for more details.) When these glands see a rise in testosterone, they send a *stop production* message to the testes, believing that the testes are being overworked. As a result, the testes actually *shrink* in size, and the steroid user's natural testosterone levels dramatically drop. Even when he stops using the steroids, the user's testosterone levels can remain far lower than normal for years after use. A twenty-two-year-old male who bodybuilds today with the help of steroids may be in for a shock when he's thirty-two and suffering from low testosterone levels linked to steroids he stopped using when he was twenty-five.

5. Personal Hygiene Habits

It's too bad our reproductive organs don't come with an owner's manual that tells us how to care and maintain all parts. Many basic hygiene habits can have a dramatic effect on both male and female fertility.

Women

As a woman, I don't have to tell you that we're prone to both vaginal and urinary tract infections. These infections not only interfere with observing your cervical mucus (see chapter 4), but will also decrease the quality of your mucus. Mucus is necessary to help the sperm swim up the female reproductive tract and fertilize the egg.

One of the worst female hygiene habits is douching. Douching rids your vagina of friendly bacteria, which is important for maintaining its ecosystem. Douching is never recommended after menstruation, even though many women practice it. As long as you bathe regularly, your vagina and uterus are self-cleaning and will do everything that's necessary on their own. Finally, if you do have a bacterial or fungal infection, douching can push the bacteria or fungus higher inside your vagina, worsening the infection.

Avoid perfumes and dyes that can get into your vagina. Many of the chemicals used in these products can cause vaginal irritation and inflammation (vaginitis). Perfumes are found in many feminine products such as sprays, pads, and tampons, but you should also be careful of perfumed or colored toilet paper, hair care products that you may use in the bath or shower, certain bath or shower gels, and deodorant soaps. Here are some other hygiene tips to follow that can help you prevent vaginal or urinary tract infections:

- *Avoid wearing tight clothing around your vagina.* Tight pants, panties, and nylon pantyhose prevent your vagina from breathing and make it warmer and moister for a yeast infection to develop. Wear loose pants that allow your vagina to breathe, switch to knee-highs or old-fashioned stockings, or limit your pantyhose wearing for special occasions. Go bottomless to bed to let air into your vagina.
- *Wear only 100 percent cotton clothing and/or natural fibers around your vagina.* Synthetic underwear and polyester pants are not good ideas. All-cotton underwear, denim, wool, or rayon pants that are loose fitting are fine.
- *Don't insert anything into a dry vagina.* Whether it's a finger, penis, or tampon, make sure your vagina is well-lubricated before insertion. Dry vaginas can be prone to abrasions during insertion, which make excellent homes for yeast.
- *Avoid long car trips on vinyl seats.* New research indicates that vinyl seats increase a woman's risk of developing a yeast infection because the vinyl traps moisture and doesn't allow the crotch area to breathe. For longer car trips, sit on a towel.
- *Urinate before and after intercourse.* Experts recommend that you empty your bladder both before and immediately after sex. Urinating after sex will also help to wash out the bacteria from the urethra. Basically, the urethra can become irritated with frequent intercourse, and more bacteria may get inside the urethra, which leads to the bladder. Many women hold back their urge to urinate during intercourse, which can aggravate matters.

A word about tampons

Women use a lot of tampons. Just in North America, over 85 million women use tampons. The average woman may use as many as 16,800 tampons in her lifetime, and if she is on hormone replacement therapy after menopause, she may use as many as 24,360 tampons in her lifetime.

Since 1980, there has been a lot of press questioning the safety of tampons. The first reports that tampons may not be safe surrounded *toxic shock syndrome*, which I discuss further on. The most shocking tampon revelations arose from an independent study in 1991, which found that tampons usually contained one of the following additives: chlorine compounds, absorbency enhancers (which can be toxic), natural and synthetic fibers (such as cotton, rayon, polyester, and polyacrylate), deodorant, and fragrance.

The main concern over tampons surrounds the bleaching of the product, which produces dioxin, a chemical the EPA and the International Agency for Research on Cancer say probably cause cancer. (For more information on environmental carcinogens, see my book *Stopping Cancer at the Source*, which can be ordered from www.sarahealth.com.) The extent to which dioxins are in tampons have been a source of debate, but since dioxin is a by-product of chlorine-bleaching processes used in the manufacture of paper products, including tampons, sanitary pads, panty liners, and diapers, it stands to reason that tampons do contain dioxin. There are bleaching processes that do not produce dioxin, but unfortunately, the paper manufacturers that produce the raw materials used in tampons use either elemental-chlorine or chlorine-dioxide bleaching processes that we know do produce dioxin. The FDA, however, insists that the raw materials used to produce tampons now involve chlorine-free bleaching processes, but it also says: "Some elemental chlorine-free bleaching processes can theoretically generate dioxins at extremely low levels, and dioxins are occasionally detected in trace amounts. . . ."

As a result, women have been unwittingly exposed to more dioxin than most men because of their use of tampons and other menstrual products. According to the FDA, "State-of-the-art testing of tampons and tampon materials that can detect even trace amounts of dioxin has shown that dioxin levels are at or below the detectable limit. No risk to health would be expected from these trace amounts." But trace amounts of dioxin are not considered safe by most environmental groups and women's health groups.

The questioning of tampon safety has led the United States Congress to introduce in 1999 the Tampon Safety Research Act, which has yet to be passed. The purpose of this bill is to research the ingredients used to make tampons, such as dioxin, synthetic fibers, and other additives, to investigate the true health effects, and whether these ingredients place women at risk for cervical cancer, endometriosis, infertility, ovarian cancer, breast cancer, immune system deficiencies, pelvic inflammatory disease, and toxic shock syndrome. Futhermore, what are the health effects on fetal and childhood development?

What about asbestos?

Some women's groups have published that U.S. tampon manufacturers add asbestos to their products to promote excessive menstrual bleeding in order to sell more tampons. This isn't that crazy a claim, considering that the tobacco industry added substances to cigarettes to make them more addictive. The FDA maintains that the asbestos charges are purely rumor and that there is no evidence that asbestos is used in tampons. Nonetheless, to confirm or negate such claims, it's important that independent studies are done on tampons.

Who regulates tampons?

Tampons are considered "medical devices," and as such, should be regularly assessed, tested, and monitored as vigorously as bandages or heart valves. But they're not. The U.S. government has determined that the FDA has not adequately investigated the safety of tampons because of its reliance on safety data provided by the tampon manufacturers rather than independent peer-reviewed scientific studies on the safety of the product. And tampon manufacturers do not make their data available to the public. This is how the tobacco industry escaped as long as it did with not disclosing all the ingredients in cigarettes. In Japan, however, there are strict tests that the government applies to tampon manufacturing and testing. No level, including trace levels, of dioxin are considered acceptable by European health authorities as well as the World Health Organization. Health Canada has no position on the substance.

Aside from toxic shock syndrome, there are other problems tampons can cause. Because they actively absorb menstrual blood and do not differentiate between blood and vaginal mucus, the skin that lines the vaginal walls dries up. That can lead to micro-ulcerations and infection. Artificial fibers such as rayon, which most brand name bleached tampons contain, are abrasive; when the tampon expands, it can cause tiny cuts and imbed pieces into the vaginal tissue. To read information directly from the FDA on tampons, see www.fda.gov/opacom/catalog/ots_tss.html or www.fda.gov/fdac/features/2000/200_tss.html. Keep in mind, though, that many health experts do not feel that the FDA's take on tampon safety is accurate or acceptable. But it's worth a read.

Tampon hygiene rules

Tampons should therefore never be used between periods, during pregnancy (to absorb mucus, for example), or when you already have a vaginal infection. In the United States, to help tampon shoppers compare absorbency from brand to brand, packages use terms that determine thickness, such as "junior," "regular," "super," and "super plus."

Many women with extremely heavy flows are in the habit of using more than one tampon at the same time. If you're among them, get out of the habit. The second one can "get lost"—pushed up so high in your vagina you can't retrieve it yourself. The general rule with tampons is to change them every four to six hours. Official warnings state that tampons left for twelve to eighteen hours may put you at risk for toxic shock syndrome.

Toxic shock syndrome

Toxic shock syndrome (TSS) is defined as a group of symptoms. It is usually caused by a bacteria already present in the vagina that adheres to the tampon. The bacteria then starts producing a toxin that attacks other parts of the body. The initial symptoms of TSS are fever, nausea, vomiting, diarrhea, sore throat, and dizziness. Other symptoms include a sunburnlike rash, peeling of the skin (especially on the hands and feet), and low blood pressure. All of these symptoms are, of course, vague and can be attributed to a host of other diseases. So, if someone has TSS, she can easily be misdiagnosed, particularly if she has only a few symptoms. These days, TSS caused by tampon use is considered pretty rare now that we have warnings about it in tampon packaging. The Centers for Disease Control and Prevention (CDC) report a great reduction in tampon-related TSS. For example, in 1997, only five confirmed tampon-related TSS cases were reported; in 1980, there were 814 cases. The higher the tampon's absorbency, the greater the risk of TSS regardless of whether the tampon is made with rayon or the purest, most organically grown cotton.

A word about toilet habits

Toilet habits are one of the most common sources of bacteria in the vagina. For example, if you wipe from back to front, you could introduce fecal material into your vagina. Using a wash cloth on your vagina can transfer germs from your washcloth to your vagina. After a loose bowel movement, wet the toilet paper and clean your rectal area thoroughly so that fecal material doesn't stay on your underwear and wind up in your vagina. To prepare for less hygienic bathrooms, bring some moist wipes with you that are safe for babies' bottoms.

Men

The testicles hang below the crotch for a reason: In order for the testicles to produce enough sperm, *they need to be a few degrees cooler than normal body temperature.*

Although the "boxer shorts" story is the classic example of temperature-related infertility, this problem is more commonly seen in men who indulge in hot baths, whirlpools, or saunas. Wearing tight underwear or tight pants all the time can also reduce your sperm count, which is why boxer shorts and looser fitting pants are encouraged.

If you're exposed to an environment that has extremely hot temperatures (certain kinds of industrial plants, trapped in traffic jams with no air conditioning, and so on), your sperm count can also be reduced. Truck drivers, cab drivers, or men who sit at a desk all day are also prone to this, as well as men who live in very hot climates.

Experts suggest that cooling the testes via cool baths, ice baths, or even wearing a cool cloth inside a jock strap can dramatically improve sperm counts for temperature-related infertility.

Because your urethra is about eight inches longer than your female partner's, you're not as prone to urinary tract infections as she is, but you, too, should empty your bladder before and after intercourse (particularly after anal intercouse, which, by the way, should only be practiced with condoms), and wash your penis carefully to reduce exposure to bacteria.

A word about shampoo

In chapter 1, I discussed the problem of estrogenic chemicals and the decline in sperm count as a result. One of the most common estrogenic ingredients used today is known as alkyl-phenyl ethoxylades, which are found in many shampoos, soaps, and cosmetics. These are thought to affect sperm quality. Try to use a shampoo made from all-natural ingredients, if possible.

6. Sexual Habits

There are some common sexual habits that can interfere with conception, but there are also common doctor-recommended "rituals" that are utterly useless in improving the odds.

Oral Sex

This first piece of news probably should go under the "Eating Habits" section. Ladies, if you're in the habit of ingesting sperm, get *out* of the habit today. Experts in the field of immunological infertility (discussed more in chapters 5, 6, 7, and 9) have found evidence suggesting that women who swallow their partners' sperm may form *antibodies* to the sperm. In a sense, swallowing the sperm is synonymous with being innoculated with it, and you could wind up giving yourself a sperm vaccine!

How is this possible? When the sperm is introduced into the digestive tract, the immune system sees it as a foreign invader, forms antibodies to it, and kills it off. Later, when the same sperm shows up in the cervical canal, the immune system gets confused and attacks and kills the sperm on the spot, preventing conception. The more sperm you swallow, the more antibodies you create, so a single episode of ingesting sperm will most likely not affect your fertility. In addition, since the antibodies are created in response to one *specific* partner's sperm, past episodes of sperm swallowing with *other* partners should *not* cause your body to form antibodies to your *current* partner's sperm.

Men often ingest their own sperm when they perform cunnilingus after intercourse with their female partners. In this case, past episodes of this with other partners *can* affect your fertility today. *To avoid swallowing your own sperm, always wash your penis carefully after sex.* When a male forms antibodies to his own sperm, the antibodies may even destroy the sperm before they leave his body.

Finally, women who have anal sex with their partners should avoid getting sperm inside their rectums, which can also cause their bodies to create sperm antibodies. Anal sex may cause the tissue inside the rectum to tear, allowing the sperm easy access into the bloodstream, triggering the immune system to create antibodies.

Bear in mind that this theory is still in the research phase and has not yet been *absolutely* proven! Nevertheless, if it's true, it could be a powerful piece of preventive medicine for millions of couples.

Sexual Lubricants

Using a sexual lubricant can interfere with the sperm's survival in the vagina, as well as with the cervical mucus. If you're using a lubricant, stop.

Ejaculation Frequency

Ejaculation—in moderation—is necessary for good sperm production. Sperm that hang around too long in the *epididymis* (a section of the testicle where sperm are stored) can spoil the bunch. In other words, dead sperm will get mixed in with live, healthy sperm and contribute to decreased sperm count. Because of this, it's important to ejaculate at least once a month through either intercourse or masturbation. However, too much ejaculation will also cause a decrease in sperm count. That's why experts recommend that couples have sex every other day around ovulation. (Some couples will have sex every other day throughout the entire cycle, which may not be realistic for those of us who work for a living!)

Many men tend to masturbate between bouts of intercourse with their partners. This is fine, but tell your partner about the frequency of your ejaculations. If you masturbated yesterday, and she's ready for sex today, it's unfair to get her hopes up. You may need to time your masturbation accordingly to allow for optimum sperm count during intercourse.

Ignore All Positioning Rituals

Planning sex around an ovulation cycle is mechanical enough, but matters are made worse by many doctors who *still* recommend the missionary position, with the woman propped up on pillows. This won't hurt, of course, *but it will not improve the odds*. Have sex any way you like. The only conditions you must meet are that the sperm be deposited deep inside the vagina. In fact, the position that turns you on the most is the one to go with; the vagina will be better lubricated, and the male orgasm will be optimum! And because many men can't stand the missionary position, they may not be able to ejaculate when they're in it.

Some doctors also give positioning "recipes" that optimize one's chances for boys or girls. While many fertility specialists feel this is the stuff of mythology and fantasy, it is certainly not harmful in any way. There was a recent study done in Britain that concluded that the age difference between male and female partners actually has bearing on the sex of their first child. Women whose male partners were more than five years older were more likely to have a son as their first child, while women whose partners were younger or the same age were more likely to have a girl as a first child. Age difference had no bearing on the sex of subsequent children, however.

Other studies done in this area show a rise in male births after World War II, which some thought was related to hardship, but others now relate to age differences between partners. (After WWII, many women married older men.) In wildlife, the age of many animals is related to the sex of their offspring, too.

Attention, Ladies

After intercourse, do what you feel like doing: sleep, urinate, eat, walk. You *don't* need to do the "bicycle" for fifteen minutes, or lie back with your knees up, or refrain from urinating. To avoid infection, it is wise to urinate immediately after intercourse.

However, many fertility experts report that, in some instances, lying quietly in bed for fifteen to twenty minutes after intercourse can help the conception process.

Anejaculation

This refers to men who do not or cannot ejaculate when they climax. Sometimes anejaculation occurs only with intercourse and not masturbation; often the problem exists with both sexual acts. This is obviously a cause of infertility, but it is difficult to diagnose and depends on *self-reporting*. If your partner is well lubricated, she may not realize that you have this problem either. It's also important not to confuse anejaculation with *retrograde ejaculation*, where the ejaculate goes backward rather than forward, a true structural problem that can be diagnosed and treated (see chapters 5 and 7).

Anejaculation is a problem rooted in psychological trauma and is an indication that you need counseling. If you suffer from this, you must report it to avoid long, involved workups. Either a primary care doctor or a urologist can refer you to a therapist who specializes in this problem.

A Word About Arousal

Getting yourself aroused when you're having sex by the calendar can be a challenge. Feel free to use as many visual aids as you like: videos, magazines, stripteases, soft lights, and so on. Research indicates that when a woman reaches orgasm at the time of ejaculation (but not before), her orgasmic contractions also help to propel the sperm upward, toward the uterus. If a woman reaches orgasm prior to ejaculation (that is, during foreplay), the contractions may keep sperm away. Try to time your orgasms if you can. You should also avoid alcohol, marijuana, cocaine, and all the other no-no's mentioned in the "Bad Habits" section. You should probably avoid flavored sex jellies or other lubricant concoctions, since they may interfere with sperm quality or cervical mucus. Vibrators and dildos are fine as long as they're clean! Finally, avoid intercourse in the shower, pool, hot tub, whirlpool, or bathtub: water may interfere with either sperm quality or cervical mucus; heat will interfere with sperm production.

7. Work Habits

In the "Coping Habits" section, I touched on the issue of work-related stress, which can interfere with ovulation as well as reduce sperm count. Job stress is caused either by working too many hours or by having to perform well under rigid scrutiny (this scrutiny is often self-imposed). But often these two conditions are combined, creating impossible schedules and goal setting for the worker, spawning a new addiction known as "workaholism," discussed below.

The physical position (that is, sitting all day) you maintain as you perform your job function can also affect fertility, while the level of toxins you're exposed to in the workplace is a major factor in reducing both male and female fertility. These issues are discussed separately in the "Occupational Hazards" section.

Workaholism

You are considered a workaholic when your job takes priority over your personal life or when you spend more time at your work than you do at home. The term *workaholic* has unfortunately come to have *positive* connotations in our society. Many companies and firms pride themselves on employing workaholics, devaluing employees who want to work reasonable hours. As a result, a new term, *work addiction*, has come to replace *workaholism*. People who are self-employed or who run businesses are also classic workaholics.

We now know that there is a real *physical* addiction that workaholics experience, as well as common personality traits. (Being called a "Type A" personality is used interchangeably with the term *workaholic*.) Workaholics tend to be overachievers, often setting goals that are so high they are unreachable. Working to reach the goal sets off a complex chain of adrenaline rushes that feed the work addiction. The workaholic actually gets high on that adrenaline rush and misses the rush when he or she is not at work. This is why workaholics prefer to spend their weekends at work rather than at home and typically work a 5 to 9 schedule rather than 9 to 5.

Many people hide from personal problems by overworking. In fact, personal stress can often *trigger* a work addiction. This is particularly common when couples experience a delay in conception. To avoid dealing with possible infertility, one or both partners will often become "too busy" to really try, using their "impossible" schedules as a cover for a real physical problem. Women who have infertile male partners will often become work "widows" as the male partners develop work addictions to avoid going home and facing their feelings of inadequacy. This issue is addressed more in chapters 5 and 7.

Whether you use the office as a refuge or you thrive on the rush of overachieving, the lack of quality time at home will affect your desire for sex as well as your reproductive capacity. In addition, work addiction will often foster other bad habits: poor nutrition, smoking, drinking, overexercising, and so on. The group *Workaholics Anonymous*, listed in your local white pages, offers a twelve-step program designed to help work addicts lead healthier personal lives. Your primary care physician can also refer you to a counselor or therapist who can help you break your addiction.

Occupational Hazards

While there are numerous things we can do to purify our bodies and our food intake, many of us face daily toxins in our workplace that can affect our fertility.

Of the roughly sixty thousand industrial chemicals used, only three have been documented as absolutely affecting human reproduction: metallic lead (still found in many gasolines and exhausts), the pesticide dibromochloropropane (DBCP), and a pharmaceutical solvent called ethylene oxide. Several other chemicals have been linked to impaired fertility, causing either reduced sperm counts or ovarian failure. These chemicals include mercury, chlordecone (another pesticide), vinyl chloride (do you work in a hard-plastics plant?), a variety of paints, solvents, stains, and varnishes, and manganese (used in steel, glass, ink, ceramics, paints, welding rods, rubber, and wood preservatives). Some of the industries where harmful chemicals are commonplace are agriculture, laboratories, oil, chemical and atomic industries, pulp and paper, and textiles.

As discussed in chapter 1, new evidence suggests that several chemicals break down into an "estrogenic" by-product. In other words, many chemicals actually "leak" a substance identical to the female hormone estrogen. This is being linked to reduced sperm counts, a rise in male anatomical problems such as undescended testes, and a rise in certain reproductive cancers, including breast cancer.

The list of damaging toxins is dizzying, overwhelming, and upsetting. The best thing you can do is to inform yourself about your workplace hazards by consulting the appropriate departments within the EPA in the United States or within Environment Canada. You can also go directly to the industry in question (such as the Department of Agriculture). Environmental groups such as Greenpeace have information on a number of industry hazards. In the meantime, you can review Tables 3.2, 3.3, and 3.4 for more information. These tables list suspected occupational hazards as of 1982.

Table 3.2 Some Chemical Hazards That May Affect Reproductive Health

Hazard	Workers at Risk	Potential Reproductive Effect	Protective Measures
Anesthetic gases (including halothane, nitrous oxide, methoxyflurane)	health care workers in hospitals and dental clinics, veterinary surgeons and assistants, researchers in animal laboratories	*male workers*: sperm abnormalities; wives/female partners of exposed male workers may experience an increased evidence of miscarriages, premature deliveries, and offspring with birth defects; *female workers*: same as wives/female partners of male workers; *the fetus*: birth defects	install scavenger units to collect stray gases; monitor air in operating theater to ensure low levels
Benzene	workers producing or using solvents, plastics, rubbers, glues, dyes, detergents, paints, petroleum, and other products containing this substance	*male and female workers*: chromosome changes, linked with leukemia and genetic effects in offspring; *female workers*: prolonged menstrual bleeding and postpartum hemorrhage after chronic exposure; *the fetus*: birth defects, higher incidence of leukemia, illness from contaminated breast milk	substitute nontoxic or less toxic products; take regular workplace air samples; ensure proper ventilation and safe engineering processes
Beryllium	ceramic makers, electronics workers, jewelry makers, laboratory workers, nuclear technologists	*female workers*: pregnancy may exacerbate symptoms of beryllium poisoning and cause death; *the fetus*: may cross placenta and affect fetal development	monitor workplace levels regularly; install proper ventilation and dust collection devices in the work environment
Carbon disulfide	degreasers, glue makers, paint removers, rubber makers, rayon viscose makers	*male workers*: decreased libido, impotence, sperm abnormalities; *female workers*: irregular menstrual cycle, decreased fertility, frequent miscarriages; *the fetus*: higher incidence of miscarriage	monitor workplace levels and reduce to minimum; ensure that prolonged worker exposure is prohibited
Hormones (including androgens, estrogens, progestogens, and synthetic products such as DES)	workers involved in the extraction, manufacture, and use of hormones, including pharmaceutical workers, laboratory workers, farmers, and veterinarians	*male workers*: sexual impotence, breast enlargement, infertility; *female workers*: irregular menstruation, infertility, ovarian cysts, breast lumps, cancer of the reproductive system; *the fetus*: may develop enlarged breasts and other signs of	monitor regularly to ensure low levels of airborne hormones; isolate the process through engineering design

Substance	Workers exposed	Health effects	Preventive measures
Lead	auto manufacturers, ceramic and pottery makers, electronics workers, farmers, pesticide makers, paint makers and users, and typographers	sexual maturity as well as abnormalities of the skeletal system, heart, and windpipe; DES may cause cancer in female offspring, genital and sperm abnormalities in male offspring *male workers:* decreased libido, decreased sperm count, atrophy of the testes; wives/female partners demonstrate adverse effects such as infertility, menstrual disorders, miscarriages; *female workers:* infertility, miscarriages, stillbirths, menstrual disorders; *the fetus:* higher incidence of miscarriages, stillbirths, neonatal death; mental retardation can occur; newborns can be affected by contaminated breast milk	sample workplace air frequently; provide adequate ventilation; clean work areas regularly
Mercury	battery makers, ceramic workers, commercial fishermen, dental workers, farm workers, jewelry makers, lithographers, pesticide makers, photographic chemical makers and users	*male workers:* reduced fertility; *female workers:* miscarriages, stillbirths; *the fetus:* linked with severe brain damage, mental retardation, increased rate of miscarriages and stillbirths	regular air monitoring and good ventilation; enclose mercury processes; check frequently for spills and vapor leaks
Pesticides (including carbaryl, dibromochloropropane, kepone, malathion 2,4,5-T)	agricultural workers, commercial and household gardeners, pesticide manufacturers	*male workers:* chromosomal changes, impotence, loss of libido, decreased sperm counts, atrophy of the testes; *female workers:* miscarriages, chromosomal changes; *the fetus:* miscarriages, birth deformities	design processes to prevent worker contact with substance; monitor air levels in workplace and keep to a minimum
Vinyl chloride	workers involved in the production of vinyl chloride and polyvinyl chloride and its related products	*male workers:* genetic damage of the sperm, leading to adverse pregnancy outcome in wives/female partners; *female workers:* genetic damage to ovum, miscarriages, stillbirths; *the fetus:* higher incidence of miscarriage, fetal death, and birth defects	monitor workplace regularly; use proper ventilation and safe design to keep levels at a minimum

Source: The Canadian Advisory Council on the Status of Women. Reprinted with Permission.

Table 3.3 Some Biological Hazards That May Affect Reproductive Health

Hazard	Workers at Risk	Potential Reproductive Effect	Protective Measures
Brucellosis (undulant fever)	animal breeders, farmers, health care workers, meat handlers, veterinarians	*male and female workers:* brucellae may lodge in reproductive organs, leading to local inflammations and infertility; *the fetus:* miscarriage, developmental defects	control infection in animals; use caution in handling diseased animals and their products as well as the urine and feces of infected humans
Chicken pox (varicella)	child care workers, pediatric nurses, teachers, laboratory workers, parents	*the fetus:* prematurity, retardation, muscular, skeletal, and heart defects, increased incidence of neonatal death	isolate infectious person and handle contaminated articles using aseptic techniques; pregnant women should avoid exposure
Cytomegalovirus	blood bank workers, health care workers, dental workers, laboratory workers	*the fetus:* infection leading to jaundice, enlarged spleen and liver, heart, eye, and central nervous system damage in the newborn	use care in handling sputum, urine, semen, blood, and other secretions of the human body; pregnant women should avoid exposure
Hepatitis (infectious and serum)	blood unit workers, kidney dialysis technicians, laundry workers, laboratory workers, sterilization unit workers	*the fetus:* infection leading to miscarriage, prematurity, stillbirth, and jaundice; enlarged spleen, increased death rate in newborns	isolate infectious individuals; label potentially infectious specimens visibly; use disposable needles, syringes, lancets where possible; pregnant women should avoid exposure
Herpes virus hominus	health care workers, hospital staff, laboratory workers, research scientists	*male and female workers:* transmissible genital infections; *the fetus:* fetal death, miscarriage, liver and eye diseases, central nervous system damage	isolate infected persons or specimens; use caution in handling infected objects

Mumps (infectious parotitis)	child care workers, hospital staff, laboratory workers, restaurant workers, teachers, parents	*male and female workers*: inflammation of testes and ovaries, leading to infertility or sterility; *the fetus*: miscarriages, stillbirths, developmental defects, hydrocephalus	isolate infectious persons, handle specimens with care; alert all workers potentially in contact; promote immunization
Rubella (German measles)	child care workers, hospital personnel, laboratory staff, restaurant workers, teachers, parents	*the fetus*: placental infection may lead to severe congenital abnormalities including deafness, blindness, heart defects, mental retardation	promote immunization; isolate infected person; handle contaminated material with care; pregnant women must avoid exposure
Syphilis	blood unit workers, health care workers, laboratory workers	*male and female workers*: secondary lesions in organs of the body including reproductive organs, infertility or sterility; *the fetus*: embryal death, infection leading to liver and spleen enlargement, developmental defects	avoid contact with infected lesions; exercise caution in handling infected equipment
Tuberculosis	dairy farm workers, health care workers, laboratory workers, laundry workers	*male and female workers*: tubercular infection of the reproductive organs; *the fetus*: can be infected through blood transfer from the mother or by aspiration of amniotic fluid	promote immunization; test animals regularly; handle infected specimens with caution

Source: The Canadian Advisory Council on the Status of Women. Reprinted with Permission.

Table 3.4 Some Physical Hazards That May Affect Reproductive Health

Hazard	Workers at Risk	Potential Reproductive Effect	Protective Measures
Ionizing radiation	atomic radiation workers, dental and chiropractor office workers, hospital employees, scientists	*male and female workers:* sterility, premature aging of the sex cells, altered genetic material; *the fetus:* damage resulting in prenatal death, mental retardation, birth defects, increased incidence of leukemia and other cancers	reduce workplace levels to a minimum; use proper shielding techniques; monitor individual exposures using film badge dosimeters and other mobile measuring devices; leave contaminated workclothes at the worksite; maintain exposure records for workers
Noise and vibration	assembly line workers, airline attendants, construction workers, garment and textile workers, machinists, motor vehicle drivers, pneumatic drill operators	*male workers:* sexual dysfunction and decreased fertility; *female workers:* disturbances of the menstrual cycle, increased rate of premature births and complications during labor; *the fetus:* disturbances of uterine circulation in the mother may lead to miscarriage, low birth weight, perinatal mortality	design machines to ensure minimal noise and vibration; use proper preventive maintenance for equipment; isolate noise using noise absorbing partitions; use sound and vibration absorbing material in floors, walls, and ceilings; install mufflers on all motorized equipment, provide frequent rest periods and job rotations to decrease worker exposure
Nonionizing radiation	flight attendants and pilots, food service workers, health care workers, radio navigation, radar communication workers	*male workers:* degeneration of the testes, decreased libido, lower sperm count and motility, abnormally shaped sperm; *female workers:* changes in menstrual cycles, decreased lactation in nursing mothers; *the fetus:* miscarriage, retarded fetal development, congenital defects such as club foot and Down's syndrome	shield or isolate operations using nonionizing radiation; check sources regularly for production of X rays
Temperature (heat)	workers in bakeries, canneries, foundries, garment and textile factories, laundries, mines, smelters	*male workers:* decreased sperm count, atrophy of the testes; *female workers:* decreased fertility; *the fetus:* increased embryal death, low birth weight	provide adequate training and acclimation, properly designed clothing, and frequent rest periods; enclose heat producing operations as much as possible; ventilate the work area

Source: The Canadian Advisory Council on the Status of Women. Reprinted with Permission.

Ladies only

If you work in a dental office as a dentist, dental hygienist, or dental assistant, it's now known that nitrous oxide can dramatically affect your ability to either conceive or sustain a pregnancy. Although nitrous oxide is also used in veterinary clinics, ambulances, and hospitals, dental office workers are exposed to higher levels because no masks are placed on patients' mouths. If you're exposed to five or more hours of "unscavenged" (unmasked) nitrous oxide, your fertility can be dramatically compromised. One study found that women exposed to these amounts experienced a 60 percent drop in conception rates with each menstrual cycle, while 50 percent of the pregnant women in the study exposed to these levels miscarried.

Since the first edition of this book, the results from one of the first female occupational risk studies has been published, done by the University of Iowa College of Medicine. This Iowa study has concluded that some further occupational hazards can damage a woman's fertility. Solvents, chemical dusts, pesticides, and video display terminals (VDTs) have all been listed as hazards that may double or even triple the risk of infertility.

Researchers found that women who were exposed to organic solvents, pesticides, or chemical dusts had a higher risk of developing the following problems, all discussed at length in chapter 2.

- Scarring on the fallopian tubes
- Ovulation failure
- Endometriosis (which may account for the fallopian tube problem)

As for VDT hazards, endometriosis and/or poor cervical mucus were much more common in women using VDTs than in those who did not. Women working around VDTs had a 3.69 times greater risk of endometriosis and a 2.65 times greater likelihood of having cervical-factor infertility.

While many of these hazards are related to occupation, a number of them are related to household products and hobbies involving painting, woodworking, and gardening. For example, solvents are found in paint, cleaners, resins (manufacturer-related), and hair sprays. Commercial wood is also loaded with chemicals to protect it from mold, fungi, and insects. And agricultural dusts also contain a variety of chemicals including pesticides and aflatoxins—which have been linked to birth defects. So next time you're watching a craft guru on cable, beware the phrase: "You can find this paint in most craft stores."

Occupational hazards you can do something about

One of the chief occupational workplace hazards is being exposed to secondhand smoke. No one today should put up with this. Many workplaces are now smoke free, but there are a disturbing number of companies that are not, or do not enforce smoke-free policies. Most states and provinces now have rigid legislation regarding smoking in the workplace. You can arrange to have an occupational health and/or safety representative inspect your workplace and fine your employer if the company isn't complying with state or provincial laws. Most of these agencies accept anonymous complaints so your job is not compromised. In most states and provinces, employers have a legal responsibility to provide a clean workplace; if you feel that you must leave your workplace because of secondhand smoke, you are in a good position to sue your employer.

Similarly, long hours of overtime work must be compensated with either equal time off or overtime pay. You should not be expected to endure repeated episodes of double shifts or twelve-hour days without compensation.

If you're in a sedentary job where you sit for long periods of time, schedule time out for stretching and walking around. Again, males may be prone to reduced sperm production due to raising the temperature of their testes (see the "Personal Hygiene" section on page 56).

Finally, anyone who works around radiation, such as health care professionals and technicians, should arrange to wear a shield over his or her pelvic region to protect the reproductive organs.

Little-known hazards

Don't underestimate the damage done by seemingly invisible occupational stresses, such as the noise and vibration associated with heavy machinery (like that used in car plants), which can affect menstruation. Continuous vibration can lead to miscarriage in pregnant women. Other not-so-obvious occupational hazards include

- heat exposure (bakers, laundry workers, or workers in heavy manufacturing);
- physical work (causing injury or fatigue);
- traveling (which can affect menstrual cycles);
- exposure to infections (teachers, child care workers, agricultural workers, health care workers, or vets).

As I stated at the beginning of this chapter, it's crucial to assess whether your lifestyle habits are posing any hazards to your fertility. If you and your partner are trying to conceive, you should clean up your act in terms of bad habits, exercise, and nutrition *before* you begin charting the menstrual cycle and timing intercourse. Otherwise, you could be wasting a lot of time and energy—something an infertility investigation is dependent on. The next chapter is the next step in the fertility journey. Understanding your individual ovulation cycle as a *couple* is a must if you're trying to conceive.

4

Zen and the Art of
Menstrual Cycle Maintenance

WHEN IT COMES to understanding the female menstrual cycle, there is a great deal of Zen involved. In a word, Zen boils down to *acceptance*. Most women of reproductive age today haven't learned to accept the timing of their natural cycles because many women have been trained to medicate in an attempt to alleviate the uncomfortable premenstrual symptoms that precede or accompany their periods. Often, women will be put on oral contraceptives in their teens and twenties, not as a form of birth control, but as a way of altering the cycle to make it more regular or bearable. Many of these women will simply stay on oral contraceptives (OCs) until they want to conceive. In extreme cases, some women who suffer from premenstrual syndrome (PMS) are put on a hormonal therapy, which may include danazol. Danazol actually *shuts down* ovarian function, mimicking menopause. And there are published case studies in which some women have been recommended for a hysterectomy as a way to treat PMS.

The bottom line is that many women planning to conceive have no idea what kind of menstrual cycle they have because the cycle has been masked for so long. This means that most couples need to formally introduce themselves to the female menstrual cycle. This chapter is designed to tell you everything you need to know about the female menstrual cycle to plan conception. Obviously, much of the information in this chapter will be better understood by women than by men. However, I have included a special section at the end of the chapter for men. Observing the menstrual cycle can be a challenging task, and there is a role the male can play in the charting process. The male hormonal cycle is discussed in chapter 5.

An Unremarkable Menstrual Cycle

Remember that lecture in health class, when the teacher warned all the girls that they could get pregnant at *any* time—during their periods, after their periods, and so on? *Well, it's not true.* Young women are told this because it's assumed that most teens are *not* aware of their menstrual cycles. In addition, because many teenage women have *irregular* menstrual cycles (extremely common from the time of *menarche*, the first period, until about age eighteen or nineteen), practicing natural birth control isn't a practical option for them. So, for a sexually active seventeen-year-old, warning her that she "can get pregnant during her period" is still a good idea.

Once you reach your mid-to-late twenties, your natural menstrual cycle will probably have established itself and will become fairly regular. But what's regular for one person may be irregular for someone else.

Your menstrual cycle is actually a "hormonal cycle." It's driven by a symphony of hormones that trigger one another, stopping and starting, flooding and tapering in a regular rhythm each month. Every woman's hormones dance to a different tune, but rarely does this pattern correspond to the English calendar. This is because the word *month* comes from the root word *moon*. The Greek word for moon is *mene*, and *menstruation* actually means "moon change." This is why some women have shorter and longer cycles. In fact, female roommates who have completely different cycles in the beginning may synchronize their cycles over time. Some experts suggest that women may produce pheromones (a sexual odor) that other women can unconsciously smell. At any rate, women's cycles are often more "in tune" with the moon and with each other, on levels not completely understood.

The Hormonal Cycle

A five-month-old female fetus has cells that can produce roughly seven million eggs. But by the time that baby is born and reaches puberty, only four hundred thousand of those eggs will be viable. That number dwindles throughout the thirty-odd years that she menstruates. Any eggs that remain dissolve into the ovarian tissue, and at this point the woman officially enters menopause. Low levels of sex hormones are continuously produced during a woman's reproductive years. But it is the continuous *fluctuation* of hormones that establish the menstrual cycle and the understandable premenstrual symptoms.

The main organs involved in the cycle are the hypothalamus (a part of the brain), the pituitary gland, and the ovaries. The hypothalamus is like the symphony conductor, controlling and signaling each hormonal "instrument" to do its solo, duet, and so on. It tells the pituitary gland to start the hormonal "program," which signals the ovaries to begin their performance by producing estrogen and progesterone. The hypothalamus is sensitive to the fluctuating levels of hormones produced by the ovaries. When the level of estrogen drops below a certain level, the hypothalamus turns on gonadotropin-releasing hormone (GnRH), which stimulates the pituitary gland to release follicle-stimulating hormone (FSH). FSH triggers the growth of ten to twenty ovarian follicles, but only one of them will mature fully; the others will start to degenerate some time before ovulation. As the follicles grow, they secrete estrogen in increasing amounts. The estrogen affects the lining of the uterus, signaling it to enter the proliferatory, or growth, phase. When the egg approaches maturity inside the mature follicle, the follicle releases a burst of progesterone (progesterone is also referred to as the propregnancy hormone) in addition to the estrogen. This progesterone/estrogen combination triggers the hypothalamus to release more GnRH, which signals the pituitary gland to secrete FSH and luteinizing hormone (LH). When FSH and LH levels peak—known as the *LH surge*—this signals the follicle to release the egg, resulting in ovulation. Home test kits are now on the market that will detect the LH surge in your cycle.

Under the influence of LH, the follicle changes its function and becomes a *corpus luteum* (meaning "yellow body" because it actually *turns* yellow), secreting decreasing amounts of estrogen and increasing amounts of progesterone. The progesterone influences the estrogen-primed uterine lining to secrete fluids that nourish the egg (the secretory phase). Immediately after ovulation, FSH returns to normal, or base levels, and the LH decreases gradually as the progesterone increases. If the egg is fertilized, the corpus luteum continues to secrete estrogen and progesterone to maintain the pregnancy. The corpus luteum is stimulated by human chorionic gonadotropin (hCG), a hormone secreted by the developing placenta. (hCG secretion is what a home pregnancy test detects in the urine.) If the egg isn't fertilized, the corpus luteum degenerates until it becomes nonfunctioning, at which point it is called a *corpus albicans*. As degeneration progresses, progesterone levels decrease. The decreased progesterone fails to maintain the uterine lining, which causes it to shed. The shedding of the lining is menstruation. All the cramps that may accompany your period are caused by uterine contractions, which help squeeze out the lining. Then the whole cycle starts again.

To simplify this, imagine listening to Beethoven's Fifth Symphony. It begins with "G-n-R-H. G-n-R-H." The next octave starts with "F-S-H-F-S-H-F-S-H-F-S-H," which continues until the symphony changes again, this time with "LH." As you hear bursts from some instruments and longer solos from others, imagine estrogen and progesterone pulsing and bursting into the bloodstream in precise, controlled amounts. When the symphony is over, the woman menstruates. Then the symphony starts over again. As we all know, however, each conductor has a different *interpretation* of a piece of music. Some use more strings, while others use more horns; some quicken the pace of the music, while

Figure 4.1 Female Ovulation Cycle

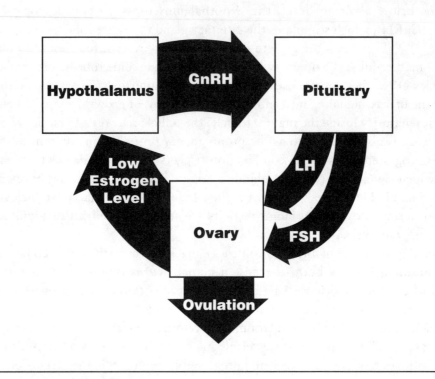

others slow it down. All women's hormonal cycles play the same piece of music, but the rhythms, timing, and pace of that music will vary from conductor to conductor. (The cycle is illustrated in Figure 4.1.)

The first period, called *menarche*, usually starts in the middle of puberty, at around twelve or thirteen years of age. The first few periods are sporadic, and it's not uncommon for periods to be irregular for a couple of years. Periods continue until about forty-eight or forty-nine years of age and then start to get sporadic again, tapering off as menopause sets in. Few cycles are actually twenty-eight days. Where does the number 28 come from? The figure is only an average representing the cycle length of thousands of women added together and divided by the number of women. It is therefore a statistical average, not a figure that refers to the typical number of days in a woman's cycle. Menstrual cycles range anywhere from twenty to forty days, and the bleeding lasts anywhere from two to eight days, four to six days being the average.

There's a big difference between your own cycle and a calendar month, however. Because your cycle length may be shorter or longer than the thirty- or thirty-one-day calendar month, the calendar date of your period may vary from month to month. That's why it's a good idea to keep a written record of your periods. (Charting is discussed later in this chapter.) Each month has a different number of days, so unless you were consistently irregular, you couldn't menstruate on exactly the fifteenth of each month.

It's important to count *the first day of bleeding as day one of your cycle*. Although many women count the first day of clear discharge after their periods as day one, this is not as accurate. What's the difference? Because ovulation always takes place roughly fourteen days before your next period, five days off in your counting could radically interfere with your family planning. When you're on OCs, the first day of bleeding is *always* counted as day one. So, when you go off the OCs, your cycle is more accurately tracked by using the same counting method. Also, doctors always count the first day of bleeding as day one of the cycle, and it's crucial to accurately establish the date of your last menstrual period prior to conception when you are pregnant.

By the way, many women assume that their menstrual flow is made up of only blood, but this is not so. The menstrual fluid consists of a variety of ingredients: cervical and vaginal mucus, degenerated endometrial particles, and blood. The fluid does not smell until it makes contact with bacteria in the air and starts to decompose.

Irregular Cycles

One of the most common fertility problems is an irregular menstrual cycle. But before you jump to the conclusion that you're irregular, it's important to remember that being regular doesn't mean your cycle is the same number of days each time. One month your cycle may be twenty-nine days, and the next month it may be thirty-one days. This is still considered the norm. It's also normal to be lighter one month and heavier the next. As long as you're menstruating every twenty to forty days, it's a sign that you're ovulating. Another common misconception about irregular cycles is that unless you have a period every four weeks (again, the statistical average) you're irregular. This is not true. Some women menstruate every three weeks; some menstruate every five weeks. The only times you should be concerned is if your period consistently yo-yos: three weeks, then four weeks, then five weeks, then three weeks, and so forth. When this happens, it's usually a sign that you're not ovulating regularly. This is common in young girls after they first begin menstruating, but it is not normal in women who are in their mid-twenties or older. If your period jumps around once or twice a year, you don't have anything to worry about. Occasional stress is usually the culprit when this happens. However, poor nutrition, overexercising, and indulging in some of the lifestyle vices discussed in chapter 3 can cause a menstrual cycle to yo-yo.

When you've skipped a period

Obviously, skipping a period when you're trying to conceive may be due to pregnancy. But women may skip a period from time to time and then experience a heavier flow with their next period. This is extremely common. Women who are trying to get pregnant, however, often fear that this is a mild miscarriage—so mild that it simply feels like a heavy period. This usually is not the case. Although it's possible for a pregnancy not to take and expel in the menstrual flow, it's rare and occurs in less than 1 percent of women. If it were to occur, it would be so early a pregnancy that the term *miscarriage* would be totally inappropriate; it would simply be a pregnancy that wasn't yet established, technically called a "blighted ovum." Skipping one period in most cases is caused by stress. The flow is heavier after a skipped period because the estrogen has been building up in the endometrium longer, and there is more lining than usual that needs to be shed. In essence, you would have built up two cycles' worth of lining, so the flow is naturally heavier than normal.

It's also common to skip a period altogether and not experience a heavier flow the next time around. This means you actually skipped an *ovulation* cycle and had not produced a lining in your endometrium that would support a pregnancy. In this case, there wasn't a lining to shed.

Causes of irregular or missed cycles

The number-one cause of a skipped period is pregnancy. Other causes of irregular or skipped periods are emotional stress or what I call "nutritional abuse." These problems are discussed in detail in chapter 3.

For some women, the cause of irregular cycles could be a thyroid disorder of some sort. The thyroid gland regulates your metabolism by secreting thyroid hormone. When the gland is overactive and secretes too much thyroid hormone, known as *hyperthyroidism*, you can either miss periods or have a much longer cycle than normal, and your period is shorter, with a scanty or light flow. On the flip side, when the gland is underactive and doesn't secrete *enough* hormone, known as *hypothyroidism*, your cycles can become shorter, while the period itself is longer with a much heavier flow than normal. Thyroid problems occur in about one in twenty people worldwide but affect women about seven times as often. If this is the cause of your menstrual irregularity, it is easily remedied. Once your thyroid problem is treated, your periods will simply return to normal.

Finally, irregular cycles may be normal for your *age*. For example, it often takes young women several years before they establish a regular menstrual cycle, which is why many young women will be put on oral contraceptives to regulate their periods. Women beyond forty could begin menopause at any time, and irregular cycles may be a sign of perimenopause, which is addressed in chapters 6 and 7.

Amenorrhea: No Menstrual Cycle

There *is* such a thing as having no menstrual cycle; however, if you don't begin menstruating by the age of eighteen, you probably have a hormonal imbalance that can be easily remedied with hormone supplements. If you're menstruating regularly and are between twenty and forty years of age, it's unusual to simply stop menstruating. If this does occur, nutritional abuse is the most common cause. When the female body is malnourished, it stops ovulating because it can't sustain a pregnancy. (See chapter 3 for more details.) Athletes in intensive training may also experience amenorrhea.

Amenorrhea can be caused by either an overactive or underactive thyroid gland. If this is the case, once your thyroid problem is treated, you should begin menstruating again. In all other cases of a stopped or stunted menstrual cycle, progesterone supplements will remedy it.

Why you need to bleed

Today, because there are fewer pregnancies and a longer life cycle, women have to deal with more periods in their lifetime than did women in the past. Also, in the past century, women have experienced a radical change in their diet, environment, stress levels, career, and family expectations. Understandably, the combination of all these factors has affected the hormonal cycle of women, which, in turn, impacts the menstrual cycle.

Again, it's fine to skip a period once in a while or experience some occasional fluctuation. But if you've missed more than two periods and know for certain that you're not pregnant (confirmed by either a pregnancy test or the absence of any sexual activity), then you need to see your doctor and have your period "induced." You'll simply be given a progesterone supplement, which will kick-start your cycle again. It's dangerous to go longer than three months without a "bleed." If the uterus isn't regularly "cleaned out," you can be at risk of developing uterine cancer.

When You Have a Heavy Flow (Menorrhagia)

If you have an extremely heavy flow, it may be normal for you. This is known as *primary menorrhagia*, which means that your flow has been heavy since you first began menstruating. If this is the case, there isn't anything to worry about. You should have your blood levels checked about every six months, however, because a consistent heavy flow is the number-one cause of anemia.

If a light flow slowly develops into a heavy flow, this is known as *secondary menorrhagia*. When this happens, as long as you're having annual pelvic exams and biannual blood tests, you shouldn't be concerned. If your flow *suddenly* becomes unexplainably heavy, see your doctor. This kind of menorrhagia may signify other problems such as fibroids or tumors. Flows are considered dangerously heavy if you need to change your pad or tampon every hour.

When You Have Painful Periods (Dysmenorrhea)

Primary dysmenorrhea means that you've had painful periods ever since you started menstruating. *Secondary dysmenorrhea* involves periods that have become more painful over time. In either case, painful periods are common, and there are medications that can alleviate cramps. Cramps are simply caused by uterine contractions, which push out the lining; some uteri contract more than others. Taking an anti-inflammatory medication such as *naproxen sodium* (Anaprox), for example, *before* your period starts, can help. (Younger women will often be placed on OCs to help alleviate painful periods.) It's also important to judge normal cramping from unusual, debilitating pain during your periods. Endometriosis, a serious disease, is often the culprit behind severe pain during your period. When your pain keeps you from participating in pleasurable activities, there's about a 40 percent chance that your pain is caused by endometriosis. (See chapter 7 for more information.)

If You've Been on Oral Contraceptives

It's common for younger women, in particular, to be placed on OCs as a way of controlling severe PMS symptoms, irregular cycles, or dysmenorrhea. When you're on OCs, periods are a dream come true. Cramps are relatively mild, flow is medium to light, and the periods are punctual to the point where you can set your watch by them. However, many women are surprised to find that when they go *off* OCs, their menstrual problems return. If their cycles were irregular before the oral contraceptives, they will continue to be irregular after they go off them; if they suffered from painful periods before, they probably will have painful periods after. Oral contraceptives are only a temporary panacea for menstrual cycle problems.

Some women will remain regular when they go off oral contraceptives, though. This is usually because when they initially went on them, they were younger and had less mature ovulation cycles. *Ovulation cycles mature as you get into your twenties and thirties, which is why the cycles will normalize.* But often the original cycle, however flawed, returns. Furthermore, it can take up to *six months* for your ovulation cycle to kick in and return to normal. When you're planning to conceive, allow at least that much time. Doctors will advise you to wait until you get two natural periods before you try to conceive. This is fine, but don't panic if you don't conceive after your third, fourth, or fifth cycle. There is a delusion that as soon as we go off oral contraceptives we'll get pregnant. This is just not true. Perfectly fertile couples having intercourse every other day can wait a year before conception actually takes place.

Fertility Awareness 101

Fertility awareness techniques, which have been around since antiquity, gained popularity in the 1970s so women could practice natural birth control. By the 1980s, these same techniques were used for the opposite purpose: to plan conception. Yet, in the 1990s, no woman outside of a monogamous, HIV-negative relationship has the luxury of practicing natural birth control because of the risk of being exposed to STDs. So, unfortunately, learning to read the menstrual cycle has become a lost art. In fact, most women are menstrually "illiterate" until they decide to have a child.

As discussed above, few menstrual cycles are an exact number of days each month. Some women may have a thirty-three-day cycle one month, a thirty-six-day cycle the next, and a thirty-one-day cycle the next. In my own case, I have cycles that run anywhere between thirty-five and forty-five days, and I *never* know how many days to expect between cycles. And I am *not* an unusual "menstrual cycle statistic" by any means. Cycles like these create problems for women trying to conceive, because there is a very small time frame within our cycle when we actually *can* conceive.

We are fertile during ovulation, which takes place about fourteen days before our *next* period begins. Women with predictable menstrual cycles can easily use a calendar to "catch" the fertile peak in their cycles. For example, a woman with an average twenty-eight-day cycle would circle day fourteen of the cycle on her calendar and begin having frequent intercourse between day twelve and day sixteen. Women with unpredictable or irregular cycles will have a much harder time doing this. Fortunately, there are several fertility awareness techniques for women who are not born "calendar girls." You'll get the best results if you combine *all* of these methods together!

Charting Your Menstrual Cycle

There's no way of knowing how regular your cycles are until you start to actually chart them. A classic case for charting exists when women decide to conceive after being on hormonal contraception for years.

For other women planning to conceive, charting serves some useful purposes. First, by charting your cycle, you'll become aware of your body's premenstrual symptoms, which are useful "precursors" to your period and hence, signs of when your fertile stage has begun or *passed*. For instance, if you suffer from tender breasts roughly a week *before* your period, you might begin to notice a pattern of premenstrual breast pain that can *assist* you in establishing a pattern of fertility. Symptoms such as mood swings or bloating can be used in this way as well.

Second, charting your cycle will alert you to the problem of an irregular cycle, which could mean that you're ovulating irregularly or not at all. Correcting the underlying problem that's causing your irregular cycles may prevent delayed conception and save you needless frustration. Charting should be done for at least four cycles before an accurate pattern can be established.

A PMS refresher

Premenstrual syndrome (PMS), which has recently been revised in the psychiatric literature to *premenstrual dysphoric disorder* ("unhappy before your period"), is a real medical condition that affects about 40 percent of all women in their childbearing years. But because of the media circus that's made PMS famous, women have been bombarded with misinformation about the condition.

PMS is an extremely vague label. Because virtually all women experience some kind of premenstrual symptom (bloating, tender breasts, and so on) women who have *true* PMS have been lumped together with women who experience premenstrual symptoms that don't bother them all that much or affect their ability to function on a daily basis. In fact, 90 percent of women who menstruate experience premenstrual symptoms of some sort. It's all part of the normal, hormonal changes that are occurring. Yet 10 percent of menstruating women experience no symptoms before their period. Of the 90 percent who do experience PMS, half will experience the more traditional symptoms such as breast tenderness, bloating, food cravings, irritability, and mood swings. For many women, these symptoms are welcomed because they indicate that all is well and alert them that their period is on the way. These symptoms are the natural, outward signs for the remarkable fluctuations in hormone levels that a woman undergoes every month when she menstruates (or even after a hysterectomy if her ovaries are still in place).

Out of the remaining 45 percent of women who experience premenstrual symptoms, 35 to 40 percent suffer the same symptoms of the first group, but in a more severe form. Their breasts are so sensitive that they hurt when lightly touched. They have severe bloating to the extent that they gain about five pounds before their periods. Instead of just food cravings, they may suddenly find that they have voracious appetites; instead of just being irritable, they may find that they become impossible to be around. Believe it or not, even these more severe symptoms are considered very normal.

The remaining 5 to 10 percent of women who experience premenstrual symptoms suffer from incapacitating symptoms, the kind the media has overreported. So it's perhaps more accurate to say that out of the 90 percent of women who experience some form of

PMS, 80 percent experience *premenstrual symptoms*, and only 10 percent suffer from an actual premenstrual *syndrome* that has a real, negative effect on their lifestyle.

When doctors refer to *true* PMS, they are referring to both the severe premenstrual *symptom* group and the group that is incapacitated by their symptoms to the point where it is a true *syndrome*. PMS is a kind of umbrella term that refers to a cluster of physical and emotional symptoms that occur one to fourteen days before the period that significantly interfere with a woman's interpersonal relationships and daily activities, and that disappear at or during menstruation. The symptoms are diverse and affect almost every part of the body. The following list of physical symptoms is only a sample of what some women report: breast swelling and tenderness, weight gain and abdominal bloating, constipation or diarrhea, headaches, acne or other skin eruptions, eye problems, joint and muscle pain, backache, sugar and salt cravings, increased appetite, fatigue, hoarseness, heart pounding, clumsiness and poor coordination, nausea, menopausal-like hot sweats and chills, shakiness, dizziness, changes in sex drive (either more or less), sensitivity to noise, restlessness, insomnia, and even asthma and seizures.

The *emotional* symptoms of PMS often cause the most problems. They include sudden mood swings, melancholy, anxiety, irritability, emotional overresponsiveness, anger, rage, loss of control, depression, suicidal thoughts, nightmares, forgetfulness, confusion, decreased concentration, withdrawal, unexplained crying, inward anger, and physical or verbal aggression toward others. Some women report increased energy levels, increased sexual drive, and bursts of creativity during this time. Even increased levels of anger and aggression can be viewed as constructive, particularly in business. Rents and bad debts are often collected at these times, and many women report that they are more productive in their work.

Using PMS to your advantage

If you menstruate, chances are you experience some of the physical and emotional premenstrual symptoms. Through charting, you'll become more aware of your body and emotions at various stages in the menstrual cycle. Charting your symptoms is the only way doctors can actually diagnose PMS, since there isn't any blood test or diagnostic tool that can confirm the condition.

The idea is to use your own individual PMS symptoms as a marker for certain times in your cycle. For instance, when I get bloated and have tender breasts around my period, it tends to occur about two weeks before my period, but *after* I've ovulated. Other women may notice tender breasts prior to or immediately after ovulation. It all depends on the individual. When I get weepy and irritable, my period is only a couple of days away, instead of a week away; other women may get weepy a week after ovulation, and so on.

How to create a symptom chart

On a separate daytimer, write down how you feel every day for three or four months. The chart should begin on day one of your cycle, which is when you actually start your bleed. Invent your own system for charting your symptoms. For example, you may want to separate your physical symptoms from your emotional symptoms and designate a number ranging from 1 to 10 (1 being less severe) to chart the intensity of your symptoms. You should also note any unusual activities that might increase your stress levels, such as getting laid off, moving, changing jobs, or fighting with a friend or family member. A sample follows on pages 81 and 82.

If you compare the two charts, obviously you see more than just a change in numbers. The first chart looks as though some thought and logic went into it. In the second chart, everything—whether real or imagined—is exaggerated. The woman was even irritated by her own chart! So it's clear that the woman of January 17 is in a significantly worse mood than the woman of January 14. On the 14th, she was sincerely trying to be as accurate and scientific as possible; by the 17th, she was filling it out hastily, without much care. Were her breasts really a 10 or were they in fact an 8.5? It doesn't matter. The second chart reveals a drastic change in her attitude and feelings—a strong indicator of how quickly her PMS symptoms overcame her and took hold of her lifestyle. Let's see how she feels after her period (see page 82).

The woman of February 4 is far happier, less stressed, and optimistic. She even has the wherewithal to observe how different she was acting just eighteen days ago, about thirteen days before her period. (Indeed, not all women experience PMS *exactly* fourteen days before their period. It can vary. Fourteen days is just a rough number used when discussing an average twenty-eight-day cycle.) A sample of a more clinical chart—the kind your doctor may have on hand—is featured in Figure 4.2 on page 83.

Observing Cervical Mucus

This is a crucial fertility awareness method that any woman can easily get in the habit of doing. It also has the benefit of convenience, unlike the basal body temperature (BBT) method discussed on page 87. This method is sometimes called the Billings method. Australians Evelyn and John Billings developed a way of interpreting the *changing consistency* of vaginal discharge, which is influenced by the cervical mucus bathing the vaginal walls. There are groups that now provide instruction in this technique. The most widely known is Serena, established and supported by the Roman Catholic Church. This group teaches the method only to married or monogamous couples who are Catholic. The Justisse Group, based in Canada, has consultants across the country who train women in both the United States and Canada to use this method. See the appendix for more information.

Cycle Day: 12   **Calendar Date: January 14/2005**

Physical symptoms
Appetite = 5 (10 means voracious)
Cravings = 0 (10 means you have definite cravings)
Breasts = 3 (10 means they're really tender)
Bloat = 8 (10 means you're really bloated)
Weight = 3 pounds
Backache = 0 (10 means you're back is very achy)

Emotional symptoms
Mood = 4 (1 means happy; 10 means sad, depressed, and so on)
Irritability = 6 (1 means calm; 10 means really jumpy)
Energy = 7 (1 means low energy; 10 means high energy)
Sex drive = 7 (1 means low sex drive; 10 means high)
Stress = 6 (1 means low stress; 10 means high)

Special circumstances
—Got into an argument with Lee again. The usual. I feel fine. Just a little miffed.

Cycle Day: 15   **Calendar Date: January 17/2005**

Physical symptoms
Appetite = 10
Cravings = 10 (chocolate)
Breasts = 10
Bloat = 10
Weight = 6 pounds (I'm a cow!)
Backache = 10

Emotional symptoms
Mood = 10!!!
Irritability = 10! 10! 10!
Energy = 0
Sex drive = 0
Stress = 10!

Special circumstances
—I hate my life!

Cycle Day: 5 (bleed—day 1 of cycle—occurred on Jan. 30)
Calendar Date: Feb. 4/2005

Physical symptoms
Appetite = 3
Cravings = 0
Breasts = 0
Bloat = 0
Weight = normal
Backache = 0

Emotional symptoms
Mood = 1 (feeling really great!)
Irritability = 0
Energy = 10 (I actually did the laundry!)
Sex drive = 8
Stress = 1

Special circumstances
—Read my earlier charts! Don't know what came over me a couple of weeks ago!

All you need to do is observe your toilet paper about twice a day, when you wipe yourself before or after going to the bathroom. Or, you can simply insert a finger into your vagina to collect whatever discharge is present. After your period finishes (that is, your flow stops), you'll notice several days of no vaginal discharge at all (your dry days). Your vagina will still be moist, however, as it always is. Then, your mucus days will begin. The discharge starts out sticky, then gradually becomes creamier, wet, and slippery. Finally, on your peak day, the discharge has the consistency of egg white (some women describe it as snotlike), and will drip out of your vagina, evident when you wipe yourself or take off your underwear. This discharge will also be thinner, transparent, and stretchy, and you should be able to stretch it between two fingers. *This* mucus is your fertility marker. You will be ovulating either just *before* or just *after* it appears. This mucus will last for just about two days, then it will begin to get thicker and stickier. These are your postpeak days, also known as your luteal phase. This is when PMS symptoms will begin to make an appearance. The mucus will remain on the thicker, sticky side until your period starts. Then, the whole phase begins again.

Figure 4.2 Sample Form Used for Charting PMS Symptoms

DAILY SYMPTOM RECORD

START DATE

DAY OF CYCLE	1	2	3	4	5	6	7	8	9	10	11	12	13	14	15	16	17	18	19	20	21	22	23	24	25	26	27	28
BLEEDING																												
SYMPTOMS																												
Irritable																												
Fatigue																												
Inward anger																												
Moody																												
Depressed																												
Restless																												
Anxious																												
Insomnia																												
Lack of control																												
Swelling																												
Bloating																												
Breast tenderness																												
Bowels: const. (C) loose (L)																												
Appetite																												
Sex drive																												
Chills (C); Sweats (S)																												
Headaches																												
Crave sweets, salt																												
Feel unattractive																												
Guilt																												
Unreasonable behavior																												
Low self-image																												
Nausea																												
Menstrual cramps																												
LIFESTYLE IMPACT																												
Aggressive toward others																												
Wish to be alone																												
Neglect housework																												
Time off work																												
Distractable, disorganized																												
Clumsy																												
Uneasy about driving																												
Suicidal thoughts																												
Stayed at home																												
LIFE EVENTS																												
Negative experience																												
Positive experience																												
Social activities																												
Vigorous exercise																												
MEDICATIONS																												

Your doctor may ask you to keep a diary of symptoms and their severity by filling out a chart similar to this.

INSTRUCTIONS
1. Consider the first day of bleeding as DAY 1 of your menstrual cycle.
2. Record your symptoms each evening at about the same time.
3. BLEEDING: Indicate bleeding by shading the box; indicate spotting with an X.
4. Fill in the box corresponding to a symptom by indicating the degree of severity as follows:
    MILD: 1 (Noticeable but not troublesome)
    MODERATE: 2 (Interferes with normal activity)
    SEVERE: 3 (Temporarily incapacitating)
5. MEDICATIONS: List these and enter an X on bad days when you take them.

(Modified with permission from PRISM Calendar, by Reid and Maddocks)

Reprinted with permission of Syntex, Inc., 1994.

To catch the peak, you'll need to begin having frequent intercourse (every other day) as your mucus days begin and continue frequent intercourse until your postpeak mucus appears. Mucus usually develops between three and nine days prior to ovulation. So you will probably need to have frequent intercourse for about two weeks. *Warning: This method is useless if you have a vaginal infection or untreated STD.*

You should also note your mucus observations on your symptom chart. Eventually, you should be able to link various premenstrual symptoms to a specific mucus consistency.

Guidelines for an accurate mucus chart

There are actually several steps involved in accurately observing your mucus. Since the chart depends on your observations throughout the day, record your observations before you go to bed at the end of the day. Never observe after intercourse, because you'll confuse semen and your sexual secretions with your own mucus. You should also refrain from observing if you are taking any medications to cure an infection, if you are on any hormonal medications, or if you are using any spermicides or lubricants. For example, medications that can make your mucus thicker and less abundant include antidepressants or tranquilizers; antihistamines; atropine and dicyclomine, both used to treat bowel spasms; drugs used in chemotherapy; and certain ulcer medications. Medications that can thin your cervical mucus and increase its abundance include certain asthma drugs; certain antibiotics; estrogen-containing medications; certain cough medications; and drugs used to treat bladder problems. Here are some guidelines for creating an accurate chart:

1. Wipe your vulva from urethra to anus, and note the sensation of the wipe: dry, smooth, or lubricated.
2. Observe the toilet paper for the presence or absence of mucus. Then create your own number coding system to describe the consistency of the mucus. For example: 0 = dry; 1 = damp, but not lubricated; 2 = wet, but not lubricated; 3 = shiny, but not lubricated; 4 = damp and lubricated; 5 = wet and lubricated; 6 = shiny and lubricated.
3. If mucus is present on the toilet paper, finger test it for stretchiness between your thumb and index finger. Again, use a code to describe the consistency: 7 = sticky; 8 = tacky; 9 = stretchy; 10 = pasty; 11 = gummy or gluelike. Using this coding, you can combine numbers to get an accurate picture.
4. Record the numbers you came up with in steps two and three. For example, mucus that is a 5 and 9 is your peak mucus, while a 5 and 10 would represent your cycle past your peak mucus days.
5. Use a coding system to observe the color of the mucus. For example, B = brown; W = white or cloudy; C = clear; T = transparent; Y = yellowish or off-white; R = red or pink (your menstrual flow).

6. On your peak days, note how many times you observed your clear, stretchy mucus that day: Once, twice, and so on. When you see it a few times a day, it's a good sign.
7. Note the mucus "metamorphosis" pattern. Does it change from clear to cloudy? Clear to dry? Dry to cloudy and then clear?
8. Observe any special circumstances, such as a "double peak," which can happen if you're under stress or have been ill.
9. Take special note of any lower abdominal cramping or backaches. This could be a sign that you're ovulating.
10. Record the length of "stretch" your peak mucus makes. The longer, the better.

But I don't notice any mucus!

This is a problem. Without cervical mucus, sperm can't survive or be transported to the fallopian tubes to fertilize the egg. The mucus also nourishes and protects the sperm, allowing them to live for three to five days. If you don't notice any mucus, this is a sign that you may not be ovulating, you may have a hormone deficiency, or you may even have a vaginal infection of some sort. You'll need to see your doctor to find out why you're not producing mucus. (See chapters 6 and 7 for more details.) That being said, it should also be noted that nothing is 100 percent. You could still conceive, but a lack of mucus will make conception far more difficult.

Couldn't You Just Spit?

Now you can. There are now several types of fertility saliva tests that examine the saliva throughout the cycle. Estrogen and progesterone are detectable in saliva through shifting patterns under a microscope. That means you'll be able to see the same pattern repeated every time you're ovulating. What's nice about this system is that it comes with a reusable mini-microscope (smaller than a pair of opera glasses) that you can use to examine your saliva. All you do is essentially lick the glass slide that comes with the kit, allow it to dry a few seconds, and then view it under the preset magnification level of the microscope.

Estrogen and progesterone mix with the natural salt content of the mouth, forming a fernlike pattern (as in the leaf) during ovulation. When you're not ovulating, the pattern is just a bunch of dots or spots. The ferning comes from crystallization. The kit has to be kept lint-free (use a lint-free cloth to clean) to avoid tainting the specimen with dust.

How accurate is it?

Studies have found these systems to be over 96 percent accurate as both a fertility aid and a contraceptive tool; that does not mean, however, that 96 percent of all women who use it get pregnant. It means that it will accurately display your menstrual cycle's pattern. (It does not, of course, protect you from STDs if you're using it as a contraceptive method.) Some fertility specialists feel that ovulation predictor kits, discussed next, are more accurate predictors of ovulation. Furthermore, if you have hormonal abnormalities, such as polycystic ovarian disease (see chapter 7), this kit will not work for you. To purchase PC 2000, refer to the resource list in the appendix.

The LH Test Kit (the Home Ovulation Test)

You can purchase a test kit that will detect your LH surge. This surge triggers ovulation and occurs anywhere from twelve to thirty-six hours prior to ovulation. This means that you can now accurately pinpoint when you're ovulating twelve to thirty-six hours in advance. LH is present in the blood throughout your cycle, but only in small amounts. Just before ovulation, the amount of LH suddenly increases. This test can pick up increased levels of LH in your urine up until twenty-four hours after your surge. With the aid of a specific kind of antibody, known as a *monoclonal antibody*, these kits can detect even minute amounts of LH in the urine, causing it to turn a specific shade of blue.

Unfortunately, if you have a cycle shorter than twenty-six days or longer than thirty-three days, the results of your test may not be as accurate or useful. If you're beginning menopause or are already pregnant (but don't realize it), the results will also be inaccurate.

Since the late 1980s, several LH test kits have come on the market. They take anywhere from one to thirty minutes to perform and a variety of brands are available. You can ask either your doctor or pharmacist to recommend one. All LH test kits work on the same principle. You buy the test about fourteen days before your next period. Each kit contains a chart that will suggest a good time for you to begin testing, based on the average length of your past periods. Each kit contains either a stick or test pad with a blue reference spot to compare to your test result. Either one will have monoclonal antibodies on them, which will detect any LH. If you're using the stick, you dip the stick into your urine cup and check to see if it changes color; if you're using a test pad, you drop a small amount of your urine onto the pad to see if turns blue. You then continue testing until the blue becomes its darkest shade, which will mark the surge. All kits have a toll-free number you can call if you have any questions. However, before you purchase a kit, go over the instructions carefully with either your doctor or pharmacist, and ask if he or she can show you how to use it. The kits are expensive, and the cost depends on the number of test sticks or test pads (expect either a six- or nine-day supply). You can also purchase individual refills that cost roughly ten dollars per refill.

Using the kit along with your mucus observations, menstrual cycle chart, and the BBT chart (discussed below), you should get a very clear picture of your fertility. This kit may also be useful in timing various diagnostic tests (see chapter 6). The following are guidelines for accurate testing:

1. Whether you're leaving a strip stick in a solution or underwater, the timing must be *exact*. Use a stop watch or timer if you have one. (I often stick a cold glass of water in the microwave, turn on the microwave for a specific time, and use *that* for a timer.)
2. Don't drink too many fluids before you collect your urine. It may water down perfectly "surged" urine and give you a false negative reading.
3. Don't reuse your test equipment by trying to wash it out. It won't work.
4. Make sure you check the expiration date on the box before you purchase your kit.
5. Refrain from testing if you have an infection or if you are on medication to treat an infection. Similarly, if you're taking any kind of hormonal concoction, fertility drug (see chapter 8), or steroids (do you have asthma?), don't test. The results won't be accurate.

Personal Contraceptive System

This is a computerized system that uses information from your previous cycles along with urine testing to give you an accurate profile of your fertility, helping you predict your most fertile time. Consequently, it can also be used as a contraceptive! This device detects the LH surge and is considered about 94 percent accurate for women who have regular cycles (that is, a period every twenty-three to thirty-five days). Different colored lights are displayed for your fertile and infertile times, as well as a light for a repeat urine test. As of this writing, these systems should be available at your local pharmacy. They have been popular in the United Kingdom since 1996.

Basal Body Temperature Chart (Symptothermal Method)

This method is a real nuisance, but it's a good way of charting exactly when you're ovulating. A basal body thermometer is an ultrasensitive thermometer that tracks your body's *exact* temperature. A digital thermometer is your best bet. These are fairly cheap and can be purchased at any pharmacy. Each thermometer kit comes with a blank graph

Figure 4.3 Sample Basal Body Temperature Chart

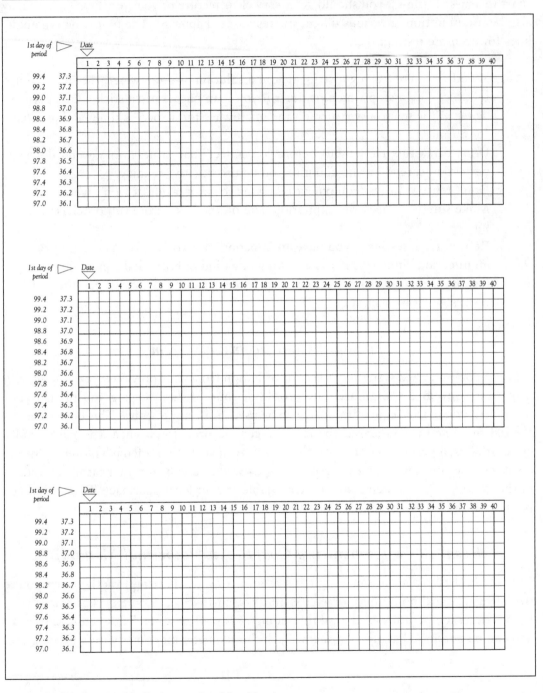

Reprinted with permission of the Infertility Awareness Association of Canada.

Figure 4.4 Sample Basal Body Temperature Chart

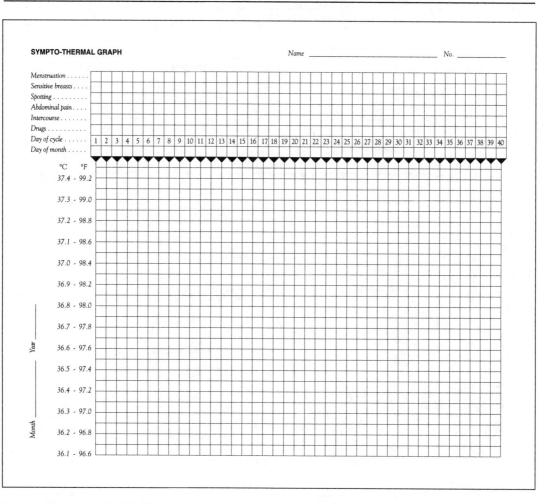

Reprinted with permission of the Infertility Awareness Association of Canada.

that may resemble Figure 4.3 (on page 88) or Figure 4.4 (above). These graphs may have space for you to record PMS symptoms. A sample chart, such as the one shown in Figure 4.5, may also accompany your BBT kit.

Most BBT kits are the same. At the top of the graph are the days of your cycle from 1 to 40, but you add more days if you need to. Underneath each cycle day you write the month and actual calendar date. Vertically listed are temperatures from 99.4° to 97.0° Fahrenheit. (In Canada, the readings would be in metric units, from 37.3° to 36.1° Centigrade.)

Figure 4.5 Sample Basal Body Temperature Chart

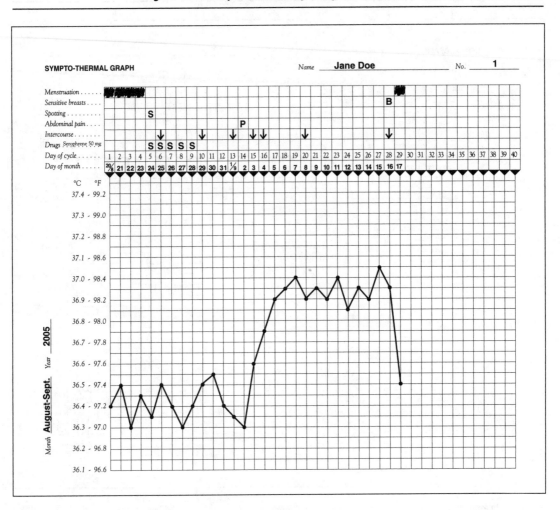

Reprinted with permission of the Infertility Awareness Association of Canada.

Each morning, before you get out of bed, you'll need to take your temperature orally (or vaginally, but orally is more accurate) and chart it on the graph. *Unless you take your temperature at the same time each morning, the graph won't be accurate! After* ovulation, your temperature rises slightly. After doing about three charts, you should notice a very distinct pattern of ovulation, which will help you time *future* intercourses and tell you whether you are indeed ovulating regularly. However, this method will not tell you *when* to have intercourse on the spot, since the temperature doesn't rise until *after* ovulation.

Yet, many couples make the mistake of planning their intercourse around this chart. This is a bad idea and can create stress over sexual intimacy. The purpose of the chart is to help you plan future intercourses and assist you in observing your own unique fertility pattern.

There is debate among gynecologists about the accuracy of these charts. Some women don't experience any sharp differences in temperature, yet are ovulating anyway; some women have an even, or "flat," pattern throughout their cycle, yet are still ovulating. If you're one of them, the absence of a pattern should tell you that you may not be ovulating, but *you must also be observing no change in your cervical mucus and no LH surge from an LH home test kit to suspect that you're anovulatory.* The next step is to have your doctor perform blood tests to check your hormonal levels or do an *endometrial biopsy* (discussed in chapter 6), a test that determines whether you're ovulating or have a hormonal imbalance.

Guidelines for an accurate BBT chart

1. The first day of your menstrual flow is day 1 of your BBT chart. Do *not* include spotting prior to your period as day 1. Your temperature should drop when your menstrual flow starts. Record your temperature throughout your period. This information is important.
2. Make sure you note the actual day of the month in the space provided on your chart.
3. Use an oral, digital, or basal body thermometer only. A regular thermometer won't do!
4. Take your temperature each morning before you get out of bed. Place the thermometer under your tongue for at least two to three minutes.
5. Don't eat, drink, or smoke before you take your temperature (this includes ingesting sperm!).
6. Record your temperature by using a dot, not an X or a checkmark.
7. Use a down-pointing arrow to indicate the days you had intercourse.
8. Record any premenstrual symptoms if there is space on the chart. Otherwise, use your symptom chart to help link a certain temperature to a symptom.
9. Note any special considerations like true illness or fever.
10. Change charts when you get your period again.

Finally, on one of your charts, record what you're eating, how much you're exercising, and whether you're under any unusual stress. Coffee, alcohol, dieting and exercise, and emotional stress all affect your menstrual cycle. By cutting out certain foods or vices, you can see if your menstrual cycle changes.

The BBT Computer

Although the point of doing a BBT chart is to get a visual graph of your cycle, a new product, which is a *computerized* BBT thermometer, is now on the market. Known as a BBT computer, this thermometer is essentially designed for the same purposes as an LH surge kit: to predict ovulation for either timing intercourse or various diagnostic tests, discussed in chapter 6.

The way the BBT computer works is similar to any other BBT thermometer, except it flashes a red light during the fertile stage of the cycle and a green light when you're infertile. In order for it to work, you still need to take your temperature daily and at the same time of day. You can take the thermometer to the pharmacy and get a printout of your cycle, but critics argue that the point of BBT is for you to do your *own* charting and, hence, gain control over the rhythms of your cycle. Furthermore, when you do a computer printout, you can't observe symptoms or mucus on the same chart, which critics say is a crucial element in BBT charting.

Attention All Men

Behind every good menstrual chart is an attentive male partner. Help your partner make her observations. Read this chapter, ask her questions, and so on. Help facilitate time for her to do the charting accurately. Sit down with the charts yourself and "proofread" them, making sure that recordings seem accurate.

You can also take part in many observations and even establish a counterchart, observing your partner's premenstrual symptoms such as irritability and weepiness. Ask her to show you her cervical mucus. Test it every day with your own fingers to get to know her pattern. Ask your partner to show you her panties or panty liners so you can observe colors and consistency of mucus. You might ask to look at menstrual discharge to observe the colors and consistencies of the flow. (I know men who do this out of sheer curiosity.) You can also take her temperature and record many of her BBT readings yourself. Finally, you can create a personal chart to observe your own fertility markers.

The Male Fertility Awareness Chart

Pattern a chart after your partner's daily symptom chart and record the following:

1. Ejaculation: Record when you've had an ejaculation on a daily basis, and record the number of ejaculations in any given day. Also note any long periods of abstinence. (Abstinence may place more stress on your prostate gland and affect your ejaculate.)

2. Fevers, colds, and infections: Your sperm count can be affected by illness. Even if you're fighting off a minor infection, increased levels of white blood cells can kill off healthy sperm.

3. If you're not monogamous, record sex you've had with other female (and particularly male) partners. You may need to be tested for STDs.

4. Record any aches or pains in your groin area and any drips or discharge from your urethra.

5. Record any change in your urine color (dark or bloody) and record any burning sensations in your urethra. This could be a sign of kidney problems, a urinary tract infection, or an inflammation caused by an STD.

6. Record any warts or sores on your genitals. This could be a sign of STDs.

7. Feel your lymph nodes under your ears and around your groin. If they're enlarged, you could be fighting off an infection, which will affect your sperm.

8. Record exposure to high temperatures, such as hot baths, saunas, and sitting in a hot car. This will affect your sperm count (see chapter 3).

9. You, too, should also be recording what you're eating, drinking, and smoking. All these factors can affect your sperm count.

When to Seek Out a Specialist

All this charting should go on for about six months before you start to "try" to conceive. Although it's fine to have as much sex as you like in the beginning, you really won't be able to technically plan your sex by your chart until you have about six cycles' worth of charts.

After your first six charts, your official "trying" phase can begin. You should be having intercourse every other day *around* the time of ovulation. That means you should try a few days before and keep going until a few days after you ovulate. Women under thirty-five should try this for about a year. After a year, if you've been unable to get pregnant this way, you should consult your "weed doctor" (see chapter 2) and send your partner off for a semen analysis, detailed in chapter 5. Women over thirty-five should not wait longer than six months before initiating a fertility investigation. Again, the male partner will need to start the workup process with a semen analysis.

The male workup is the next step when you're not getting pregnant using fertility awareness techniques. This workup usually starts with an initial consultation with your weed doctor. A fertility specialist is not yet necessary at this point. Bring all six of your charts to your weed doctor. Make sure your doctor understands your coding methods, and have him or her assess whether you've done the charts accurately. If you haven't, you may need to redo them before an official workup is ordered, but a semen analysis can be done in the meantime just to save time.

In some cases, the charts may reveal an obvious hormonal imbalance that warrants a monitored cycle or some of the tests discussed in chapter 6. Even if there is an obvious, undisputed female hormonal imbalance, get the semen analysis done *first*. Why? If there is a male factor problem that coexists with the female problem, it will need to be corrected or confirmed anyway, which will save the woman from undergoing a grueling workup. For example, even though your menstrual charts reveal a luteal phase defect, if the male has no sperm at all, fixing the luteal phase defect will do you no good. If the semen analysis is done *first*, the two of you would immediately progress to either donor insemination (see chapter 9), adoption, or making a decision to live childfree (see chapter 12). Time is everything in a fertility investigation. You don't want to waste it.

5

The Male Workup

INFERTILITY HAS LONG been perceived as a "woman's problem," even though causes of infertility are evenly split between male and female factors. Yet, no matter which partner has the problem, the woman, who ultimately carries the fetus, is often the one who undergoes treatment.

It's impossible to change the basic facts of life, which is why these workups tend to be kinder to men than to women. Delivering numerous sperm samples and possibly urine and blood samples is just about as invasive as it gets for most men. Occasionally, imaging tests and biopsies involving the testicles are needed, but this is not the case in the majority of male workups.

The average, basic female workup consists of invasive, time-consuming procedures, discussed in chapter 6. Understandably, when fertility is in question, the man should *always* be the first to undergo any testing, even if a female factor is suspected. This is because 20 percent of all infertility involves *both* partners. In this case, if a male factor is untreatable, you can go on as a couple to assisted reproductive technology (ART), which may include donor insemination (see chapter 9), or you can decide on either adoption or childfree living.

This chapter discusses the kinds of tests men will undergo in a fertility investigation and the purpose of each test. To fully explain this, a brief refresher on how the male reproductive organs work and contribute to fertilization is also provided.

Forty-five percent of the time, the male workup will end after one or more normal semen analyses, but it's important for a man to deliver at least two samples, for reasons I'll explain in the next section. An abnormal semen analysis will turn up 55 percent of the time, but 30 to 40 percent of the time, no cause for the abnormal semen will be found.

Although the various causes of male factor infertility and the emotional consequences of a diagnosis are covered in this chapter, the treatments are discussed in chapter 7. In many cases, if no treatments exist for your problem, procedures may be available that can still enable you to *father* a biological child through new reproductive technologies. If you are not able to father a biological child, there are only three solutions: *donor insemination* (DI), adoption, or childfree living. All ARTs are discussed in chapter 9; alternatives to biological parenting are discussed in chapter 12.

The Semen Factor

Assessing the quality of the semen is the most important aspect of a male workup. Whether the problem is hormonal or structural, all clues to a male factor problem are found within the semen. Before you can grasp exactly what's being analyzed when you deliver that sperm sample, here's a brief refresher on what happens to your sperm from the time they're produced until fertilization. Also, review Figure 5.1, for a *visual* refresher!

The Sperm Cycle

The male reproductive hormonal cycle controls semen production. The hormones involved are almost identical to those involved in the female cycle, except that *testosterone* is flooded into the bloodstream instead of estrogen and progesterone. The main difference between the male and female hormonal cycles is that, in the woman, the cycle runs in a continuous loop (see chapter 4), whereas in the man, the cycle runs endlessly without any marked beginning, middle, or end. In women, the ovulation cycle peters out with age, resulting in menopause; in men, there is no time limit for semen production. This distinction in hormonal timing also causes vast differences in male and female sexual behavior, but that's another book!

Every day, a man's testes are busy producing millions of sperm. As in the female cycle, the hypothalamus starts the process by secreting gonadotropin-releasing hormone (GnRH) into the bloodstream. GnRH is released approximately every ninety minutes, triggering the pituitary gland to release both luteinizing hormone (LH) and follicle stimulating hormone (FSH) into the bloodstream, which carries the hormones to the testes. Within the testes, LH goes directly to the *Leydig cells*, which triggers the production of testosterone; FSH goes directly to the *Sertoli cells*, which triggers the production of sperm. When testosterone levels drop, this tells the hypothalamus to release *more* GnRH, which tells the pituitary gland to secrete *more* LH and FSH, which tells the body to make *more* testosterone and sperm. As we will discuss later in this chapter, this hormonal interrelationship, clinically called the *hormonal axis*, must be in tip-top shape in order for men to produce enough high-quality sperm to fertilize an egg. Trouble with either the Leydig or Sertoli cells may cause unusually high levels of either LH or FSH or unusually low levels of testosterone. Trouble in the hypothalamus or pituitary glands will cause a breakdown of the entire hormonal axis. In all cases, sperm counts will be low or even nonexistent.

The testicles are situated inside the scrotal sac, which is positioned outside the body to keep the testicles at roughly 94° Fahrenheit (35° Centigrade), a few degrees cooler than body temperature. The testicles themselves are not visible to the eye and are made up of small, tightly coiled tubes known as *seminiferous tubules*. The sperm are produced inside these tubules, where they stay until they're mature. Sperm cells have their own guardians, the Sertoli cells, also known as nurse cells, which help protect and nourish the sperm until they're mature. These are the cells that respond to FSH. There is one nurse cell for roughly every 150 sperm.

Figure 5.1 Male Reproductive Organs

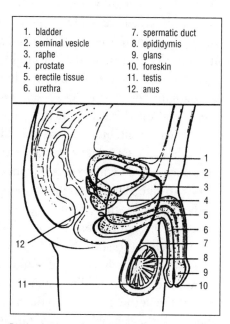

1. bladder	7. spermatic duct
2. seminal vesicle	8. epididymis
3. raphe	9. glans
4. prostate	10. foreskin
5. erectile tissue	11. testis
6. urethra	12. anus

Reprinted with permission of Serono Symposia, USA, 1994.

It takes two to three months (about seventy-four days) for sperm to mature. Mature sperm gather in the center of the tubules, while the immature sperm remain on the outer edges of the tubules. The nurse cells continuously "sweep" sperm into the center as they mature. When the sperm mature, they leave the tubules and enter the *epididymis*, a coiled, tubular organ attached to the testes. Here, the mature sperm learn to "swim" and fine-tune their motility (movement). Mature sperm resemble microscopic tadpoles. They have an enzyme-coated *head*, a *tail*, and a thinner portion of the tail, called an *end piece*.

Once inside the epididymis, mature sperm wait to be ejaculated into the vagina—not unlike the scene depicted in Woody Allen's satirical film, *Everything You Always Wanted to Know About Sex*, where the sperm are waiting to "parachute" out of an aircraft and complete their mission. What happens to the sperm if no ejaculation takes place? They die and are reabsorbed by the body. This is as close as a man comes to having a "period."

Getting Ready to Jump: Ejaculation

The penis is equipped with sensory receptors that tell the brain to make the penis erect. The erectile tissue that lines the penis fills with blood, causing the penis to grow and elongate.

The sperm get ejected from the body through one of two parallel sets of tubes, known as the *vas deferens*, an artery that serves as a canal. The vas deferens carries the sperm above the pubic bone, past the bladder. (If you've had a vasectomy, the vas deferens does *not* carry the sperm anywhere, and the sperm are quickly reabsorbed by the body.) The vas deferens takes the sperm to the ejaculatory duct, which serves as a holding area. Until now, the sperm, along with small quantities of fluid (present to help propel the sperm along) are the sole ingredients to the ejaculate. In the holding area, seminal vesicles, small organs nearby, add large quantities of fructose, a sugar solution, to the ejaculate. The fructose nourishes the sperm and turns it into semen. The semen is then dumped into an enlarged section of the urethra called the bulbous urethra. The prostate gland is connected to the bulbous urethra through a separate duct system. At this point, the prostate gland adds an alkaline fluid to the semen, which will protect it from the acidic environment of the vagina. This, by the way, is the prostate gland's main function in life. A tiny amount of lubricating fluid is then added to the semen by the *Cowper's gland*. The ejaculate is now complete. The fluids are then forcefully ejected by contractions of the pelvic floor muscles and prostate gland. The bladder neck closes to stop sperm from going back into the bladder. An average ejaculate contains forty to one hundred fifty million sperm, out of which only a few hundred will even come *close* to the egg. The semen measures between a half to a full teaspoon and is ejaculated through the urethra. (To the naked eye, semen without sperm is indistinguishable from semen with sperm, which is why males who produce little or no sperm do not realize it.)

Survival of the Fittest: Fertilization

Once inside the vagina, the semen immediately coagulates, for reasons not yet understood. Because the vagina is acidic, only about 10 percent of the sperm will survive the first ten minutes inside the vagina. After about twenty minutes, the semen becomes fluid again, enabling the surviving sperm to swim up the reproductive tract. Here's where the cervical mucus enters the picture. When a portion of the surviving sperm reach the cervical mucus, they will find tiny strands of protein within it that will carry them toward the uterus. *This protein is present only in mid-cycle mucus, which has an egg-white consistency*. The mucus is a sign that ovulation has just taken place or will be taking place shortly. The woman's egg remains viable for about twelve to twenty-four hours; the sperm can live up to forty-eight to seventy-two hours. This creates a reproductive window of roughly four days.

As discussed in chapter 3, new research indicates that when a woman reaches orgasm *at the time* of ejaculation (but not before), her orgasmic contractions also help to propel the sperm upward, toward the uterus. However, if a woman reaches orgasm prior to ejaculation (during foreplay, for example), the contractions may help to keep the sperm away.

Once the sperm reach the uterus and continue upward, they number in the hundreds. Some of these sperm will get lost or will become embedded in the lining of the fallopian tubes. The enzyme cap that coats the head of the sperm is covered with a net of membranes that protect it. This membrane is almost completely worn away by this point, so when the sperm reach the egg, the enzymes are "naked" and can easily penetrate the egg. During many of the assisted conception procedures discussed in chapter 9, this membrane is artificially worn away through a process known as *sperm washing*. The clinical term for this membrane wear and tear is known as the *capacitation process*.

When the sperm enters the egg's outer layer, a biochemical change in the egg takes place, making it impossible for any other sperm to penetrate it. The sperm and the egg at this point merge genetic material. The entire fertilization process takes about twenty-four hours, and the fertilized egg takes about four days to reach the uterus. The egg then secretes a hormone called *human chorionic gonadotropin* (hCG). In a home pregnancy test kit, this hormone causes the stick to change color.

Sometimes the egg will not travel to the uterus to develop, but will instead grow inside the fallopian tube. This is known as an *ectopic,* or *tubal pregnancy*, and is more common in women who have a history of STDs or intrauterine device (IUD) use.

Rarely, some freakish versions of fertilization can result in a *molar pregnancy*, where there is either no developing embryo or an embryo that will not be able to survive at birth. There are three ways this can occur: Two sperm can fertilize one egg, with the loss of the mother's chromosomes; one sperm can enter the egg and then divide, delivering a double dose of chromosomes to the egg instead of its usual single dose; or an abnormal sperm carrying two sets of chromosomes can fertilize the egg.

The Semen Analysis

As discussed in chapter 2, when you and your partner suspect infertility, the semen analysis begins the workup for both of you. A normal series of semen analyses will prompt a female workup; an abnormal series will prompt a male workup. This test can be handled by your primary care doctor, your partner's gynecologist, or your own urologist or andrologist. In short, whoever has been handling your preconception screenings and "weedings" until this point will manage the semen analyses.

This same doctor should also ask you questions about your medical/surgical history and perform a thorough physical exam, including an examination of your external genitals. This helps the doctor rule out infection, structural abnormalities, and so on. The doctor may order general lab tests to rule out other diseases, such as a urine test for diabetes or kidney infection; blood tests for complete blood counts, ruling out syphilis, anemia, or leukemia; and screenings to rule out viral or bacterial infections. Your doctor should also do a thyroid function test. In general, bloodwork is not routine, however.

You should also be asked about your sex life: How old were you when you reached puberty, first erections, viral infections after puberty (such as mumps or high fevers), previous paternity, how often you have intercourse, how often you masturbate, whether you use lubricants, and whether you have any of the lifestyle habits discussed in chapter 3 that may interfere with your fertility. Sometimes this more probing look at your personal life isn't done unless your semen analysis is *abnormal*, or unless you're referred to a urologist or andrologist. Detailed physical exams of the testes and rectal exams that evaluate the prostate gland and seminal vesicles aren't done unless you're referred to a urologist.

If you have diabetes or (had) testicular cancer

After you produce your semen sample, ask your doctor to perform a *urinalysis* (urine test) *next*. A common problem for men with these conditions is *retrograde ejaculation*, where the ejaculate is propelled backward into the bladder. Men with diabetes may gradually lose nerve function at the bladder's opening, causing sperm to shoot backward during ejaculation. Men who have had lymph nodes removed in the testicles may have nerve damage that may interfere with the closing of the bladder neck during ejaculation.

In these cases, semen would be present in your urine. In order to diagnose retrograde ejaculation, you must collect your urine immediately *after* an ejaculation. Doing the urinalysis first can save you a lot of time. Occasionally, antihistamines may improve sperm ejaculation because they help to close the sphincter muscle between the urethra and the bladder.

Otherwise, while there is no specific treatment for retrograde ejaculation, there is a procedure your doctor can do that will enable you to biologically father a child. It involves extracting live sperm from your urine and then depositing it into your partner. Success rates for this procedure are high. (See chapter 7 for more details.)

You *can* do this test at home. Once your doctor gives you a requisition for a semen analysis, you can take the requisition to any lab. All labs are equipped with take-home semen analysis kits. As long as you live within a half-hour drive of the lab, you can produce the sample at home and drop it off at the lab. Sperm can survive for at least that long in the cup. It's important to keep the specimen warm. Placing it in a front pants pocket, tucking it into the waistline of your pants, or tucking it under your arm is the best way to transport it. If you spill any of the semen during or after collection, you'll need to repeat the test. Do *not* put the collection in the fridge or freezer overnight.

The kit includes some of the instructions I'll go into, perhaps a small questionnaire with your name, address, insurance information, and some brief medical history questions and a *sterile* specimen cup. (A clean glass jar is also fine, but don't go the Dixie cup route.) If your doctor has a laboratory in his or her office building or clinic, you could produce your sperm sample in the office bathroom or another private room. This is certainly the simplest route.

Home semen test

There is currently a home semen test on the market called FertilitySCORE™ which can determine whether your sperm "has normal or less than normal activity." This means that it will identify if you have a lot of sperm or insufficient or no sperm, but it won't tell you anything about the characteristics of your sperm, such as how well they move, the shape, and so on. In short, this test looks at quantity, not quality.

The test takes roughly sixty minutes to do (if you can figure out all the instructions), and if you test positive (meaning, "yep, looks normal") then there's an 87 percent chance that your sperm is normal. If you test negative (meaning "hmm . . . this looks strange"), there's an 87 percent chance that your sperm is not normal. In other words, this test has a roughly 10 to 15 percent false positive/false negative rate.

This home kit comes with two tests, since results can vary depending on activity, diet, environment, and so on. Urologists feel that this test is really more of a marker for normal or abnormal results, but it cannot replace the high quality of a laboratory semen analysis.

Guidelines for good samples

You'll need to wait at least two full days after your last ejaculation to do the test.

If you've taken any medications (such as antibiotics, for example) prior to the test, you'll need to wait at least four months after you swallow your last pill before you can produce a sample. It can take three to four months for your sperm count to come back to normal levels. You can either masturbate into the specimen cup, or your partner can bring you to orgasm through petting. Some labs tell you it's fine for your partner to help you ejaculate via oral sex or coitus interruptus (pulling out), but saliva or vaginal mucus may interfere with the test results. If you're doing it through intercourse, don't use collected sperm from a regular condom. There are special condoms that may be used, known as "semen collection devices" (SCDs). Your doctor can tell you where to purchase them. If you are masturbating, avoid using creams or lubricants because they can poison the sperm.

What's normal?

There are several elements your doctor will look for in your lab results. *Because semen is extremely volatile and changes daily, you'll need to deliver at least three semen specimens so your lab can establish a semen baseline.* Since numbers and percentages vary from man to man, sample to sample, minimal limits of "normal" have been set. Your sample needs to meet these limits on at least two occasions to be truly considered a "normal" result. *Warning: If your doctor sends you off for a female workup after only one normal semen analysis, you should seek a second opinion or request that your doctor order another semen analysis.* If your doctor is satisfied that you're "normal" after only one sample, this indicates that your doctor doesn't know what he or she is doing. Two normal semen analyses are enough proof that you are indeed "normal."

On the flip side, if your sample comes back "abnormal" the first try, don't accept this finding until you do at least another test. Two abnormal semen analyses that are *consistent* are enough proof that there's a problem. If no sperm was found in your sample, immediately request that your doctor do a urinalysis to rule out retrograde ejaculation.

The semen analysis checks for a few things (see Table 5.1).

- *Sperm count.* There is debate among the medical community about what a healthy number of sperm is. The World Health Organization (WHO) considers twenty million sperm per milliliter to be fertile; the International Society of Andrology (ISA) considers forty million sperm per milliliter to be fertile. Generally, anything below twenty million is considered a low sperm count. Anything between twenty and one hundred million sperm is considered normal. Keep in mind, however, that sperm numbers can change daily, weekly, and monthly. Colds, flus, STDs, infections, antibiotics, temperature, and ejaculation frequencies all will affect the number. Also keep in mind that men with sperm counts of well below twenty million have often been able to father children.
- *Motility.* This refers to the sperm's ability to swim and move quickly. Again, infection, illnesses, or gonadotoxins such as marijauna or tobacco can affect movement. Just because the sperm are produced in high numbers and are shaped well doesn't mean they're all on the Olympic swim team. Motility is one of the most important determining factors in the sperm's ability to fertilize the egg. At least 60 percent of your sperm need to be motile in order to be considered "normal." At least 65 percent of the sperm must be alive. They also need to be moving *forward.* When you find out your motility percentage, this is the percentage of sperm that are moving. For example, 75 percent motility means that 75 percent of your sperm are moving.
- *Morphology.* This refers to the shape and maturity of the sperm cells to determine the quality, *viscosity of semen* (consistency—thickening is a bad sign), *volume of semen* (amount of semen produced—about 1 teaspoonful is normal), and the *pH balance* (it should be slightly alkaline). Some examples of poor

Table 5.1: An Unremarkable Semen Sample

The following are the usual parameters for a normal semen sample:

Count	More than 20 million sperm/ml
Motility	More than 50% motile
Morphology	More than 50% normal morphology
Semen Volume	2–5 ml
White Blood Cells*	Less than 1 million/ml

Source: Adapted from the *Consumer Journal of Infertility Awareness Association of Canada* (October 1996).

* Note: A high white blood cell count in a sperm sample usually indicates infection, and is often treatable.

morphology would be large numbers of sperm with two heads, no tails; two tails; no heads; deformed tails and heads; and so on. Again, infection and gonadotoxins can affect morphology, and again, at least 60 percent of your sperm need to be formed normally in order to meet the "limits of adequacy." Your volume needs to reach between 1.5 and 5 cubic centimeters in order to meet these same limits.

- *Clumping.* Sperm that clump together are unhealthy and could be a sign of *immunological* infertility, in which your body is making antisperm antibodies.
- *White blood cell count.* High levels of white blood cells in the semen may indicate infection. Treatment for infections ranging from *prostatitis* (inflammation of the prostate gland) to *orchitis* (inflammation of the testes) is discussed in chapter 7.
- *Red blood cell count.* High levels of red blood cells in the semen aren't normal. You'll need to be evaluated for underlying conditions such as infections.

Finding out the results

A significant percentage of all semen analyses will have flaws in them. Men tend to be more in the dark about their test results than women, who usually have some symptoms that hint at a problem. Men usually have no symptoms that would indicate male infertility, whereas women often experience pain or irregular cycles that indicate a female factor.

If you don't hear from your doctor's office within two weeks after your test, you can assume that the results are normal. The results are categorized into two basic groupings:

normal or abnormal. You should also request a copy of the lab report so that you can study it yourself and ask questions about terminology you don't understand. Having a copy of the report will allow you to make copies for the next specialist(s) you encounter. (Don't count on your doctor to send the results.) A normal test series ends the male workup here. You and your partner will then go on as a couple to a gynecologist and/or reproductive endocrinologist to begin the female workup.

An abnormal test could involve any one of the above categories. You could also have sperm that meet the limits in one category but not the other. For example, you could have excellent motility but a low sperm count. In this case, you would be classified as subfertile, which means you're not as fertile as you could be. Many men make the assumption that a diagnosis of being subfertile is the same as being infertile. *This is not true.* A subfertile faces *lower odds* of conceiving a child in any *one* cycle. This is quite different from being infertile, which is a complete inability to father a child. For example, if a normal couple has a 20 percent chance of conceiving each month, subfertile men have *less* than a 20 percent chance of conceiving each month. As one urologist told me, "It's like Las Vegas. If you roll the dice often enough, most of the subfertile couples will conceive. It may just take longer."

If your results came back showing you produced no sperm at all, a condition known as *azoospermia*, all categories in the sperm analysis would be affected, and you would be considered infertile. A diagnosis of azoospermia must always be followed up by a urinalysis to rule out retrograde ejaculation. Again, don't accept this diagnosis until two more semen analyses confirm it. In other cases, abnormalities may be found in several categories, such as motility, morphology, and volume, while the sperm count may be normal.

If after three collections your results are indeed abnormal, you'll be referred to a urologist and/or andrologist for further diagnostic tests. Before initiating more complicated lab work, though, your specialist will have you repeat the semen analysis at least twice over a three-month period. Again, fevers, infections, or viruses can affect the sperm count for months afterward. If two more collections come back abnormal, the male workup continues and will now focus on discovering why your results are abnormal.

Statistically, most male infertility revolves around structural problems. Roughly 40 percent of all male infertility is due to *varicoceles*, a varicose vein in the leg that moves up into the scrotum. Two to 3 percent of all male infertility is due to obstructions (blockage). Out of this group, 5 percent of the obstructions are in the ejaculatory ducts, 2 to 3 percent is due to post-testis obstruction ("bad plumbing"), and 95 percent of the time the blockage occurs in the epididymis. In these cases, microsurgery can remedy the problem (see chapter 7). About 10 percent of all male infertility is caused by infections. About 5 percent of all male infertility is caused by immunological problems, where your body produces antisperm antibodies that kill off the sperm. About 2 percent of male infertility is due to hormonal factors, while another 5 percent of all male infertility is caused by various anatomical defects, such as torsion or undescended testicles, discussed in chapter 7. The remaining percentage is caused by a hodgepodge of genetic problems (discussed below), congenital abnormalities (covered in chapter 7), and retrograde ejaculation.

Finding the Cause

Investigating male factor infertility works differently than most diagnostic processes because you have a diagnosis *before* you have the cause. With other diseases, the diagnosis is made when the cause behind your symptoms is *found*. When you're referred to either a urologist and/or andrologist, your abnormal semen analysis report will have at least one of these diagnostic labels:

- Low sperm count—*oligospermia*
- Poor motility—*asthenospermia*
- Poor morphology—*teratospermia*
- No sperm—*azoospermia*
- High white blood cell count—*pyospermia*

The next test you undergo will depend greatly on your lab report. Since most explained male infertility (versus unexplained) is structural in origin, common structural problems such as varicoceles or blockages may be sought out first. (See Figure 5.2.)

Finding Varicoceles

If all your sperm characteristics are abnormal, chances are the culprit is a *varicocele* (varicose vein in the testicle). Any experienced urologist or andrologist (and some primary care physicians) can find this common structural problem, which afflicts 15 percent of the male population and accounts for at least 40 percent of all male factor infertility. Usually the doctor can find a varicocele just by feeling your scrotum with his or her fingers. In fact, 80 percent of all varicoceles are discovered this way. You'll need to be in a standing position for several minutes before your doctor can find them, however. If a varicocele is suspected, you may need to have either an ultrasound done via a Doppler ultrasonic stethoscope, or a *venography*, which is an X ray of your testicular veins, to confirm the diagnosis. In a venography, a contrast dye is injected into the renal vein outlining the spermatic vein to see how well the blood flows around the testes. *Scrotal thermography*, which uses infrared light to detect temperature gradients in the

Figure 5.2 The Male Factor Breakdown

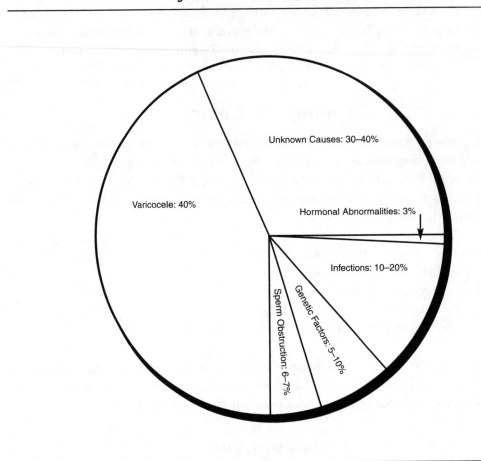

Source: Adapted from the *Consumer Journal of Infertility Awareness Association of Canada* (October 1996).

testicles, can also confirm a varicocele. In some cases, varicoceles are too small to pal-pitate by hand.

Varicocele is a particularly common problem for men who are experiencing secondary infertility, where they have already fathered one or more children but cannot father additional children. Varicoceles cause low sperm counts and poor morphology and may even interfere with testosterone levels. Varicoceles are treatable with microsurgery and are discussed further in chapter 7. Pregnancy rates typically soar from 6 percent per year prior to treatment to 40 percent per year after treatment.

Finding Other Anatomical Problems

As your doctor feels your penis, scrotum, and testicles for firmness and size, he or she will be able to detect less common anatomical problems immediately, such as *torsion*, where one testicle is twisted; inflammation, where one or both testicles may be infected (*orchitis*); undescended testicles; and other congenital problems (see chapter 7). During this exam, honest answers to tough questions may also help to pinpoint sexual disorders that interfere with ejaculation.

Checking Out Azoospermia and Oligospermia

Azoospermia or oligospermia are often caused by structural problems that exist within the seminal vesicles and testes. In azoospermia, the first step is always a urinalysis to rule out retrograde ejaculation. Normal seminal vesicles should also add fructose to the semen. When there's no sign of fructose, this indicates that there's a problem with the vas deferens or seminal vesicles, or it could also be a sign of retrograde ejaculation. Fructose in semen with no sperm indicates a variety of other structural problems that could be at work: blockage in the ejaculatory ducts, a cyst in the pouch of the prostate, or an inflamed prostate gland. Problems within the seminal vesicles or the prostate gland are confirmed by a thorough *digital rectal exam*, possibly followed by a *vasography*. This is an X ray of sperm transport ducts. Radiopaque dye is injected into the vas deferens and ejaculatory ducts, and then an X ray of the dye flowing through the tubes is taken. This test is similar to the *hysterosalpingogram* performed on women (see chapter 6). The vasography results confirm blockage, which may be repaired through surgical techniques.

Hormonal testing

If no structural problem is found, there could be a hormonal imbalance at work. Simple blood tests will check your FSH, LH, prolactin, and testosterone levels, giving your doctor a clear picture of the hormonal axis. For example, high levels of FSH mean that there's trouble within the seminiferous tubules, where the Sertoli cells live. One of the most common male endocrine problems is to find normal levels of LH and testosterone but very high levels of FSH. High levels of FSH is the body's way of shouting at the seminiferous tubules, telling them to *work*!

When your FSH levels are too high and your testosterone levels are low, this is testicular failure; there is no treatment. Donor insemination, adoption, or childfree living are your only options.

High levels of LH indicate problems with the Leydig cells, which make all the androgens, including testosterone. Although Leydig cell problems are almost always associated with a sperm-producing problem, sperm-producing problems rarely involve the Leydig cell. Levels of androgens and estrogens need to be checked as well.

When levels of either FSH or LH (and consequently testosterone) are low, it's a sign that there is a pituitary gland problem. This can be remedied with fertility drugs. Human menopausal gonadotropin (hMG) (Pergonal), which is pure FSH, can be used to stimulate the seminiferous tubules, or clomiphene citrate (Clomid), which is pure LH, can stimulate the Leydig cells. Both these drugs are discussed in chapter 8.

Sometimes *hyperprolactinemia* is the culprit. This is more commonly a problem in women, but men may have high prolactin levels due to a benign tumor in the pituitary gland, which will interfere with testosterone levels. This tumor can be removed, or the drug *bromocriptine* (discussed in chapter 8), may be prescribed to block prolactin secretions.

In more extreme cases, *hypogonadotrophic hypogonadism* may be discovered. Here, very low levels of FSH and LH with possibly normal testosterone levels may be found. This means that there is no hormone stimulation taking place at all, causing no testicular or sperm development. This problem is usually caught well before a man ever considers having children, because he will remain boylike. He will have small testes, have missed puberty, and have extremely low levels of FSH and LH. This disorder indicates *Kallmann's syndrome* (curiously, these men also lack the ability to smell). Hormone injections will take care of the problem. If, for some reason, this syndrome was never diagnosed, it is usually detected during a physical exam.

Thyroid disorders are also common hormonal culprits. Your thyroid gland is responsible for maintaining cell function throughout your body. When your thyroid is overstimulated (hyperthyroidism) or understimulated (hypothyroidism), the result can be a low sperm count and poor libido. This problem is easily treated by an endocrinologist.

Genetic testing

Genetic testing is often done if no sperm are found. Here, a chromosome (karyotype) study is done on a blood sample. This study will reveal possible defects, such as *Klinefelter's syndrome*, where a man carries an extra X chromosome, resulting in no sperm within semen and no sperm production in the testes. Some men have mosaic Klinefelter's syndrome, in which some cells are normal and others have an extra X chromosome. Although these men may have some sperm, they are usually infertile. Klinefelter's syndrome afflicts one in four hundred men—not as uncommon as you may think.

Young's syndrome is another genetic disorder of the *cilia*, small hairs that exist throughout bodily tubes and ducts. Men with Young's syndrome will have no sperm as well as respiratory problems. Here, the epididymis gets plugged up with mucus, which normally is cleaned by the cilia. The lungs will be blocked because of a mucus plug as well. *Intracytoplasmic sperm injection* (ICSI), a "hybrid" of in vitro fertilization (IVF), can be used in these cases to help produce offspring. (See chapter 9 for details.)

Recently, scientists at the University of Minnesota School of Medicine in Minneapolis identified another possible genetic defect related to male-factor infertility. This defect involves a missing piece of DNA along the Y chromosome, which is believed to be necessary for sperm development. Men with this particular defect can be infertile, regardless of their sperm count. And even if these men eventually conceive with assisted reproduction, there is a strong chance that this genetic defect can be passed along to a son.

This Minnesota study found that 7 percent of the men in their study had this defect, and a good portion of them had normal sperm counts. While fertile men can also have this genetic defect, it is believed by the authors of this study that in infertile or subfertile men, this defect is the most likely cause of the condition.

This study may also explain why some men with varicoceles (see earlier) also have difficulties conceiving children. Even if the initial diagnosis was varicoceles, this defect may be present.

Since a good portion of males will not be able to find a cause for their infertility, this study may help to pinpoint that cause sooner, whereupon affected men may wish to conceive through new reproductive technologies, discussed in chapter 9.

The testicular biopsy

This is the procedure men fear the most when they hear the phrase *infertility testing*. When there's no sperm, but all the diagnostic tests seem to check out normally, a testicular biopsy is an important part of the male workup. This biopsy will determine whether the problem originates in the sperm *production* process or sperm *transport* system.

To have the biopsy done, you'll report to the hospital as a day patient and undergo either a general or a local anesthetic. During the procedure, a small piece of testicular tissue, which contains both the seminiferous tubules (which house the Sertoli cells) and the Leydig cells, is removed so it can be examined by a pathologist (see Figure 5.3). You're then sewn up with stitches that gradually dissolve into the body. The procedure takes fifteen to thirty minutes, and you'll be able to go home the same day. This is considered very minor surgery, and the only postoperative side effect you'll likely experience is some pain and tenderness, which a painkiller will take care of. Very rarely, some men may experience bleeding or swelling, usually caused by an infection in the incision.

There are four common results to a testicular biopsy. "Normal" means that your testicles are operating just fine and are producing healthy sperm, but there is an obstructed or missing duct leading from the testicle to the prostate. This abnormality is preventing

Figure 5.3 Testicular Biopsy

a. After a small incision is made in the scrotal skin, an incision is made into the testicle through which the tubules protrude.

b. Extruded tubules are removed. They are placed in a special solution and examined microscopically. The small incisions in the testicle and scrotum are then closed with absorbable sutures.

Reprinted with permission of Serono Symposia, USA, 1994.

the sperm from getting into the ejaculate. Microsurgery techniques can be used to treat an epididymal obstruction, and sperm aspiration can be done when there are absent ducts. Endoscopic surgery can be performed if there is an obstruction in the ejaculatory ducts.

Maturation arrest patterns means that your seminiferous tubules, which contain the Sertoli cells that nurse the sperm, aren't working properly. Something stops the sperm from developing into fully normal, mature sperm. This may be treated with medications. When hypospermatogenesis is found, it means that there are also problems within the seminiferous tubules. Here, while sperm are produced, the number of normal sperm produced represent a small fraction. Sometimes a hormonal imbalance is behind this, which may be treatable. Often the causes are *idiopathic*, meaning "we don't know."

Germinal cell aplasia means that your testicles do not have the germ cells within them that produce the sperm. (Both the sperm and egg start out in the body as tiny germ cells, which then go through a maturing and dividing process.) There is no known cause of this, and there is no treatment available. Options in this case are donor insemination (see chapter 9), adoption, or childfree living (see chapter 12).

Other results a biopsy may find are problems within the Leydig cell, indicating a testosterone deficiency, evidence of inflammation or infection of the testicles, or, *very* rarely, cancer, which interferes with sperm production. It's important to remember that a testicular biopsy is never performed as a first procedure and is reserved for situations where every other possible diagnostic test for an absent sperm count has been exhausted.

Checking Out Asthenospermia, Teratospermia, and Pyospermia

When sperm counts are normal but motility and morphology are poor, your workup will move in a slightly different direction. The first step is to rule out varicoceles, discussed earlier. If no varicoceles are found, infection is the next best explanation, particularly when poor motility is the *only* factor. In short, when something goes wrong *inside* the sperm, something *outside* is usually the culprit. Infections that affect motility are varied, ranging from the gamut of STDs to garden-variety flus and colds. To detect infections, cultures of the semen, urine, and possibly fluid from the prostate gland will be sent to a laboratory for examination. In some studies, up to 10 percent of infertile men have infections but show no symptoms of infection. In women, untreated bacterial infections almost always head for the fallopian tubes, causing the majority of structural problems that affect female fertility; in men, untreated bacterial infections tend to head for the prostate gland, causing prostatitis. Bladder infections (cystitis) in both men and women will also affect fertility. Treating infections is covered in chapter 7.

Whether you're infection-free or not, you'll proceed to a sperm antibody test (via blood test and semen sample) to explore whether *immunological infertility* is a possible cause of your poor motility/morphology or even a consequence of an infection. Sometimes an injury or infection can cause your immune system to react to itself, creating an autoimmune response, which means "self-attacking." Here, the immune system somehow recognizes the sperm as an invader and forms antibodies to it that coat the sperm and ultimately kill them off. This is often a cause of poor motility or visible clumping. Men who have had vasectomy reversals are particularly vulnerable to this, and men who have ingested their own sperm are now recognized as "high risk" for immunological infertility (see chapter 3).

Genetic testing may be the next step if you're infection free. Another genetic defect, *immotile cilia syndrome*, is diagnosed when the sperm tail cannot propel the sperm forward. Here, the sperm count may be high, but the motility would be very poor. Treatment is not available for this defect.

Unexplained Infertility

Many men who produce abnormal semen analyses will find out the cause of their *whateverspermia*. In 30 to 40 percent of the cases, no definite cause behind semen abnormalities will be discovered, but doctors usually will be able to speculate or at least tell you what part of the body is not working.

About 10 to 20 percent of all men with a normal semen analysis series will go on with their partners to a female workup, which will include a *postcoital test* (PCT; you have intercourse, she goes to the doctor) that checks whether your sperm is able to penetrate your partner's cervical mucus. The PCT also makes sure that your partner isn't making antisperm antibodies, killing your sperm once they're in the vagina. After all the female tests, these men may discover that nothing is wrong with their partners either. This is called *unexplained infertility* (or *idiopathic infertility*). In this case, there may be a problem with the sperm's ability to penetrate the egg—something that would *not* show up in a semen analysis or in any of the female tests.

Just to be thorough, your doctor may suggest a *sperm penetration assay* (SPA) or *hamster-egg penetration test* (via semen sample). It's important to have this test done if you have a low sperm count and are planning intrauterine insemination (IUI) or IVF, or if you're planning to do IVF for other reasons.

The test takes a million washed, mature sperm (that is, "capacitated") and leaves them to incubate with twenty to twenty-five hamster eggs. These eggs have had their outer shells removed to allow penetration but *no* development. (Don't worry—your genetic material will *not* turn up in an unsuspecting hamster!) Your doctors can determine the fertile potential of the sperm by observing how many eggs were penetrated. This test is not usually routine in a normal male workup. The test was originally developed in 1979 and since then has undergone many upgrades. A positive result (meaning yes, your sperm can penetrate) is usually reliable, but some false negatives have been reported, where the test reveals that the sperm is unable to penetrate the egg, yet a pregnancy has resulted nonetheless.

Erectile Dysfunction (Impotence)

To be considered impotent, you must have been unable to obtain or sustain an erection long enough to have intercourse—for a period of at least six months. In other words, we're not talking about one of those movie scenes where a frustrated couple lies in bed and the woman turns to the man, saying, "It happens," and the man replies, "Not to me." Premature ejaculation is also not considered to be "impotence" although it can happen when you are impotent. A small percentage of men are infertile because of impotence.

Diabetes-related impotence

Roughly 60 percent of all men over age fifty with diabetes (Type 1 or 2) suffer from impotence, which means that about 33 percent of all impotence is caused by diabetes.

Diabetes can lead to impotence because the small blood vessels responsible for causing an erection could be damaged, or the nerves controlling sexual response could be damaged. Damage to your large blood vessels can affect the flow of blood to your penis as well.

When a physical problem is at work, signs come on gradually. Over time, you'll notice that your penis becomes less rigid until you are unable to obtain or sustain an erection completely.

Diagnosing diabetes-related impotence

Just because you have diabetes, it doesn't mean your impotence is caused by it. Therefore, to diagnose physical impotence, doctors will tell you to place a paper band around your penis before you go to sleep. Since all healthy men will have erections during their sleep, if you wake up with a broken band, it means your impotence is not physical, but psychological. If your band is intact upon waking, it means that your problem is physical (although not necessarily related to diabetes—it could be hormonal).

Once it's established that you have a physical disorder at work, your doctor can rule out nerve damage versus blood vessel damage by checking out both. To check nerve damage, a test involving a painless electrical current can measure your penis's response.

To check blood vessel damage, a device similar to testing blood pressure in your arm can be used on your penis. Or a drug that bypasses your nerves can be injected into your penis to see if you can have an erection. If you can't, then blood vessel damage is indeed the problem, and it's most likely a large blood vessel problem. Ultrasound and a tracer dye can confirm impotence caused by large blood vessel damage, where the doctor can actually see whether the blood is flowing freely through the vessels into the penis.

Another physical cause of impotence can be blood-pressure-lowering medication, while smoking and alcohol are considered aggravating factors.

Treating physical impotence

One of the most popular treatments for ED is Viagra ® (sildenafil citrate). It is a pill that you take about an hour prior to potential sexual contact. You will only get an erection if you are aroused. Viagra should begin to take effect in about thirty minutes, and lasts up to four hours. Viagra works by increasing blood flow to the penis, and works in about four out of five men who take it, regardless of how long they have had ED, what caused it, or how old they are. But men over sixty-five, men who have cardiovascular problems, kidney problems, or liver problems should consult their physicians about the safety of Viagra. If you are on medications for the treatment of HIV, you should also consult your physician about the safety of Viagra. In some cases, depending on the severity of your other health problems, your doctor may okay it, but the makers of Viagra caution against it. Furthermore, if you take any drugs containing nitroglycerine or nitrates, you must not take this drug, as it can lead to a heart attack or stroke (see previous chapter). Nitrates are found in many prescription medications that are used to treat angina (chest pain due to heart disease). If you cannot take Viagra, or it doesn't work, there are older remedies such as:

- *Drug injections*. Various drugs can be injected into your penis prior to intercourse, which will increase blood flow and produce an erection for at least thirty minutes. Prolonged erection is a side effect, however. (In Europe, there is actually a problem of certain "patch" medications—intended for heart disease— being used by healthy men to prolong their normal erections!)

- *Vacuum devices.* Here, a vacuum device is used to enlarge the penis, and then a tension band is placed around the penis to maintain the erection for intercourse. Bruising can occur if the tension band is on longer than twenty minutes.
- *Penile implants.* Here, either an inflatable or semirigid rod is placed inside the penis to restore sexual function (although it will not help with ejaculation).
- *Blood vessel surgery.* Here, blood vessels that are blocking blood flow to the penis can be corrected.
- *Yohimbine.* This is a sexual stimulant that increases nerve sensitivity in the penis; if nerve damage has occurred, you may want to ask your urologist about the benefits of this drug.

The Male Factor Roller Coaster

During the workup, most men may feel isolated in the doctor's waiting room, which is filled mostly with women. Men who choose to deliver their samples at the office may dread the room where they must produce their sample. These rooms usually have a variety of *Penthouse* magazines and assorted porn videos to speed the process along. Why are there so *many* women in the waiting room if infertility is split between male and female factors? Many of those women are there for treatment after a male factor problem has been discovered; many of those women are there to get sperm requisitions and test kits to take home to their partners, who are doing all their workup tests at home; and some may be *single* and pursuing a family through donor insemination.

Every infertility situation is unique and therefore carries unique emotional and social consequences. When it is a female factor problem, men tend to play the "supportive partner" role, allowing their partners time to grieve, time to rant and rave, time to cry, and time to be angry. They will also reassure their female partners about their attractiveness and femininity. But few men will truly *feel* a female factor problem, although they obviously will be affected by it.

When a couple is dealing with a male factor problem, women who star in the "supporting role" tend to hit a brick wall. Many men will go the "ostrich" route, preferring *not* to discuss the problem, not to reveal their true feelings, and hence *not* to plan for an alternative, such as donor insemination or adoption. Many will experience depression and even sexual dysfunction as a result. Many men will turn to addictions such as work or alcohol.

The urge to repress feelings is a male tendency that is encouraged not only by our social structures and definitions of "masculinity," but often by male friends and acquaintances. After interviewing many couples who have dealt with male factor infertility, the number-one problem most men faced was admitting their infertility to another *male*, particularly close family members and friends. Psychologists and psychiatrists substantiate the finding. The psychiatric literature confirms that while women focus on the loss of a baby, putting to rest their dreams of pregnancy, childbirth, and breast-feeding, men focus on their fears of *competition*: "What will my friends say?" As a result, many men will choose silence over disclosure.

This is an understandable but emotionally unhealthy choice. In the long run, continued silence will create communication gaps in your relationship with your partner. Admitting the infertility to even one other male will help you find a "place" for your feelings. To help you break that silence, I've compiled a list of guidelines based on the experiences of many men and couples who have dealt with male factor infertility. Not one male I spoke with regretted his disclosure.

Guidelines for Breaking the Silence

1. *What are you afraid of?* Try to imagine your worst fears of disclosure: being the subject of cruel jokes at the office; being ostracized by the "guys"; being laughed at by people you respect. Try to evaluate whether your fears are justified, and think about how your lifestyle would change if these fears were actualized. For example, if your best friend laughed at the problem, this information could help you reevaluate your criteria for friends and help you form more lasting, deeper friendships. Male factor infertility tends to be like a wedding or funeral: it brings out the worst and best in people.

2. *Educate yourself.* Request literature, article clippings, or videos from your doctor on male infertility. If this fails, do your own research through organizations and libraries. The more you read about your particular problem, the less isolated and freakish you'll feel.

3. *A date for discussion.* Make a date with your partner to discuss your problem. Clear a night on your calendar and *devote* the evening to discussing your feelings and options. The more your partner feels included in your pain, the more she can support you rather than just "guess" at how you must be feeling. You can also use your partner to practice disclosure lines on other males or family members. For example, ask her advice on how to start: "There's something I need to tell you," "I'm telling you this because I think you'll understand," and so on. Ask her advice on comeback lines to rude comments such as "When are you two having a baby?" or male friends who joke, "You can't use *my* sperm!"

4. *Start a journal.* Write down your feelings instead of keeping them inside. Your journal will begin to feel like an old friend, help you sort out your feelings, and help you *monitor* them from month to month. Are you coping better today than last month? Are your coping skills getting worse? You can even read your journal entries to your partner. Or, if you're not able to talk to her, you may want to invite her to read the journal anytime she wishes. (See Figures 5.4, 5.5, and 5.6 for examples of journal notes between a real-life couple coping with male infertility.)

Figure 5.4 Note Between a Couple Dealing with Male Infertility

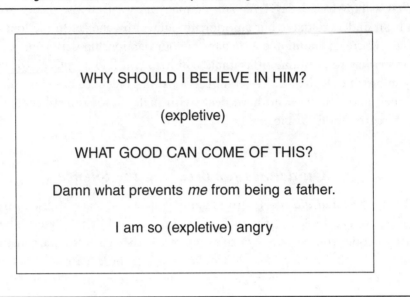

Source: Infertility Awareness Association of Canada, 1994.

Figure 5.5 Note Between a Couple Dealing with Male Infertility

He has taken a part of me that means the most. I want a child. I want a baby . . . that will never be part of me—THERE CAN NEVER BE A PART OF ME THAT CONTINUES, a fact that can never be denied, I can not handle the thought that I will not continue . . . my eyes, my thoughts, my dreams. I will never have the joy or the satisfaction of saying "this is a part of me." Yet, I see the cruelty of so many parents toward their children! Children they have never even thought of as a privilege. (Expletive) THEM FOR NOT LOVING THEIR OFFSPRING ENOUGH . . . I'm angry and very mad at God. He has taken the one thing I would have loved unconditionally.

Source: Infertility Awareness Association of Canada, 1994.

Figure 5.6 Note Between a Couple Dealing with Male Infertility

Dearest P.,

I'm so sorry you went through what you were feeling last night. It pains me to see you unhappy.

I'm sure you know that I understand and share your anger. I'm sure you also know that you are already an important part of our children. You may not be able to give them the shape of their eyes, the curve of their nose, or their beautiful thick hair, but you will give them things much more important—the shape of their beliefs, curiosity, and compassion are just a few of the things that come to mind as I picture you sharing your joy of life with them.

P., you are *very* special and I look forward to having your children.

Love always,

S.

xo

Source: Infertility Awareness Association of Canada, 1994.

5. *Find a good male friend.* You need to talk to another man about your infertility. If you don't have a male friend or close family member (brother, brother-in-law, father, cousin) you can talk to, maybe you need to rethink some of your relationships. Try to choose someone who poses no threat to you regarding workplace or community politics. Take some time to find this person. Don't rush it. All you need is one good friend. (See number 6.)

6. *Seek out a male counselor.* Again, the idea is to find another male to confide in. Someone who knows what it's like to *own* a penis and testes may be able to offer you more practical solutions to your dilemma. You don't have to sign up for long-term counseling; just a few sessions with a male social worker or male psychologist should do. In some cases, male clergy can make ideal counselors.

7. Find a good support group. All major cities have branches of infertility support organizations. You need to find other couples in your situation and hear that other men have felt what you do now. This may be where you find that one good friend to talk to.

As discussed at the beginning of this chapter, 45 percent of all men will graduate to a female workup after three normal semen analyses. The next chapter may be in order or out of order, depending on the results of your male workup. For treatment options to many male factor problems, see chapters 7 and 9. Donor insemination is covered in chapter 9.

6

The Female Workup

AFTER YOUR MALE partner has delivered two normal semen analyses, the two of you can proceed to the female workup. The female workup is infamous for its involved and invasive testing. Many of the tests require a woman to be at a certain phase of her cycle, which can result in weeks between tests and months before a reason for your infertility is found. For 10 to 20 percent of infertile couples, no fertility problem will be identified after the female workup, leaving you with the maddening diagnosis of unexplained infertility, discussed later, and in detail in chapter 7. The good news is that there is still a 70 to 90 percent chance that the cause of your infertility *will* be found during this workup.

About 30 percent of all female infertility is caused by hormonal factors. This is a significant percentage when you consider that only 5 percent of all male factor infertility is hormonal. As a result, a great deal of female factor infertility can be treated with medications. The remaining 50 to 60 percent of all female factor infertility is caused by structural problems involving infections or inflammations of the fallopian tubes or other pelvic organs. This chapter focuses on all the *diagnostic* tests involved with the female workup and discusses the appropriate procedures from least invasive to most invasive. Treatment, when available, for female factor infertility is covered in chapter 7, fertility drugs are addressed in chapter 8, and ART techniques are detailed in chapter 9.

Some women will still require a full workup even though a male factor problem has already been identified. This is because the woman is the one who will need to undergo the bulk of ART treatments. In addition, in 20 percent of the cases, both partners have problems. A fertility doctor will need to know whether the woman is *able* to conceive via intrauterine insemination (IUI), in vitro fertilization (IVF), gamete intrafallopian transfer

(GIFT), or even donor insemination (DI). As a result, this chapter introduces an option that I'll explore further in chapter 12: *Refusing treatment*.

What's the First Step?

Your primary care physician will refer you to a gynecologist who subspecializes in reproductive endocrinology. Review chapter 2, which covers guidelines for finding a good specialist and the questions you need to ask. If your gynecologist has been managing the workup so far and is skilled in reproductive endocrinology, you don't need to be referred elsewhere.

Both partners should see the gynecologist together. You should also bring in your basal body temperature (BBT) charts, and any other charts you're using to keep track of your cycles (see chapter 4). The doctor will begin by interviewing both of you. *Note: To save time, bring along your medical chart from the initial male workup and physical, as well as the results from the last three semen analyses. Otherwise, men may wind up doing everything again*!

The doctor may even request *separate* interviews, asking each of you about your relationship, how long you've been together, and how long you've been trying to conceive. A man will be asked whether he has impregnated a woman in the past; a woman will be asked whether she has ever been pregnant, has had any abortions, or has had previous pelvic surgery. These questions help the doctor determine the likelihood of either a structural problem, such as scarring on the pelvic organs, or a hormonal problem. Women will also be asked a great deal about their lifestyle, diet, and weight history. Presuming no other disorders, ovulation irregularities are usually caused by one of three things: excessive weight loss or weight gain, excessive exercise, and emotional stress (see chapters 3 and 4).

No competent infertility specialist will proceed with the workup without taking a full menstrual and contraceptive history. The doctor will be looking for a history of intrauterine device (IUD) usage as well as any signs of endometriosis or pelvic inflammatory disease (PID). The specialist will also make sure that you've been having regular menstrual cycles throughout the "trying to conceive" period for at least a year, that you've been timing your intercourse correctly, and that you've been having intercourse frequently during your ovulation peak. At this point, he or she should ask to see your BBT chart. (If you haven't been keeping a BBT chart, you'll need to start one and keep track of your cycles for at least three months. You won't see the specialist again until you have completed the charts.)

"What's the first test?" This question will have different answers depending on what your ovulation charts and medical history revealed. For an average woman who had no history of STDs and had charts revealing normal patterns of ovulation, her specialist would most likely start with a postcoital test, proceed to a hysterosalpingogram, and finally to an endometrial biopsy. If a structural problem was suspected, some specialists may *immediately* check out the fallopian tubes before doing other tests, while others may still begin with the least invasive tests first and gradually progress to the more invasive procedures. For the purposes of this chapter, I'll follow the "least invasive first" plan. Keep in mind that workup philosophy isn't necessarily better or worse, but simply a different *approach*. Finally, age does play a major role; the older you are, the speedier your workup needs to be. For a woman of average age (late twenties/early thirties), a workup should not last longer than a couple of months. If your workup is dragging on for more than three months, it's time to question your specialist.

As in the male workup, the female workup begins with a full physical: a pelvic exam, screening for STDs, Pap smear, blood work, and so on. If all goes well, you'll move on to the tests discussed throughout this chapter.

Sleuthing Out a Female Factor Problem

Because the initial interview will set the stage for your workup, there are several clues your doctor will be on the lookout for:

- *Late menarche (having your first period after eighteen)*. This is a sign that you may have a hormone imbalance.
- *Spotting between periods*. This could be a sign that you have a uterine abnormality of some sort.
- *Severe pelvic pain* or *cramping during menstruation (dysmenorrhea)*. This could be a sign of endometriosis.
- *A "heavy" feeling in your pelvis*. This could mean you have a large fibroid. Treatment for fibroids is discussed in chapter 7.
- *History of abdominal or pelvic surgery*. Even if your surgery was unrelated to a gynecological problem (such as an appendectomy or bowel repair), scarring from the surgery could still affect your ovaries. Surgeries such as cesarean sections, removal of ovarian cysts, previous ectopic pregnancies, dilation and curretage (D & C), or abortion could definitely cause pelvic adhesions and scar tissue that may be obstructing your reproductive organs.
- *History of abnormal Pap smears*. If you were ever treated for an abnormal Pap with cone biopsies, laser surgery, or cryosurgery, these procedures can interfere with your cervical mucus. Any surgery on your cervix could weaken it and may lead to an incompetent cervix, which will need to be stitched in the event of a pregnancy.

- *History of STDs.* You know this one. Again, chlamydia and gonorrhea can spell PID.
- *History of IUDs.* This device can predispose you to PID as well as an ectopic pregnancy.
- *Vaginal infections.* Any vaginal infection, such as yeast or "trich," can be toxic to sperm. It will be a "treat and repeat" situation.
- *Exposure to DES.* Are you a DES daughter?

The Pelvic Ultrasound

One of the least invasive procedures, a pelvic ultrasound is an excellent way for your doctor to get an idea of the size, shape, and dimensions of your pelvic organs. An ultrasound will also reveal whether your ovaries are producing follicles, and whether you have any unusual enlargements or inflammations that warrant specific tests. An ultrasound will also show whether your uterus is thickening accordingly, showing that you're making *enough* progesterone, which is crucial if the embryo is to implant itself in the uterus. The idea is to make sure that you don't have any obvious gynecological problems or infections at work.

There are two methods of doing a pelvic ultrasound: transvaginally and abdominally. In Canada, most doctors will want to do both for insurance purposes.

Abdominal ultrasound

Abdominal ultrasounds require a full bladder, and many women will find it an uncomfortable procedure as a result. There are ways around the discomfort. You'll be given specific instructions to drink a large quantity of water (usually about eight glasses one hour prior to the procedure). For most women, this is just too much water! Before you begin drinking, call your clinic or doctor's office and find out whether you'll be seen on *time*. If the clinic is running behind, time your drinking accordingly. If you find that you're feeling uncomfortable before you even leave for your appointment, *empty your bladder completely*. By the time you arrive at the clinic and are called in to see the doctor, your bladder will have filled up again. If you arrive at the clinic and are in pain, ask for a paper cup and empty your bladder enough to fill it about 75 percent. This should tide you over. Finally, if you know that your bladder fills up quickly, all you need to do is drink half the water you're told to, or even one mug of coffee. That should be enough to fill your bladder for the appointment without causing extreme discomfort.

Ultrasound is also called *ultrasonography*. It is the use of an echo sounder to produce a picture of the pelvic tract. High-frequency, low-energy sound waves are used to scan your abdomen, reflecting your pelvis's outline on an electronic screen through a series of bright dots. A full bladder causes the uterus (normally lying behind the pelvic bones) to be pushed outward. This makes your reproductive organs easier to find and see on the scan. Jelly is rubbed all over your abdomen, and a probe (called a transducer) is placed on the jellied area and moved around. A computer translates the sound echoes into video pictures. This picture is called a *sonogram*. The operator will point out what the patterns in the video picture mean and will probably show you your parts on the screen. The procedure takes about ten minutes.

Since the ultrasound technologist does many ultrasounds in a day, you should make a point of telling him or her that you're there to investigate infertility. This will tell the operator to take special note of unusual enlargements, cysts, scarring, fluid, and so on. Request a copy of the lab results from your doctor so you can discuss terminology and "normal variances" that may not seem so normal to *you*! For example, if you have a retroflexed uterus (tipped backward), your doctor may not bother to tell you about it (one in five women do). Some doctors believe it's more difficult to conceive with this shape. If you have fluid in your cul-de-sac (the pocket surrounding your reproductive organs), your doctor may not find this significant, but you may want to know why the fluid is present. It may be an early indication of endometriosis.

Transvaginal ultrasound

You don't need to have a full bladder for this procedure, and some women prefer it to the abdominal procedure. At any rate, a transvaginal procedure can detect more than the abdominal ultrasound. A dildo-shaped transducer, with a condom over it and lubricated with jelly, is inserted into your vagina. If you can have comfortable intercourse, you shouldn't feel any pain at all. The procedure is usually performed by a female technician or supervised by a female. If you are very modest, you may request to insert the transducer yourself, but you must have very clean hands to avoid transferring bacteria. The procedure takes about ten minutes. Again, make sure you tell the technician why you're there so he or she can keep an eye open for red flags. Request a copy of the lab results from your doctor.

Testing for a Hormonal Problem

If your ultrasound results are normal, you'll begin a series of hormone tests that will be taken at different times in your cycle. The process begins by discussing your menstrual charts with your doctor, who may have observed some unusual patterns in the cycle right off the bat. For example, some BBT charts have flat patterns, whereas others have too many peaks and valleys.

Again, roughly 30 percent of all female infertility is caused by a hormonal imbalance of some sort. Depending on what kind of imbalance you have, you'll be plagued with different symptoms that include irregular cycles, failure of the embryo to implant in the uterus, poor-quality cervical mucus, or the inability to sustain a pregnancy, causing you to repeatedly miscarry (see chapter 11). Some ovulatory problems are not obvious. For example, even though you may not be ovulating every month, you could still have regular periods. This is known as an *anovulatory cycle*.

Blood Tests

When irregular ovulation is cited as the probable culprit, you'll undergo a series of simple blood tests done at various points in your cycle (different hormones peak at different times) to find what hormone is either missing, deficient, or exploding from your body. Assuming a twenty-eight-day cycle, on day two or three of your cycle, FSH, LH, and estradiol (a type of estrogen) are measured. Then, during the luteal phase (anywhere from days twenty-two to twenty-four), progesterone levels are measured. Your doctor will check your levels of gonadotropin-releasing hormone (GnRH) and androgen levels. Prolactin levels can be checked at any time during your cycle, but it's best to do it in the morning, and for you to avoid touching your breast prior to the test. Touching your nipples or breasts, for example, may stimulate the hormone and throw off the test, causing inaccurate results. You'll most likely undergo a transvaginal ultrasound and endometrial biopsy (explained later) to accompany some of these blood tests.

Progesterone withdrawal test

This is an important test for women who have either bouts of *amenorrhea* (no periods) or chronic amenorrhea. This test determines whether the amenorrhea is caused by a uterine abnormality or a hormonal imbalance. Is the uterine lining getting thick enough to shed to begin with? If it isn't, you don't have the right amounts or combinations of hormones in your body to trigger a period. Is your uterus thickening each month but somehow not responding to your hormones, which is a signal to shed? There's an easy way to find out. Progesterone is given to you either orally or by injection to induce a period or "withdrawal bleeding." If the bleeding starts, then the problem is clearly a *hormonal* one. The hormonal problem will then need to be pinpointed by further tests. If you still do not bleed despite hormonal supplements, there's either a *uterine* abnormality at work that will need to be ruled out, or you may not have enough estrogen to respond to the progesterone withdrawl.

If you have excessive body hair . . .

During your initial physical exam, your doctor will be checking to see if you have body hair on your breasts, back, abdomen, face, and so on. Your doctor may not notice that you have excessive hair because you might be *removing* it. If you're asked this question, you should answer truthfully. There is a condition known as *polycystic ovarian (PCO) syndrome*. This is a condition where your ovaries have small cysts that interfere with ovulation and hormone production. You'll also be asked about any skin problems such as acne, and you may also have a history of irregular periods and/or a battle with obesity. Obesity, oily skin and acne, irregular cycles, infertility, and excessive hair growth are symptoms of PCO.

If you have this problem, you're probably not ovulating regularly, which will show up in your menstrual charting. Your doctor will do some additional blood tests in this case to check for any elevated levels of *androgen*, a male hormone all women secrete in small amounts. You can also have elevated androgen levels and *not* have PCO. If androgen is the problem, you may need to be put on female hormone supplements such as estrogen replacement to offset it. PCO is treated with fertility drugs and is a classic "textbook" cause of female infertility. See chapter 7 for more details.

If you're anovulatory, under five feet tall, and suffer from a variety of chronic medical problems . . .

There is a genetic condition known as *Turner's syndrome*, which affects roughly 1 in 2,500 women. Turner's women have either a missing or a damaged X chromosome (normally, women have two X chromosomes). These women are short, not growing beyond about 4 feet 7 inches, and usually have other medical problems, including ear, eye, heart, kidney, or thyroid disorders, diabetes, high blood pressure, and keloid healing.

These women also lack many secondary sexual characteristics (such as breasts or pubic hair), have irregular or nonexistent menstrual cycles, and are usually infertile. Other physical features include low-set ears, a low hairline, a webbed neck, pigmented moles, bending out of the elbows, and puffy hands and feet. Finally, while Turner's women are not mentally impaired and have the same IQ levels as the general population, many will suffer from learning disorders involving arithmetic and spatial skills (map reading, puzzles, visual problem-solving). Children with this problem may also be hyperactive.

If you suspect you have Turner's syndrome, request a *karyotype study*, or a genetic test (via blood test), from your doctor. Fertility drugs will successfully treat Turner's and may alleviate other medical problems associated with it.

Cushing's syndrome

There is another disorder you can be tested for, known as *Cushing's syndrome*, which is an abnormality of the adrenal gland. Symptoms include irregular menstrual cycles or no menstrual cycles, a distinctive hump of fat between the shoulder blades, water retention (also known as edema), high blood pressure, obesity, general muscular weakness, and easy bruising. Other characteristics include a moon-shaped face, acne, and abnormal hair growth (similar to PCO). Treating Cushing's syndrome is fairly simple. A steroid medication will return hormone levels to normal, which will reverse your infertility.

The Monitored Cycle

Some fertility specialists may want to place a woman on what's called a monitored cycle. If blood tests seem to be inconclusive, your doctor may want you to deliver a blood sample each day of your cycle, beginning on day one. This way, he or she can get a clear picture of which hormones are appearing and disappearing within specific time frames of the cycle. A monitored cycle may also involve ultrasound, which can help establish whether you're developing follicles or whether your uterus is thickening accordingly.

This is an involved process that requires daily trips to a lab or the doctor's office, but the information it yields could nail down a hormonal imbalance. For example, one of the most difficult hormonal problems to diagnose has to do with *luteal phase defects*, discussed later in this chapter.

Monitored cycles are also done once you enter treatment, so your doctor knows exactly when you're ovulating for certain procedures such as IVF, IUI, or GIFT.

The Endometrial Biopsy

This is an in-office procedure that involves placing a small plastic cylinder inside the cervix. The cylinder contains a suction device that sucks up only a small portion of the endometrial lining. The lining is then sent to a lab and analyzed. The procedure is an excellent diagnostic tool but is invasive and can be painful. Taking anti-inflammatory medication prior to the procedure will help take the edge off any cramping.

This biopsy procedure is used to investigate hormonal imbalances that can cause irregular cycles or annovulatory cycles, repeated miscarriages (see chapter 11), or even irregular uterine bleeding. It takes less than ten minutes to do and is far less invasive than a laparoscopic procedure.

For an infertility investigation, an endometrial biopsy is usually done between days twenty-two and twenty-four of the menstrual cycle (assuming a twenty-eight-day cycle). At the beginning of that cycle, your doctor will explain the importance of preventing pregnancy for that month. Abstinence or condoms are highly recommended during this interval. Prior to the biopsy, if you have any reason to suspect you're pregnant, a pregnancy test must be done to rule it out.

The purpose of the biopsy is to examine the characteristics of your endometrium to make sure it's the right consistency and thickness for that time of the month, which will indicate whether you're secreting the right *combination and levels* of hormones. Some doctors may choose to do the biopsy within the first eighteen hours of your period, but this is trickier to time and to do. The outcome of your endometrial biopsy will determine whether you have a progesterone deficiency, an estrogen deficiency, or even an LH deficiency. Depending on the hormonal imbalance, you may just need a hormone supplement.

Prior to taking the test, your doctor will want you to keep a basal body temperature chart during the cycle of test, and perhaps for one cycle following. This will help him or her to put the results into context. You will also have your progesterone levels taken via a blood test on the day of the test.

After the test, you can expect some cramping and spotting. Make sure you don't go home alone in case you have a bad time of it.

Few women will escape an endometrial biopsy during a female workup. This is a very important test that helps to pinpoint hormonal problems that may be suspected through a combination of blood tests, monitored cycles, and charting. While some of you may be recommended for treatment prior to the endometrial biopsy, most doctors will wait for the outcome of this test before recommending treatment.

Common Hormonal Problems

The results of all the above tests will probably uncover one of the following hormonal disorders (unless you have PCO, Turner's syndrome, or Cushing's syndrome).

Postoral contraceptive syndrome (also known as postpill syndrome)

It usually takes three to twelve months for your cycles to return to normal after going off oral contraceptives (OCs). Roughly 5 percent of the women who stop using OCs will not see normal cycles for over a year. (See Table 6.1.)

In these cases, fertility drugs may be suggested as well. Women who are prone to this usually had irregular cycles prior to taking their OC. It's crucial to note, however, that OCs do not cause infertility; they simply aggravate a preexisting fertility problem. Some of these women may also have hyperprolactinemia.

Table 6.1 When the Cycle Returns

Use this table to help determine when to expect the return of your natural periods after discontinuing a hormonal contraceptive.

Type of Contraceptive	Periods Return
Combination oral contraceptive	Anytime within ten days to a few weeks. Can be as long as a year, depending on your age. Women over thirty, or those on monophasic (versus triphased) pills can expect longer delays in natural cycles.
"Mini-pill" (progestin-only pill)	Within twelve hours of a missed dose; no delays in cycles returning have been reported.
"Morning after" pill (postcoital/emergency contraception)	Your next period will be a natural cycle.
Depo Provera (injectable contraceptives)	Within six to eighteen months of discontinuation.
Norplant (subdermal contraceptives)	Within four to seven weeks after removal; 80 percent of women will conceive within a year of removal.

Hyperprolactinemia

Fifteen to 25 percent of irregular ovulation is caused by secreting too much of the hormone *prolactin*, which interferes with both ovulation and embryo implantation in the uterus.

Prolactin is released from the pituitary gland and is responsible for breast milk production. When levels are high, prolactin stops the pulsing of GnRH from the hypothalamus, which interferes with the pituitary gland's release of FSH and LH, interfering with estrogen and progesterone.

Normally, prolactin levels should be high only if you're pregnant or nursing. Otherwise, high levels can be caused by emotional or physical stress, exercise, nipple stimulation, or large intakes of protein (don't get your prolactin levels tested after you've eaten a giant steak!). Surgery around the rib cage can also raise prolactin levels. Drugs such as amphetamines, tranquilizers, antidepressants, hallucinogens, and alcohol may also be the culprit. If you have either PCO or an underactive thyroid gland (hypothyroidism), you can also have hyperprolactinemia.

Thirty percent of the time, women who have too much prolactin will notice milk in their breasts (called *galactorrhea*) or will notice milk when they squeeze their nipples during a breast self-exam. Other symptoms might include decreased vaginal secretions and irregular cycles. A woman may also have light, irregular, short, or no periods.

Hyperprolactinemia can be detected by a simple blood test. At least two blood tests will show high levels of prolactin. If the problem is caused by food, you may need to fast before retesting. Often these blood tests are followed up by a CAT scan to check for a possible *benign* pituitary tumor (occurring in about 5 percent of all women who have hyperprolactinemia). In fact, with chronically high levels of prolactin, a benign pituitary tumor known as a microadenoma (small) or a macroadenoma (large) is often the cause.

The drug bromocriptine (see chapter 8) usually offsets prolactin secretion and shrinks any tumors that exist. If a tumor is found, it can be surgically removed through the nasal passage, but this procedure may not restore your fertility. Radiation may also be used to shrink a pituitary tumor, but it's rare in this case.

Premature ovarian failure

Premature ovarian failure is when your body goes into premature menopause. Your ovaries just "close shop." This is responsible for about 10 percent of all ovulation problems and, if you're under thirty, your doctor may want to do a chromosome test. This is fairly easy to diagnose through blood tests and a pelvic exam. Some causes include a decreased number of eggs at birth (they get used up earlier), exposure to radiation or chemotherapy, chromosomal abnormalities, diseases such as cancer or AIDS, and physical trauma to the area (injuries and so on). Natural ovarian failure is diagnosed when you have very high levels of FSH and LH in your blood or urine, while your estrogen levels are very low.

This is not a treatable condition, but you may be put on hormone replacement therapy (HRT) to prevent osteoporosis and menopausal symptoms. In this situation, you and your partner have three choices: adoption, surrogate parenting, or childfree living. In some instances, if your uterus is still healthy, you can have an egg donated and try IVF using your partner's sperm. Premature ovarian failure is discussed more in chapter 7.

A deficiency in GnRH

GnRH triggers the release of FSH and LH from the pituitary gland. Without this, you won't ovulate. This is easily treated by replacing the hormone synthetically with fertility drugs. See chapter 8 for more details.

Luteal phase defects

This is when you don't have enough progesterone to keep your uterus embryo-friendly. Remember how the follicle bursts and then turns into a corpus luteum, which secretes progesterone? Well, this stage of your cycle is also called the "luteal phase" and refers to a progesterone deficiency. Most women have a luteal phase that lasts ten to fourteen days. If your luteal phase lasts for less than nine days or longer than fourteen days, you may have a luteal phase defect. This is diagnosed from a blood test done during your luteal phase (the serum progesterone test) as well as an endometrial biopsy (see page 126). In this case, two endometrial biopsies are usually done to study variations on the lining's thickness in more detail. A third biopsy may be recommended if there is a question about the results. Your doctor will also look at your BBT chart and monitor your ovaries via ultrasound to try to catch your luteal phase (which will follow your follicular phase). You might want to review chapter 4 to recall how a normal cycle should work.

In a luteal phase defect, the corpus luteum stops working and doesn't produce enough progesterone to keep the endometrium thick enough for an embryo to implant itself. Luteal phase defects may also cause pregnancy loss if the embryo does implant and is a common diagnosis in the event that you have more than two miscarriages. If you conceive with a luteal phase defect, usually the embryo is shed along with the endometrium lining (when you menstruate) before you would discover the pregnancy. This is known as an *occult pregnancy*.

In general, it's common for women to have luteal phase defects at some point during their menstrual lives. During puberty, around menarche (the first period), during the postpartum phase (after childbirth), and prior to menopause are when luteal phase defects strike the average woman. In these cases, the cycle usually corrects itself. Smoking and stress may also trigger this problem.

The diagnosis of a luteal phase defect has met with some controversy. Many U.K. researchers believe that this luteal phase defect is incorrectly labeled; the reason why the corpus luteum is failing is because the follicle it originated from was a dud. In short, if the follicle was a "good egg" to begin with, the corpus luteum would not be failing. According to this line of thinking, if a good egg is produced during the *follicular phase* of the cycle, then all should go well in the second stage of the cycle. Many U.K. women will be treated with fertility drugs for this problem, in the belief that the drugs will help stimulate the ovaries to produce a *better* follicle, which in turn will develop into a better corpus luteum.

Most North American doctors, however, feel that treating a luteal phase defect with fertility drugs is akin to putting a bandage on a corpse. The feeling on this continent is that corpus luteum defects have nothing to do with how "good" the original egg is. Instead, the treatment recommended is to compensate for the failing corpus luteum by supplementing this phase of the cycle with progesterone. This will help to prime the endometrium during the luteal phase, making it more receptive to the embryo. These supplements will also help lower a woman's immune system response, preventing it from rejecting the embryo once it does implant. These supplements are given by vaginal or rectal suppository.

When you're taking a progesterone supplement, your doctor will need to monitor you via another endometrial biopsy to make sure that the supplements are working and that the dosage is correct. You'll need to be on these supplements for about four to five months before you can expect to conceive. In some cases, the supplements may continue during the first trimester of the pregnancy to reduce the chances of losing the pregnancy due to a lack of progesterone.

If the suppository doesn't work, the "British rules" for treatment are usually tried next. You'll be put on clomiphene citrate to see if your corpus luteum improves when your follicle production escalates. But clomiphene citrate, however, may *cause* luteal phase problems and even alter cervical mucus in ovulating women. In this case, intrauterine insemination can be done to compensate for the mucus problem. Some doctors will supplement either treatment (suppositories or fertility drugs) with an injection of human chorionic gonadotropin (hCG) within the third or fourth day of the luteal phase.

Hypothalamic amenorrhea

This is usually caused by a few of those seven habits discussed in chapter 3: weight loss, overexercise and stress, anorexia, and bulimia. An underactive hypothalamus or a late puberty may also trigger this problem. The symptoms include very light periods or no periods, and your blood tests will reveal very low hormones and no ovulation. You may have flat temperature readings and no mid-cycle cervical mucus.

If your lifestyle habits are the cause, your doctor will send you home and tell you to gain some weight, stop overexercising, try to relax, and so on. If this doesn't work, you will probably be prescribed a regimen of hormonal supplements or fertility drugs. Even if you're planning on childfree living, women with constant low estrogen levels are at a high risk of developing osteoporosis.

Nonspecific anovulation (oligo-ovulation)

This means "we don't know why you're not ovulating." If you're ovulating less than twelve times a year and no cause for your irregular cycles are found, you'll be given this "diagnosis." The treatment is to put you on clomiphene citrate and wait. Pregnancy rates in this case are actually quite high.

You'll be relieved to know that ovulatory problems can almost always be treated with fertility drugs. This is known as *ovulation induction*. Between 60 and 90 percent of women treated for an ovulatory disorder go on to conceive. There *are* some drawbacks to fertility drugs, though. Women on clomiphene citrate, for example, may have problems producing high-quality cervical mucus and may not be able to sustain a pregnancy beyond the first trimester due to a luteal phase defect. All the drawbacks to fertility drugs are discussed in chapter 8. Pregnancy loss is discussed in chapter 11.

As a precaution, don't begin taking *any* fertility drugs before the cause of your ovulatory problems is nailed down. Some doctors tend to prescribe these drugs as soon as they see you're anovulatory, without bothering to find out *why*. In addition, just because you do have a hormonal imbalance doesn't mean there aren't other structural problems at work.

Testing Cervical Mucus

If you haven't yet read chapter 4, read the section on observing cervical mucus. While you may be ovulating right on schedule, you may not be producing high-quality cervical mucus. This is usually an indication that there is a hormonal problem at work, but the causes of poor cervical mucus are often unexplained. You should rule out infection before your doctor concludes that you're having mucus problems. Vaginal infections such as yeast or "trich" or other STDs will *absolutely* interfere with your cervical mucus production. Get this checked out if you haven't done so yet.

The Ferning or Spinbarkheit Test

The *ferning test* is so named because it involves drying a sample of your mid-cycle mucus to see if it forms a ferning pattern when it's examined under a microscope. Prior to ovulation (anywhere from days ten to fifteen of a twenty-eight-day cycle) as discussed in chapter 4, high-quality cervical mucus changes texture to a clear, stringy, and plentiful discharge that is very stretchy. This egg-white consistency is known as *spinbarkheit*. This test involves getting into the "Pap" position, then your doctor collects cervical mucus for the test. That's it. Fairly noninvasive. Bear in mind that spinbarkheit refers to the stretchiness of the mucus when it's grasped with surgical instruments, such as clamps or forceps. The ferning test is usually done at the same time as the postcoital test, discussed next.

The Postcoital Test (PCT): Are You "Sperm-Friendly?"

This is a simple, noninvasive test that is often one of the first tests performed during a female workup. Before going ahead with the PCT, some doctors may suggest that you use an LH test kit (see chapter 4) or may want you to undergo an ultrasound, which can help pinpoint ovulation. The postcoital test is far less invasive than a hysterosalpingogram. This test is painless but may be embarrassing. You'll need to make an appointment with your gynecologist around your mucus peak day. Then, you and your partner will need to have intercourse about twelve hours before the appointment (some doctors do it two to four hours after, but this isn't the best time). The timing depends on your schedule and the doctor's. When you arrive at your doctor's office, he or she will get you into the Pap position and then insert a syringe high inside your vagina to collect your postcoital mucus. The doctor will also insert an instrument into your cervical canal to retrieve mucus. Your cervical opening should also be dilated slightly and will change in color around ovulation. Your doctor will make sure to check for this. The dilated opening allows more sperm through.

This is an important test, because it not only reveals the *relationship* between your partner's sperm and your cervical mucus, but it tells the doctor how well they're "getting along." The test also tells the doctor about your ovulation cycle. After collecting the post-coital mucus, your doctor places it under a microscope and examines it. The first thing that's checked is the cervical mucus consistency. It should be *egg*-whitelike, transparent, stretchy (stretching about 6 to 10 centimeters), have an alkaline pH balance (to match the pH balance of healthy sperm), be rich in mucin, glycoprotein, and salt. If your mucus is too dry or scanty, or lacks these properties, the sperm will not be able to survive long enough to fertilize the ovum. The doctor will also check for sperm life signs and the number of sperm present. *This is why twelve hours after intercourse is the best time for the test.* Since healthy sperm should be able to survive for at least twenty-four hours after intercourse, if there are no live sperm after twelve hours, there's a problem. The absence of sperm, or the presence of immobilized (live but paralyzed) sperm after twelve hours indicates that the mucus is rich in sperm antibodies, that sperm production is faulty—which would be an odd thing to discover after two *normal* semen analyses—or that intercourse positions are poor (ejaculating outside the vagina, or the penis is not placed high enough inside). Another reason why this test is best performed twelve hours after intercourse is because it puts far less pressure on the two of you. You can simply have intercourse the night before. This timing is preferable to some mad-dash interlude in the back seat of your car at lunch hour, and then racing to the doctor's office afterward.

If the test results are normal, you'll move on to the next step: hysterosalpingogram.

What do the PCT results mean?

Roughly 15 percent of all female infertility problems *are* caused by poor-quality cervical mucus. If *this* is what the postcoital test finds, you may be put on estrogen supplements about seven to ten days before ovulation to try to raise the quality of the mucus. This doesn't work too often, though. A somewhat odd remedy that *has* been known to work is taking *decongestant cough syrup* during the first two weeks of your cycle to increase mucus production throughout the body! In fact, this is considered the "answer" to infertility in some small towns. Some women have reported an increase in the quality and quantity of their mucus by using this method and *have* gotten pregnant as a result. (Sometimes truth really is stranger than fiction.) However, there is no definitive scientific evidence to support the cough syrup cure. In any event, many specialists will tell you to give it a try because this peculiar practice is harmless. You'll be asked to repeat the PCT a few times during your mucus Total Quality Management effort. If estrogen and cough syrups fail, the only other choice left to you is to have your partner's sperm placed high inside your uterus. This is known as *artificial insemination by husband* (AIH) (although your partner, of course, doesn't have to be your husband), or *intrauterine insemination* (IUI) with washed sperm.

If the PCT results find that the sperm are immobilized or dead, yet the semen analyses and cervical mucus are normal, your infertility may be caused by the presence of antisperm antibodies, known as *immunological infertility*, where your immune system manufactures antibodies that destroy your partner's sperm. This is also discussed in chapters 3, 5, and 7. Or, your intercourse position may have simply been a dud. With this kind of test result, you'll be asked to repeat the test. If you still get the same PCT result, immunological infertility is probably what's going on. This can be confirmed with further blood tests for both of you. There is no known effective treatment for this form of immunological infertility. Some doctors suggest clearing out all sperm from your system, wearing a condom for the next six months, and then trying again. The theory is that your body may relax once it's rid of it's "invader." Then, you can sneak the sperm back in during ovulation and hopefully become pregnant before your immune system has time to destroy the sperm. Another theory is to put you on cortisone treatments to suppress your immune system; this has a very low success rate of about 25 percent. Otherwise, your only choice is IVF, discussed in chapter 9. Treating male-produced antisperm antibodies is discussed in chapter 7.

Making the most of your PCT

As mentioned above, you must have this test done prior to ovulation (around your mucus peak day). In order for there to be ample numbers of sperm, it's advised that your partner refrain from ejaculation forty-eight hours prior to having intercourse with you. When you have intercourse, you should refrain from using any lubricants or creams, which will interfere with the test results. Some doctors may want you to refrain from urinating prior to the test, but this is an unreasonable demand if you're seeing the doctor several hours after intercourse. Some doctors suggest that you remain still after intercourse for roughly fifteen minutes to avoid losing any ejaculate, but again, this "holding-the-sperm-in" theory is highly controversial and dismissed as rubbish by most experts.

The PCT Cup Test

If the results from either your first or second PCT were ambiguous, your doctor may progress to the highly controversial PCT cup. Your partner delivers a semen sample while your cervical mucus is collected. Then, a small portion of both samples are placed on a glass slide to see what happens. If the sperm penetrates the mucus, the rest of the semen is put into a plastic cup and placed over your cervix for about two hours (you can move around normally during this period). After two hours, *another* sample of mucus is collected, and survival rate of the sperm is assessed. Whether or not this test reveals anything terribly significant is in debate.

Penetrak Test

This test, also known as the bovine cervical mucus test, crosses back into the male workup domain, but the results could pinpoint whether the problem is your mucus or his sperm, or a little bit of both. If the PCT result showed that the sperm had trouble penetrating your cervical mucus, the sperm may be placed inside thin tubes with cervical mucus from cows. The sperm is given about ninety minutes with the cows' mucus to see if the sperm can penetrate it. If the sperm react the same way to this mucus as they did to yours, then the problem is with the sperm. If, however, the sperm react differently to the cows' mucus than to yours, then the problem is truly with your cervical mucus and not his sperm.

Checking for Structural Problems

This is where the workup gets quite invasive. The procedures below may cause cramping and discomfort for a few hours. You'll need to arrange for appropriate time off when you have these procedures done. In other words, immediately heading to work after these tests isn't a good idea. Many specialists will perform the following tests in the late afternoon (3 to 5 P.M.) so you can return to work the next morning.

Looking into the Tubes: Hysterosalpingogram (HSG)

If your ovulation cycle is normal and you've passed your PCT with flying colors, it's time to check out the fallopian tubes. Basically, this test checks for symptoms of *salpingitis* and other signs of inflamed fallopian tubes caused by chlamydia or gonorrhea (see chapter 2), scarring from *endometriosis* (discussed in chapter 7), or scarring from past ectopic pregnancies. Your tubes can also become inflamed from previous abdominal surgery or a ruptured appendix. An HSG will also be done on women who want a tubal ligation reversed.

This test is invasive but quick. At best it's uncomfortable; at worst you'll feel *extremely* painful cramping. The pain *is brief*, however. Done in the first half of your cycle (after your period but prior to ovulation or days seven to eleven of a twenty-eight-day cycle), you'll get into a Pap position, and your doctor will place a clamp on your cervix, which is uncomfortable. Your doctor injects a dye into the uterus, which should fly through your tubes and come out the other end. X rays are taken as the dye is injected and can detect whether the dye passes through the tubes' open ends or not. If the dye passes through, your tubes are open; if it doesn't, your tubes are blocked, which will make the test more painful.

Because this dye is a foreign substance, to prevent any risk of infection you may need to take antibiotics for about three days before undergoing this test. However, this is only done if you have a high risk of developing an infection. In addition, an allergy to iodine should be checked out prior to undergoing the test. Some doctors recommend that you take anti-inflammatory medication prior to the test to reduce cramping. Even if your tubes are open, the dye can cause discomfort. It will be expelled as a sticky discharge from the vagina, and the rest will be absorbed by your body.

What do the results show?

This test can be inconclusive. For example, if the dye flows through your tubes freely, you may *still* have a problem with the quality of your *cilia* (small hairs that line your tubes and cavities). This may prevent smooth delivery of the egg through the tube into the uterus.

The test may not be successful in picking up pelvic adhesions, endometriosis, or problems with the *fimbria* (fringes at the ends of the tubes). It will usually pick up abnormalities affecting the tubal block or uterine structures, endometrial polyps, fibroids, and adhesions in the uterus itself.

Are there any risks?

The HSG can cause pelvic inflammatory disease (PID) by carrying bacteria into your tubes. Because of this, you should be given antibiotics prior to the test. If your tubes are blocked, your doctor may want to do a laparoscopy (discussed next). Or, he or she may suspect PID and treat you with an aggressive antibiotic regimen (see chapter 7). Laparoscopy will also find other structural problems caused by PID, cysts, or endometriosis. Repair surgery is discussed in chapter 7.

Hysteroscopy (a telescope that's passed through the cervix) and falloposcopy (a telescope passed through the fallopian tubes) can apparently show a little more than an hysterosalpingogram, but as of this writing, more studies into the validity of these tests are warranted.

Laparoscopy and Hysteroscopy

Laparoscopy and hysteroscopy are the most invasive procedures of all, done under a general anesthetic. (See Figures 6.1 and 6.2.) While many women will have laparoscopic or hysteroscopic surgery to treat a number of gynecological procedures, these procedures are usually used as diagnostic tools only in an infertility workup. The only difference between a laparoscope and a hysteroscope is that a laparascope is used to look outside the uterus, fallopian tubes, ovaries, and internal pelvic area; the hysteroscope is used to look inside the uterus. This test is usually considered the last one done in a female workup. If, however, your doctor strongly suspects endometriosis, this may be one of the first procedures you undergo. The only way to absolutely diagnose endometriosis is through a laparoscopy.

For this test, you'll need to check into a hospital as a day patient. Under a general anesthetic, a long thin tube, called a laparoscope, is inserted into your abdominal cavity. This cavity is inflated with carbon dioxide to force the walls away from the organs so that the doctor can get a good look inside your abdominal and pelvic cavity. Light from a projector outside the tube is passed through the cables containing hollow glass wires. The sur-

Figure 6.1 Laparascopic Procedure

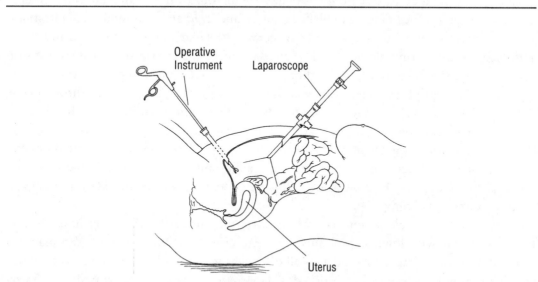

Reprinted with permission by The American Society for Reproductive Medicine, 1209 Montgomery Highway, Birmingham, Alabama, 35216-2809, (205) 978-5000.

Figure 6.2 Hysteroscopic Procedure

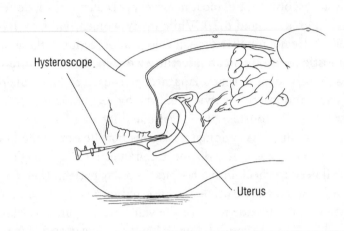

Hysteroscope

Uterus

Reprinted with permission by The American Society for Reproductive Medicine, 1209 Montgomery Highway, Birmingham, Alabama, 35216-2809, (205) 978-5000.

geon can now get a clear, three-dimensional view of your ovaries, fallopian tubes, uterus and peritoneum (pelvic lining), gall bladder, spleen and liver, and large and small intestines.

Sometimes referred to as "keyhole surgery," the laparoscope is inserted into your abdomen through a tiny incision in the belly button. Sometimes a second small incision is made above the pubic bone, and a thin probe is inserted to help move organs around.

A more in-depth HSG may be done at this point, as a blue dye is passed through your fallopian tubes, giving your doctor a better idea of the condition of the tubes. In addition, some minor corrective procedures may be done, such as burning away spots caused by endometriosis. Your surgeon may also do a hysteroscopy. Here, a device is inserted directly into your uterus, which will hunt for tumors, adhesions, and congenital abnormalities. Finally, a tuboscopy may be done as well, in which a scope is put right inside your fallopian tube to examine its lining.

The laparoscopy takes about twenty to thirty minutes. After the procedure, the carbon dioxide gas will slowly escape through the incision prior to stitching. You may feel discomfort in your chest or shoulders if all of the gas was not released. Don't worry about this. The gas will eventually be absorbed. A laparoscopy reveals nothing unusual 50 percent of the time. If you have any tumors, cysts, endometriosis, pelvic adhesions, or scarring, laparoscopy will find it. Most women need to be off work for a few days after the procedure. You may have a bad reaction to the anesthetic and need to rest. You may also feel nauseated and tired for a couple of days following the procedure. You should expect some cramping and mild abdominal discomfort; however, many women find they have no symptoms and can return to work the day after surgery.

If you're experiencing extreme discomfort and pain and/or have a fever, report this to your doctor immediately. You may have contracted an infection.

What are the risks?

Overall, 2 percent of the women who undergo laparoscopy or hysteroscopy will experience some type of minor complication.

The most serious risk of any laparoscopic procedure is damage to surrounding organs (bowel, bladder, ureters, uterus, blood vessels, and so on) during the insertion of various instruments through the abdominal wall. This kind of injury occurs in roughly 4 out of every 1,000 laparoscopic procedures. If you have (a history of) any of the following conditions, you are at greater risk of serious injury:

- bowel surgery (e.g., for ulcerative colitis)
- previous abdominal surgery
- pelvic adhesions
- severe endometriosis
- pelvic infections or pelvic inflammatory disease

Women who are obese or too thin are also at greater risk of serious injury.

Less serious but still uncommon risks such as bruising or pooling of blood (called a hematoma) within the abdominal wall, pelvic infections, bladder infections, and infection at the incision site may also occur.

The most common risk involved with a hysteroscopy procedure is puncturing the uterus (called perforation), which can be painful but usually heals on its own. Other complications are related to the liquids used to distend the uterus, which can cause fluid on the lungs and breathing problems, blood clotting problems, allergic reactions, and decreased body temperature.

What's the Next Step?

For most couples, a female workup will finally reveal the cause of your infertility. For others, it may reveal that a female factor problem exists *along* with a male factor problem (discovered in the event that treatment is sought for a male factor problem). Or, the infertility may be unexplained. Whatever the results, you will need to move on to the next part of the fertility journey: treatment. Fertility drugs can usually treat any hormonal problems that exist for a female factor problem. However, when the problem is structural, many microsurgical techniques have poor results and may not increase your chances of conceiving. Under these circumstances, it's important to truly educate yourself about your options, the costs, the time involved in treatment, and the emotional investment you'll need to make. All these issues are discussed in chapters 7, 8, and 9.

Unexplained Infertility

Ten to 15 percent of couples will not find an identifiable cause for their infertility. Of those, 20 percent will get pregnant each year for three years. It may be a relief that nothing is "technically" wrong with you, but it's also a maddening predicament. The situation can create tension in your relationship and may be aggravated by rude or tactless remarks from outsiders.

Just because your infertility is unexplained doesn't mean you cannot seek treatment. Fertility drugs and a number of ART procedures can be ideal solutions to this problem. See chapters 7, 8, and 9 for more details.

Refusal of Treatment

Some of you may not want to go beyond this point. You may have discovered a problem that isn't treatable, or you may have discovered that a female factor problem exists along with a male factor problem. You may have unexplained infertility, or you may have a treatable problem, but you may not *want* to be treated.

For many people, the idea of not treating a fertility problem seems incomprehensible. How could you not want to *fix* the problem? Remember that just because a problem *is* treatable, there is no guarantee that you'll conceive. For some, the idea of refusing treatment is an ideal option.

Treatment involves repeating various aspects of both the male and female workup, investing a great deal of time and energy (including time off work), and investing a great deal of money. Couples with limited financial resources may not be able to make the stretches and compromises that treatment demands. Other couples who are financially secure may just feel comfortable accepting what nature has in store: "If we get pregnant spontaneously, great. If we don't, that's fine, too." Again, the next chapter may be in order or out of order, depending on what you decide.

7

What's the Problem
and How Do We Fix It?

IN THE PREVIOUS two chapters, I discussed the diagnostic journey involved in finding either a male or female factor cause for your infertility. This chapter addresses the course of treatment for your infertility. For many of you, the buck stops here. Whether your problem is hormonal or structural, once the problem is fixed you may conceive without difficulty. For others, fixing the problem may not be that simple, and conception delays may persist. Under these circumstances, you may need to move on to further treatments involving assisted reproductive technology (ART), discussed in chapter 9.

For many female fertility problems, treatment entails fertility drugs such as clomiphene citrate, human menopausal gonadotropin, and several others. These drugs are powerful and potent. Some women will experience side effects, and some may be reluctant to use fertility drugs because of studies that suggest a link between them and ovarian cancer. Some men may also be placed on fertility drugs if their fertility is linked to a hormonal problem. Chapter 8 covers fertility drugs in detail.

Female Factor Infertility

Roughly 30 percent of all female factor infertility is caused by hormonal problems. Common hormonal disorders revealed by the female workup (see chapter 6) can be treated with fertility drugs or hormone supplements. Polycystic ovarian syndrome, a more complicated hormone disorder, carries a variety of treatment options. Ovarian failure, another disorder, is a consequence of many cancer therapies as well as exposure to certain environmental toxins. Both are discussed next.

The remaining 50 to 60 percent of all female factor infertility is caused by a structural problem, and pelvic inflammatory disease (PID) or endometriosis is usually the culprit. Both conditions, along with less common structural problems, are discussed as well.

Polycystic Ovarian Syndrome

Polycystic ovarian syndrome (PCO), also known as polycystic ovarian disease or Stein-Leventhal syndrome, is a classic female infertility problem. About 4 percent of the general female population suffers from PCO, which accounts for half of all hormonal disorders affecting female fertility.

With PCO, your body secretes far too much androgen, which counteracts your ovaries' ability to make enough progesterone necessary for a normal cycle. Your estrogen levels are fine, though, and your levels of lutenizing hormone (LH) are higher than usual, working overtime to try to kick-start the cycle. But the androgen levels interfere with your follicle stimulating hormone (FSH), which you need to trigger progesterone. As a result, your follicles never develop, and instead turn into small, pea-size cysts on your ovaries. Your ovaries can then enlarge. The elevated androgen levels can also cause you to develop facial hair, hair on other parts of your body (this happens in 70 percent of the cases and is called *hirsutism*), or even a balding problem. Acne is another typical symptom, as well as obesity, although women who are thin or of normal weight can also have PCO. Your periods will be irregular, and as a result you might be at greater risk for developing *endometrial hyperplasia*, in which your uterine lining thickens to the point of becoming precancerous. (If you have endometrial hyperplasia, progesterone supplements will be given to you to induce a period, or a dilatation and curettage [D & C] may be done to eliminate the lining.) Because of your high levels of androgen, you may also be at an increased risk for cardiovascular disease. Diet can help reduce the onset of heart problems.

If PCO was caught early on in your menstrual history, you simply would have been put on combination oral contraceptives to induce normal withdrawal bleeding and pump your system with normal levels of estrogen and progesterone. Or you would have been put on progestin, a synthetic progesterone supplement, and would have been instructed to take it about mid-cycle.

If you were treated earlier with progestin, you won't experience problems with your cycle unless you go off the drug for some reason. But women who were treated with oral contraceptives for irregular cycles at a very young age may not know *why* they suffered from irregular periods to begin with (see chapter 4). When these women go off contraception to conceive, they will be plagued by the same symptoms that initially warranted oral contraception. Sometimes women with normal cycles may develop PCO later in life. In this case, they will suddenly develop irregular cycles (called *secondary amenorrhea*).

Why are estrogen levels normal in PCO women?

Normal estrogen levels come as a surprise to women with PCO. In normally fertile women, estrogen is made from the follicles. In this case, however, your body converts the *androgen* into estrogen. If you're obese, estrogen will also be stored in fat cells. This constant estrogen level confuses the hypothalamus, which assumes that high estrogen levels are present because of a developing egg inside the follicle. The hypothalamus will then tell the pituitary to slow down the release of FSH. Without FSH, your follicles won't mature and burst and hence you won't ovulate.

Who's at risk for PCO?

PCO is hereditary and is more common among women of Mediterranean descent. It's also uncommon to develop PCO later in life, although it can happen. Generally, a PCO woman will begin to experience menstrual irregularities within three to four years after her menarche (first period). Women who are obese can be predisposed to PCO because their fatty tissues produce estrogen, which can confuse the pituitary gland. Women who are diabetic or who have a problem with their adrenal glands, thyroid gland, or pituitary gland can develop symptoms of PCO, but technically not have the condition. Make sure you ask your doctor to rule out these conditions before you begin any treatment for PCO. In some cases, PCO may coincide with these conditions.

Reversing infertility

To reverse infertility in women with PCO, doctors will use the fertility drug clomiphene citrate (Clomid or Serophene) in tablet form. You'll start clomiphene citrate on day five of your cycle, then go off the tablet on day ten. If you've had long bouts of amenorrhea, your period will be induced via a progesterone supplement before you start on clomiphene citrate. An average dosage of clomiphene citrate in this case ranges between 25 and 50 milligrams. In some cases, an antiestrogen drug called *tamoxifen* (also used as treatment in certain kinds of breast and gynecological cancers) may also be used with clomiphene citrate. Roughly 70 to 90 percent of all PCO women on clomiphene citrate will ovulate, but pregnancy rates vary; 30 to 70 percent of PCO women on clomiphene will conceive.

If you're still not ovulating after taking clomiphene, human chorionic gonadotropin (hCG) may be added to your hormonal "diet" during the luteal phase of your cycle, roughly one week after your last dose of clomiphene citrate.

If this regimen fails, you'll graduate to FSH therapy. (During menopause, FSH naturally soars in the body to compensate for tired ovaries.) Prior to starting FSH therapy, you'll need to have a hysterosalpingogram (see chapter 6) to make sure that your fallopian tubes are clear. You may also need a pelvic ultrasound to rule out other structural abnormalities. PCO women don't fare as well on FSH therapy as they do on clomiphene citrate. While 70 to 80 percent will ovulate with FSH therapy, only 20 to 40 percent will conceive. While receiving FSH therapy, you'll also need to be monitored through blood tests (to check estrogen levels) and ultrasound (to check follicle growth). The side effects, costs, and risks associated with clomiphene citrate and FSH therapy are discussed in chapter 8. Multiple births are also common with both drugs.

Other treatments for PCO

In many PCO women, weight loss is considered the "cure." However, when infertility is a concern and a PCO patient wants to conceive, weight loss is not really a realistic short-term treatment because it's a slow, time-consuming process. If you have PCO and are being treated with fertility drugs, you may be able to reverse your infertility through natural weight loss for future pregnancies. You'll need to see a nutritionist and design a weight loss program that's in tune with your lifestyle.

If the ovaries have large cysts on them, some fertility specialists may want to try to cauterize the ovary in about eight to ten small spots through laparoscopic surgery. Roughly 62 percent of PCO women who undergo this surgery successfully go on to conceive, and when the surgery is combined with fertility drug therapy, the pregnancy rates are as high as 80 percent.

In some PCO women, androgens are also produced in the adrenal glands. Under these circumstances, your doctor may want to put you on a corticosteroid to suppress the adrenal gland, lowering the production of androgens. This will help induce ovulation as well.

Bromocriptine (discussed in chapter 8), which suppresses prolactin, will be given to 15 to 20 percent of all PCO women. The high levels of estrogen associated with PCO commonly cause hyperprolactinemia (see chapter 7).

Treating hirsutism

Because one of the unpleasant symptoms of PCO is hirsutism, which results in excessive male-patterned hair growth on the face, navel, or breasts, many women will want treatment. An antiandrogen drug, which is available in pill or cream form, will take care of the hair growth problem. You'll need to discuss the exact dosage of this drug with your doctor. Hair growth should slow down after about five months on the drug. For more information, consult my book, *Women and Unwanted Hair*.

In the interim, electrolysis is the most effective treatment for hair growth on the face, navel, or breasts. Make sure you go to a reputable clinic and ask to talk to past clients.

The insulin connection

It has recently been discovered that insulin resistance and polycystic ovary syndrome go hand-in-hand. Women with insulin resistance are either at risk for, or have been diagnosed with, Type 2 diabetes. Lowering insulin in women with polycystic ovary syndrome seems to help restore menstrual cycles and lower male hormone levels. Oral hypoglycemic agents used to treat Type 2 diabetes are now being used to treat PCO. Only about half the women diagnosed with PCO have insulin resistance, which means that your body is not responding properly to the insulin produced by your pancreas gland.

Before you're placed on an insulin-lowering drug, ask your doctor about how diet and exercise can help your body use insulin more efficiently. You should also ask how insulin-lowering drugs affect pregnancy, and make sure you're aware of all the side effects of these powerful drugs. For more information, consult my book, *The Type 2 Diabetic Woman*.

Premature Ovarian Failure

As discussed briefly in chapter 7, ovarian failure is when your ovaries shut down, resulting in a premature menopause. Depending on the degree of ovarian failure, ovulation induction may be attempted with fertility drugs. If this fails, there is no way to treat the condition, although hormone replacement therapy may be suggested to prevent *menopausal* symptoms. There are several options available to women at risk for this, however.

Who's at risk?

Any woman undergoing chemotherapy or radiation therapy to her abdominal or pelvic region is at risk for premature ovarian failure. Hodgkin's disease, non-Hodgkin's lymphoma, and leukemia are classic cancers that strike women in their teens and twenties. Breast cancer, rare in women under the age of thirty-five, may result in infertility for women who have delayed having children until their mid-to-late thirties. Disturbing increases in a variety of skin cancers, such as melanoma, can strike women who overexpose themselves to the sun while they are still in their childbearing years. Keep in mind that not all chemotherapy treatments will result in ovarian failure. Dosages in some cases have been refined to the point where ovarian function resumes uninterrupted, although an early menopause (prior to age forty) is often the consequence.

Women exposed to occupational hazards, including chemicals and radiation, or to radiation from environmental fallout are also at risk for premature ovarian failure. See chapter 3 for more details.

In some cases, premature ovarian failure is due to natural causes (being born with a limited number of eggs), congenital abnormalities, and so on. If your mother went into an early menopause, you may be at risk for premature menopause yourself.

Options to maximize your fertility

No woman will undergo chemotherapy or radiation treatments without being informed about the risks to her fertility. Although in most cases the loss of fertility may be a secondary concern over the potential loss of one's life, there are a few options you can consider if you want to have a biological child. Depending on your situation, none of these options may be possible or feasible, but it doesn't hurt to ask.

- Discuss the idea of retrieving some of your eggs *prior* to your treatment. These eggs can be frozen and used later for an in vitro fertilization (IVF) or a gamete intrafallopian transfer (GIFT) procedure with your partner's sperm when you're well again. (You still may be able to carry a child if your uterus is intact and healthy.) You can also use these eggs in a "host uterus" of a surrogate mother who is impregnated with an embryo resulting from your egg and your partner's sperm. Bear in mind that this procedure is still in the experimental stage, though.
- If you're receiving external radiation therapy to your pelvic region, investigate whether an *oophoropexy* can help prevent ovarian failure. This is a surgical procedure that moves your ovaries out of the path of the radiation beam. Then, after the treatment, the ovaries are repositioned and your ovarian function can resume. If you're receiving chemotherapy either alone or in conjunction with radiation therapy to the pelvic region, an oophoropexy will be ineffective.
- Discuss the risks of *delaying* your treatment for one year so that you can get pregnant prior to your therapy.
- After treatment, get pregnant as soon as possible. You'll usually be cautioned to wait two years after chemotherapy before you can try to get pregnant. Depending on your dosage of chemotherapy, ovarian function may resume for a few years before menopause sets in. Try to get pregnant as soon as your doctor considers it safe. If you're not married and are not in a position to have a child yet, you may want to consider having your eggs retrieved and frozen for later use just in case ovarian function shuts down earlier.

What Can You Freeze?

There are a variety of techniques that involve cryopreservation, meaning freezing embryos, eggs, sperm, and now even ovarian tissue, which can sustain your fertility if you're at risk for ovarian failure. When you're well again, these procedures can help you mother a biological child. As of this writing, here's what freezes well, or what one day soon may freeze well.

Eggs

Either mature or immature eggs can now be successfully frozen and thawed, but fertilizing thawed eggs hasn't yet "matured" as a science. It's getting there. When the first edition of this book was published, freezing the egg was experimental; today, the eggs freeze well, but it is getting them to fertilize that is the challenge. As of this writing, some births have resulted from formerly frozen mature eggs, or frozen immature eggs that were matured in a laboratory. Techniques such as intracytoplasmic sperm injection (ICSI), where the sperm is injected directly into the egg, could be used to optimize fertilization.

The problem with mature egg-freezing is that you need roughly 100 unfertilized eggs in order to ensure that one of them will fertilize. Relatively small numbers of eggs are available with each menstrual cycle—even when fertility drugs are used—making it pretty difficult to get 100 mature eggs from one woman. The promise in egg freezing will likely result from removing ovarian tissue (discussed next), which contains hundreds of immature eggs. Through this process, hundreds of potential eggs could be harvested from one woman, frozen for as long as twenty years, and then matured in a lab, known as in vitro maturation. Experts believe this will be widely available in the next few years, which can help to establish egg banks.

Ovarian tissue

Small pieces of ovarian tissue may contain several hundred follicles. Grafts of frozen ovarian tissue have already spawned baby mice and sheep in animal experiments. (And a sheep has even been cloned, which I'll discuss more in chapter 9.) Freezing human grafts of ovarian tissue is still in the experimental stages, but the advantage is that wedges of ovarian tissue can be collected via laparoscopy from each ovary at any stage of the menstrual cycle without compromising a woman's health or fertility. The tissue can be frozen and then used to produce mature eggs for IVF.

Single women who do not have a life partner, but who don't want to get caught later in life in the biological clock game, may also benefit from this procedure.

Embryos

Embryo freezing is pretty routine these days. You can have your eggs harvested and fertilized with your partner's or a donor's sperm, and have the embryo frozen and then transferred at a later date when you're well. The pregnancy rate with two to three embryos transferred is around 15 to 25 percent; the odds increase with each repeated transfer.

If cancer is the reason why you want to preserve embryos, it will only be possible if you are "cleared" for having your ovaries stimulated with fertility drugs. The high levels of estrogen involved may be absolutely *unsafe* if you're undergoing therapy for breast cancer or a gynecologic cancer. This may also be a problem for women with severe endometriosis or fibroids, discussed further on. There is also a risk of transferring cancer cells together with the embryos. Make sure the embryos are checked for cancer cells before they are transferred back into the uterus.

As another alternative, *immature egg harvest*, discussed in chapter 9, can be a way of obtaining eggs without stimulating your ovaries with fertility drugs.

Pelvic Inflammatory Disease (PID)

PID is a general term that refers to infection and inflammation of one or more of your pelvic organs: your cervix, uterus, fallopian tubes, or ovaries (known as your *upper genital tract*). These infections can also spread to other parts of your body, infecting your abdominal cavity, kidneys, liver, lungs, and so on. PID is a serious condition that affects well over one million women each year in North America. In the United States alone, about three hundred thousand women are hospitalized because of PID; one thousand women die from PID annually; and over $4.2 billion is spent on treatment. This disease is also a major cause of female factor infertility in North America. Because of the availability of ultrasound and laparoscopy, PID is also a newly recognized disease that wasn't really diagnosed until the early 1970s. Prior to the 1970s, women with PID were often misdiagnosed or branded hypochondriacs when they complained of chronic pelvic pain or other PID symptoms.

What causes PID?

Bacteria is the cause of PID. Normally, the cervix acts as a barrier, preventing bacteria from getting inside the upper pelvic region. But when the uterus is invaded by a STD or is dilated for any reason, bacteria can enter and do a lot of damage. For example, when certain bacterial STDs—primarily gonorrhea and chlamydia—remain untreated, the infection can spread and cause PID. Bacteria can also enter your pelvic region through intrauterine device (IUD) insertion, the second major cause of PID in countries that use IUDs. Douching, certain pelvic surgical procedures such as abortions, D & Cs, amniocentesis, or natural phenomena such as miscarriages and childbirth can also cause PID. Smoking increases a woman's risk of PID. Both current and past smokers were found to be twice as likely to develop the disease. The reasons why are not known, however. The irony is that in the majority of cases, PID is preventable.

Symptoms

Because PID is a general label that doesn't tell you where the infection is, the symptoms can vary depending on what organ is infected. Although there are several symptoms associated with PID, the common pattern is to experience only one or two of them. Some women have only mild symptoms, some women have symptoms so severe they can't function, and other women experience no symptoms at all and may discover they have PID only when they investigate infertility.

The most common symptom is lower abdominal pain. It may be sporadic or chronic and may occur only during or after intercourse, menstruation, or ovulation. The pain is often on one side of the abdomen and increases with movement, such as walking or climbing. The pain is always present during a pelvic examination, when your doctor feels your pelvic region manually to check for enlargements or abnormalities. Sometimes the pain is present when you urinate or move your bowels.

Other symptoms include lower back pain, nausea and dizziness, a low fever, chills, bleeding between periods, bleeding after intercourse, heavier menstrual cramps and flows, frequent urination, burning during urination or an inability to empty the bladder, unusual vaginal discharge with a foul odor, constantly feeling like you have to move your bowels, a general feeling of ill health, and abdominal bloating.

It's most common for PID to localize in the fallopian tubes, causing *salpingitis*, or inflammation of the fallopian tubes. The tubes close up or scar as a result, which is why infertility is often the result (it's often reversible, however). Ectopic pregnancy can also result from PID for the same reasons. PID is divided into three categories of infection: *acute*, meaning severe; *subacute*, meaning less severe; and *chronic*, meaning that you have a fresh acute infection or that scarring has developed as a result of a previous infection.

Diagnosing PID

For many women undergoing a female workup, PID is suspected when a hysterosalpingogram reveals blocked tubes. However, prior to undergoing a hysterosalpingogram, PID can often be diagnosed during a normal pelvic exam. In this exam, your doctor should always perform what's known as a *bimanual examination*. Two fingers are inserted into your vagina, while your abdomen on the outside is felt with the other hand simultaneously. This procedure is comparable to fitting a comforter inside its cover: one hand on the inside, the other on the outside to adjust and feel for contours and abnormalities. Pain and swelling are classic signs of PID that an experienced gynecologist or primary care physician will notice immediately. Then, during the speculum examination, your doctor will look for pus that might be coming out of the cervix, a symptom of *cervicitis* (inflammation of the cervix). If your cervix is red or swollen for any reason, a Pap test might be done as well. If pus is found, a sample will be sent to a lab for analysis, and a vaginal swab will also be taken to look for bacteria. At this point, the bacteria causing your pain (and PID) might be identified right off the bat, and the appropriate antibiotic medication will be prescribed. You could conceivably be cured at this point. Your partner will also need to be treated to prevent reinfecting you or someone else.

A blood test can also indicate whether you're fighting an infection of some sort. If you are, you'll have increased levels of white blood cells and an elevated sedimentation rate. An ultrasound test is also helpful. It can show whether an abscess has developed on the fallopian tubes or ovaries.

Finally, if all else fails, a laparoscopy can be performed which will definitely confirm a PID diagnosis. A laparoscopy might also be done if the doctor suspects that you have abscesses (resulting from severe inflammation) that have burst, a potentially life-threatening situation.

Once your PID is diagnosed, successfully treating it is dependent on identifying the right bacteria responsible for the infection in the first place, so you can be treated with the *right* antibiotic! This isn't always easy. There are three procedures used to obtain a culture of the PID bacteria. The first is obtaining a cervical culture. The second procedure is called a *culdocentesis*, similar to amniocentesis, where fluid is taken out of the cul-de-sac, an area in your pelvic cavity where fluid tends to collect. A long needle is used to withdraw the fluid, which is then sent to a lab. The procedure is done under a local anesthetic in a hospital. The third procedure used is a *tubal sample*. Here, fluid and tissue samples from your fallopian tubes are obtained during a laparoscopy procedure and sent to a lab for bacterial analysis.

Antibiotic therapy: the PID treatment

The beauty of bacterial infections is that they can be destroyed with antibiotics. Antibiotic therapy is the most common treatment regimen for acute and subacute PID. Even chronic PID can be treated successfully with antibiotics. Since PID indicates such a serious infection, antibiotics are given intravenously as a therapy; they're more potent this way and work faster. When several different types of bacteria are identified in PID, this is known as a *polymicrobial* infection. If this is the case, you may either be treated with more than one kind of antibiotic simultaneously, or you might be treated with a single, broad-spectrum antibiotic, which is less effective.

By far, the best treatment approach is intravenous antibiotic therapy. To receive intravenous antibiotics, you'll need to be admitted into the hospital for about four days, the usual treatment duration. Ten to fourteen days of oral antibiotics may follow in conjunction with bed rest.

What are the recommended antibiotics?

There are many different kinds of antibiotic regimens that work. The following is a sample regimen. For PID caused by gonorrhea and/or chlamydia, 100 milligrams of doxycycline by IV (intravenous) twice a day, plus 2 grams of cefoxitin (an antibiotic used to cure gonorrhea) four times a day by IV is the standard treatment for about four days, followed by 100 milligrams of doxycyline twice a day for about fourteen days.

For PID caused by chlamydia and/or anaerobic bacteria (a certain strain of bacteria), treatment is 100 milligrams of doxycycline by IV, plus 1 gram of metronidazole twice a day for about four days, followed by the same dosages of both drugs orally twice a day for about fourteen days.

For PID caused by anaerobic bacteria or facultative gram-negative rods (other strains of bacteria), 600 milligrams of clindamycin four times a day by IV, plus gentamicin or tobramycin at a dosage of 2 milligrams for each kilogram of body weight, followed by 1.5 milligrams per kilogram three times a day for four days, then 450 milligrams of clindamycin four times a day orally for about fourteen days is the treatment.

If you're already pregnant but don't know it yet or if you have other health problems, other antibiotics will be recommended. The above antibiotics are prescription only, and these doses are generally recommended for women who aren't pregnant and who are otherwise healthy.

What are the side effects of these antibiotics?

Yeast infections are a main side effect, because antibiotics interrupt the vaginal ecosystem. However, each antibiotic carries individual side effects. *Doxycycline* can cause nausea, yeast infections, allergies, liver damage (particularly in pregnant women), and brown discoloration of teeth in children. *Cefoxitin* (fine for pregnant women but not always for women allergic to penicillin) can cause allergies and kidney damage. *Metronidazole* (Flagyl) results in nausea, headache, loss of appetite, metallic taste, dark urine, abdominal pain, constipation, inflammation of the tongue or mouth, yeast infections, and deposits in breast milk (*therefore unsafe for pregnant women*) and cannot be combined with alcohol. *Clindamycin* brings on diarrhea, colitis, allergies, and temporary abnormalities in liver function.

What should I do after my antibiotic treatment?

Get rechecked by your doctor to make sure you are indeed cured. Request another bacterial culture to make sure it's been destroyed, and make sure your partner is treated for the same bacterial infection. Otherwise, you could be reinfected. You should also abstain from intercourse until you are pronounced cured. Intercourse can spread pus in your pelvic cavity while you're healing.

Reversing infertility

Most cases of reversing infertility from PID involve reopening the fallopian tubes. This is known as a tuboplasty. The surgery is delicate and is done through laparoscopy. If your PID is severe and your tubes are badly scarred, a tuboplasty may not be possible and you'll need to seek out ART options that do not require healthy fallopian tubes but can be done if your ovaries and uterus are intact. If your tubes are intact but scarring exists elsewhere, your scarring may be removed through laparoscopy. The one problem with having a tuboplasty or other pelvic repair surgery is that fresh scarring may result. The risk of ectopic pregnancy can also increase. Because of this, a "second look" laparoscopy may be recommended, which is discussed toward the end of this section.

In some cases, PID results in abscesses that *must* be surgically removed before they burst and spread infection throughout your pelvis and upper abdominal region. This surgery would be performed as a life-preserving measure rather than a fertility repair procedure.

Surgical treatment for PID

Inflammation is one thing, abscesses are another. An abscess occurs when the inflamed tissue forms a collection of pus. The abscess can then rupture and spread the bacterial infection, causing your PID to infect other parts of your pelvic region. In many cases of PID, abscesses may not even develop. But when they do, surgical removal of the abscess may be necessary, and even surgical removal of the badly abscessed *organ* may be an option. In either case, surgery is either emergency or elective.

If your abscesses have ruptured or are about to rupture, your doctor will schedule emergency surgery. *Emergency surgery need not be major surgery* and can involve simply removing the adhesions through laparoscopy or even laparotomy, a procedure similar to laparoscopy, where a four-inch incision is made in the abdomen, resulting in very little scarring. However, it's crucial that you discuss exactly what *kind* of surgery to expect, and take every precaution to preserve your reproductive organs if possible. Both laparoscopy and laparotomy procedures are considered major surgery, and you'll be required to go under a general anesthetic. A laparotomy is also performed if a *salpingectomy*, surgical removal of the fallopian tubes, is necessary. Depending on the severity of your PID and the location of the infection, this might actually be the best option for you. As mentioned above, it's most common for PID to localize in the fallopian tubes, which can cause a host of uncomfortable and painful symptoms for you. If the tubes are badly infected and have abscessed, removing them may just be the answer.

Removing the tubes is often done to preserve your ovaries and uterus, preventing the PID from spreading further and facilitating ART techniques that do not involve the tubes.

If abscesses have formed in the uterus or on the ovaries, more drastic surgery may be necessary in the form of either a hysterectomy or *oophorectomy* (surgical removal of the ovaries), or both.

If surgery is being recommended to relieve your pain, but there are no active infections, abscesses, or inflammations present, a procedure known as a *presacral neurectomy* is an option. In this operation, the sensory messages from the organs of the pelvis, carried along the presacral nerve, are eliminated by removing the nerve itself. Hence, the pain is also eliminated. This is also major surgery and requires a very skilled surgeon, since the nerve is close to large blood vessels. It is also a more difficult operation to perform than a hysterectomy, but the surgery is about 75 percent effective in eliminating pelvic pain (a promising statistic) and does not affect fertility. One interesting side effect is that if a woman gets pregnant after the procedure, she will experience less pain during labor or childbirth! The procedure can interfere with bowel and bladder function (which usually clears up on its own). To what extent this procedure affects sexual sensations or even menstrual cramps has not yet been statistically tracked. A presacral neurectomy is considered a last resort for relieving pelvic pain associated with PID and is only a *palliative* solution, not a cure.

Prevention

The good news is that in almost all cases, *PID is a completely preventable disease*. The number-one cause of PID in North America is an untreated STD; chlamydia and gonorrhea are the two STDs that are considered "principally implicated" in causing PID. Translation: You can prevent STDs by practicing safe sex. Currently, vaccines for chlamydia and gonorrhea are being researched and may soon be introduced as standard vaccines available to the general public. In addition to choosing uninfected partners, postponing intercourse with new partners for as long as possible, and using barrier methods, notifying sex partners after discovering any STD is an important step in primary prevention. In fact, women are not considered cured of PID unless their partners are treated for the initial PID-causing STD as well. Partners of women with PID have infection rates as high as 53 percent for chlamydia and 41 percent for gonorrhea, and a large percentage of these infections are asymptomatic.

Another crucial step in preventing PID is educating yourself about the risks involved with certain contraceptives. It is an undisputed fact, for example, that women who use IUDs are three to nine times as likely to develop PID. Why? First, bacteria, normally screened by your cervix, can enter your uterus during IUD insertion. (Some experts counter that taking doxycycline prior to insertion will reduce the risk of infection.) Second, even if no bacteria enters during insertion, the IUD can irritate your uterus later on, causing a local infection.

As a rule, whenever your cervix is dilated for *any* reason (childbirth, miscarriage, D & C, abortion, IUD insertion), avoid getting *anything* into your vagina for about six weeks, or *until your cervix has closed up again*. This means no baths (showers are fine, though), no swimming, no intercourse, sex toys, douching, or tampons! See your doctor to make sure that the cervix has resumed its usual shape and appearance.

There is also evidence that hormonal contraceptives affecting your cervical mucus may increase your chances of contracting an STD during unprotected sex. Apparently, the mucus is not as effective in screening out harmful bacteria as "untampered" or natural mucus is.

Douching is also a factor in primary prevention. Douching may alter the vaginal environment and make it less protective against harmful bacteria, and douching might flush vaginal and cervical bacteria into the upper pelvic region, causing infections.

Finally, basic vaginal hygiene habits, discussed in chapter 3, in addition to good overall nutrition, can also help prevent PID. Even if you can't afford proper health insurance, you can improve your overall nutrition and hygiene regimen.

If you're not practicing safe sex, request a screening for chlamydia and gonorrhea before you have sex with a new partner.

If you notice any kind of unusual symptom that may indicate an STD, see your doctor and request a diagnosis or prompt antibiotic treatment for suspected STDs. Never self-diagnose! Treating an STD quickly will prevent it from causing PID.

Endometriosis

Another cause of painful periods is *endometriosis*, a disease affecting women in their reproductive years—which, until recently, was widely undiagnosed. The name, as you've probably guessed, comes from the word *endometrium*. The clinical definition of endometriosis is "abnormal growth of endometrial cells." Roughly 5.5 million women throughout North America have endometriosis. Endometriosis was at one time coined "husbanditis" because the pain that characterizes endometriosis was seen as women simply inventing pain to get out of their marital duties. In the past, treating women who complained of pelvic pain ranged from tranquilizers to flat-out hysterectomies. The bad news is that many women may still find that they're told their symptoms are "in their head" when, in fact, endometriosis is a physical disease causing real physical symptoms. It is now known that exposure to environmental estrogens is responsible for most endometriosis. A wide variety of man-made chemicals are breaking down into the environment that mimic estrogen, contributing to more estrogen-dependent conditions such as endometriosis and fibroids, as well as estrogen-dependent cancers. In addition, there are questions surrounding the link between dioxin exposure (dioxin residue is in most tampons—see further on) and endometriosis. See my book *Stopping Cancer at the Source* for more information.

What is it?

What happens here is that endometrial tissue is found outside the uterus, in other areas of the body. Then, this tissue develops into small growths or tumors. (Doctors may also refer to these growths as "nodules," "lesions," or "implants.") These growths are usually benign (meaning noncancerous) and are simply a normal type of tissue in an abnormal location. (There are now some cancers that are being recognized in conjunction with endometriosis, however.)

The most common location of these endometrial growths are in the pelvic region, affecting the ovaries, fallopian tubes, the ligaments supporting the uterus, the perineum, the outer surface of the uterus, and the lining of the pelvic cavity (40 to 50 percent of the growths are in the ovaries and fallopian tubes). Sometimes the growths are found in abdominal surgery scars, on the intestines or in the rectum, and on the bladder, vagina, cervix, and vulva. Rarer locations include the lung, arm, thigh, and other places outside the abdomen.

The problem

Since these growths are in fact pieces of uterine lining, they *behave* like uterine lining, responding to the hormonal cycle and trying to *shed* every month. These growths, in essence, are blind—they can't see where they are and they think they're in the uterus. This is a huge problem during menstruation; when the growths start "shedding," there's no vagina around for them to pass through, so they have nowhere to go. The result is internal bleeding, degeneration of the blood and tissue shed from the growths, inflammation of the surrounding areas, and the formation of scar tissue. Depending on where these growths are located, they can rupture and spread to new areas, cause intestinal bleeding or obstruction (if they're in or near the intestines), or interfere with bladder function (if they're on or near the bladder).

Signs of endometriosis

The most common signs of endometriosis are pain before and during periods (much worse than "normal" menstrual cramps), pain during or after intercourse, infertility, and heavy or irregular bleeding. Other symptoms may include fatigue, painful bowel movements with periods, lower back pain with periods, diarrhea and/or constipation with periods, and intestinal upset with periods. If the bladder is involved, there may be painful urination and blood in the urine with periods. Irregular menstrual cycles and heavier flows are also associated with endometriosis, but, usually, women with severe endometriosis continue to have regular, but painful periods.

There are some women with endometriosis that have no signs of endometriosis at all, but infertility affects about 30 to 40 percent of endometriosis sufferers, and as the disease progresses, the infertility is often inevitable.

It's important to note that the amount of pain is not necessarily related to the extent or size of the growths. Tiny growths (called "petechial") have been found to be more active in producing prostoglandins, which may explain the significant symptoms that seem to occur with smaller growths. (Prostoglandins, mentioned earlier, are hormonelike chemical substances that are manufactured by the endometrium. They are thought to be the culprit behind many of the classic signs of endometriosis.)

Since endometriosis usually includes so may seemingly unrelated symptoms, it's no wonder that it's so often missed or simply misdiagnosed. Here is a list of some of the most common signs and symptoms of endometriosis, which would appear during or before your period:

- pelvic pain and/or painful intercourse (in one survey, 78 percent of women with endometriosis reported pain severe enough to wake them up at night or else interfere with their falling asleep)
- infertility (this is often the *only* symptom women experience—even with Stage IV)
- abnormal cycles or periods
- nausea and/or vomiting
- exhaustion
- bladder problems
- frequent infections
- dizziness
- painful defecation
- lower backaches
- irritable bowels (loose, watery, and often bloody diarrhea; many women diagnosed with Irritable Bowel Disease (IBS) really have endometriosis)
- other stomach problems
- low-grade fever

A questionnaire distributed by the Endometriosis Association revealed that 100 percent of respondents experienced pain one to two days prior to their periods. In addition, 71 percent reported pain mid-cycle; 40 percent reported pain other times; 20 percent reported pain throughout their cycle; while 7 percent reported intermittent pain with no particular pattern. The pain in this questionnaire was mostly abdominal pain.

The stages of endometriosis

Endometriosis can really vary in terms of severity. So like other diseases, it's categorized into four stages—the higher the number, the more severe your endometriosis is. Stage I is when your endometriosis is minimal, where your endometriosis is still very thin and "filmy," hence easier to treat. Stage II means you have mild endometriosis, where the endometriosis is still on the thin side, but is situated more deeply into your surrounding tissues. Stage III is when you have moderate endometriosis; here, your endometriosis is denser mixed with some Stage I or Stage II endometriosis. Stage IV means that you have severe endometriosis. In this case, the endometriosis is dense and deep—a bad combination.

A laparoscopy is the only surefire way to diagnose endometriosis, but if you suspect you have it, you should request a pelvic exam be performed *during* your period—when endometriosis is in full "flare." This may help your doctor to find certain clues that will send you into the right diagnostic direction, since so many women are misdiagnosed. For example, transvaginal ultrasound versus abdominal ultrasound is very useful in finding many of the physical clues that endometriosis leaves behind, such as cysts or masses. You may want to even request a transvaginal ultrasound even when your doctor doesn't order it.

Treatment

Natural progesterone therapy has been found to help some women, but treatment for endometriosis has varied over the years, and there is still no absolute cure. If you don't have any symptoms and you've decided on adoption, surrogacy, or childfree living, then no treatment is necessary, just regular checkups. If you have only mild symptoms and infertility is *not* a factor, simple painkillers like aspirin or Tylenol may be all that is necessary.

To reverse infertility, *operative laparoscopy* is the best approach. Through a laparoscope, surgery is done with either a laser, cautery, or small surgical instruments. Endometrial implants can be burned off with the laser. However, recurrence is common with this procedure, so you may need to have it repeated if you want future pregnancies. About 40 percent of women who have an operative laparoscopy procedure will go on to conceive. Even after this more conservative surgery, however, between 20 and 50 percent of endometriosis patients will need more radical surgery done.

There is a nonsurgical treatment for endometriosis appropriate for women who've decided on childfree living, adoption, or surrogacy. It involves creating a pseudopregnancy with hormonal therapy used to stop ovulation. This *does* work for as long as you're taking the synthetic hormones, and sometimes the therapy can force endometriosis into remission for months or years. Often, though, when you go off the hormones, the disease comes right back. The hormonal recipe here can include estrogen and progesterone, progesterone alone, *danazol* (a testosterone derivative), and GnRH (gonadotropin-releasing hormone), which creates a pseudomenopause.

For severe symptoms, depending on where the growths are located and their size, your doctor may recommend hysterectomy and removal of the ovaries. This may be an unnecessary procedure and warrants a few separate opinions from other doctors before you agree. Although hysterectomy is considered a "definitive" cure, research has shown that women who undergo a hysterectomy for endometriosis sometimes experience a recurrence of the disease.

Pregnancy as a cure

Pregnancy, believe it or not, does cause endometriosis to go into a temporary remission because you don't ovulate when you're pregnant. Furthermore, permanent remission of endometriosis has been known to happen after childbirth; the growths in this case shrink, and the pain associated with the disease stops. The problem is that the longer you have endometriosis, the greater the chance you have of becoming infertile. Furthermore, even under the best of circumstances, women with endometriosis have a higher risk of ectopic pregnancy and miscarriage. One study has found that full-term pregnancies and labor are more difficult when the mother has endometriosis.

Menopause as a cure?

Menopause does generally cure endometriosis (which is why hysterectomy is performed). But a severe case of endometriosis can be reactivated if you begin hormone replacement therapy or continue producing hormones after menopause, which is common. In fact, the oldest woman in whom endometriosis was diagnosed was seventy-eight years old. Some doctors suggest no replacement hormone be given for about three to nine months after menopause or a hysterectomy procedure.

Fibroids

The medical term for fibroids is *leiomyoma uteri*. Roughly one in four North American women will develop a fibroid at some point in her thirties or forties. Fibroids are benign muscle tumors within the uterus. These are harmless growths that can cause a range of symptoms that include pelvic pain and heavy bleeding during periods. But only about 2 to 3 percent of all female factor infertility is actually caused by fibroids. Many women with symptomless fibroids experience uncomplicated pregnancies and childbirth. If a fibroid is large enough that it is truly interfering with the implantation of an embryo or the successful duration of a pregnancy, the fibroid can be surgically removed, leaving your reproductive organs intact. Surgical removal of fibroids is called a *myomectomy*. You may need to hunt around for a surgeon that performs this procedure. The best bet is to contact Hysterectomy Educational Resources and Services (HERS) at (888) 750-HERS (4377) for the name of a surgeon in your area. The HERS Web site is http://ccon.com/hers.

If your fibroids are the culprit behind your infertility and you've decided to adopt or live childfree, you may not need to treat them. Symptomless fibroids can coexist peacefully in your uterus, and since they depend on estrogen to grow, they *will* shrink after menopause (as long as you do not take estrogen therapy). Symptomatic fibroids, however, will probably affect your quality of life and will therefore warrant treatment. You could look into hormone therapy, which involves drugs that block estrogen. For severe fibroids, a hysterectomy will be recommended, but often a myomectomy can be done instead, which will preserve your reproductive organs.

Tubal Ligation Reversal

The same surgery that corrects a blocked tube from PID or endometriosis can be used to reverse a tubal ligation in about 60 percent of the cases. (This procedure was demonstrated on The Learning Channel's "The Operation.") As long as the *fimbria* within the tube are intact, and there is enough of the tube left for cutting and stitching, the procedure can be a success. The inner canal is sutured, and the outer layer of the tube is reattached. You'll need to have a hysterosalpingogram done about six weeks following the procedure to make sure that the blocked tube is now corrected. Microsurgical techniques in tubal ligation reversals are improving by leaps and bounds. Therefore, the success rates are improving dramatically, too.

Other Structural Abnormalities

Because of the complexity of female anatomy, there's a long list of congenital anatomical defects that can affect a woman's capacity to conceive or sustain a pregnancy. These defects include a double uterus, a double vagina, a separated uterus, an abnormally shaped cervix, uterus, or vagina, and closed or even fused fallopian tubes. All these defects may not be detected until a fertility workup reveals them through ultrasound or a manual pelvic exam.

Every anatomical oddity is unique and carries options that include reconstructive or repair surgery, or certain kinds of ART procedures that can facilitate biological offspring. You'll need to weigh your options and have a frank discussion with your gynecologist.

Follow-Up Care After Surgery

If you've undergone repair surgery for PID, endometriosis, or other structural abnormalities, you will most likely need to have a second hysterosalpingogram done, and possibly a second-look laparoscopy procedure that can check to make sure you're healing properly and that no fresh scarring has occurred.

Most women can expect to feel soreness, have gas, and experience bloating after surgery, but these go away in a few days. You can resume having intercourse once you feel less tender. Pregnancies have been known to occur within the first two cycles after surgery, but many women may continue to experience delays.

Male Factor Infertility

As discussed in chapter 5, close to half of all explained male factor infertility is caused by a structural problem that is *fixable through surgery*. These problems include a varicocele, a varicose vein within the scrotum (contributing to roughly 40 percent of all male infertility); a blocked tube (accounting for about 3 percent of all male infertility); and other anatomical defects, such as retrograde ejaculation (about 5 percent). Infections are occasionally the reason behind poor motility or morphology when a varicocele is ruled out and are treatable through antibiotics.

When male factor infertility is caused by immunological factors (accounting for about 5 percent of all male infertility) or hormonal factors (about 2 percent), treatments are far more tentative and experimental. In these cases, improving sperm quality through various ART techniques may be the only treatment options available. Techniques for improving sperm quality and artificial reproductive technology for males are discussed in chapter 9.

Varicoceles

A varicocele occurs when a varicose vein develops in the spermatic veins leading from the testicles. This happens when the valves in the spermatic veins are damaged and blood ascending to the heart flows backward instead of engorging the vein. Varicoceles are more common in the left testicle because the veins connect to the renal vein at a right angle, placing more pressure on it.

Infertility is usually the result of a varicocele because the collection of blood surrounding the total area raises the temperature of the testes, which prevents them from producing sperm. Low sperm count, poor motility, and poor morphology are the results. Diagnosing varicoceles is discussed in chapter 6.

Varicocele repair surgery

This is by far the most common surgical procedure performed to reverse male factor infertility. There are a few different methods available, however, to repair a varicocele.

The least invasive procedure is really an alternative to traditional surgery. It involves the use of an *occlusive*, a device that blocks or plugs up the troublesome vein. In this procedure, an intravenous-like needle is placed through the skin into a large vein in the *neck*, which leads directly to the varicocele, and a springlike coil is dropped down into the vein, which essentially repairs the varicocele. Sometimes a small balloon is used instead of a spring coil, and occasionally a solution is used instead of a coil or balloon, which purposely irritates the varicocele, causing it to scar shut. The procedure is done under a local anesthetic, and you can usually go home a few hours after it's done. You may need to be on a mild painkiller for a few days, and you may need to refrain from sexual activity for two to three days following surgery.

Varicoceles can also be repaired under a general anesthetic. Here, you'll go into the hospital as either a day patient or an overnight patient, and you'll have the varicocele repaired through an incision in your groin (called a *transinguinal* or *subinguinal* approach). After surgery, you may be uncomfortable for a few days, and you may need to refrain from sexual activity until your incision has healed. Roughly ten days after your surgery, your doctor will want to check your incision to make sure it's healing properly. Then, after about three months, your doctor will request a semen analysis and may want you to deliver a monthly sample until about the twelfth month after your surgery.

About 67 percent of all men who undergo surgery to repair their varicoceles will see a dramatic improvement in the quality of their semen. Pregnancy rates following surgery are approximately 40 percent per year, and conception usually occurs within six to nine months after the surgery. In short, pregnancy rates triple after a varicocele repair.

Infections and Inflammations

Poor motility or morphology is occasionally caused by infections when a varicocele has been ruled out. When men get infected with STDs such as chlamydia or gonorrhea, if left untreated the infection can either spread deeper inside the reproductive tract or can cause inflammations of the prostate gland (prostatitis), epididydmis (epididymitis), or the testes (orchitis). Other viruses and bacteria that are *not* sexually transmitted can cause inflammation, too.

Prostatitis

Prostatitis literally means "inflammation of the prostate gland due to infection." Most urologists see at least one case of either acute or chronic prostatitis a day. Acute prostatitis means you have a fresh infection and the symptoms come on suddenly. In chronic prostatitis, the condition has existed over a long period of time. Classic symptoms include painful urination, painful ejaculation, and pus and/or blood in the urine. One of the most common causes of prostatitis is coliform bacteria. (*Escherichia coli*, or *E. coli*, is a strain of coliform bacteria.) Coliform bacteria can travel from your colon (where there are always large amounts) into your bladder, urethra, or prostate. When you're constipated, you're especially vulnerable to higher levels of the bacteria, which will hitchhike to your reproductive organs through your lymphatic system or bloodstream.

Another major cause of prostatitis is STDs. Chlamydia, gonorrhea, Trichomonas vaginalis ("trich"), and even vaginal yeast infections (which are technically not STDs but can be passed on to the male) can cause this infection. Bacteria such as staphylococcus (causing common colds and a garden variety of ailments) accounts for roughly 5 percent of all prostatitis.

Prostatitis will affect your fertility for as long as you're infected, causing poor motility and poor morphology. Treatment is simple: antibiotics. Your doctor will first need to culture your infection by either taking some prostatic fluid (done during a rectal exam, where the doctor puts pressure on the gland and causes the fluid to come out of your urethra), or in some cases, a culture can be obtained from a urine and a semen sample. Once the right bacterium is identified, you'll be placed on antibiotics for about three to six weeks and will then need to repeat your semen analysis and urinalysis to make sure the infection has cleared. Your partner must also be treated to make sure that you aren't passing bacteria back and forth.

Epididymitis

When the epididymis becomes inflamed, it causes swelling, pain, burning urination, and even discharge from the urethra. Blockage of the ejaculatory ducts can result, causing either low or no sperm counts. The most common causes of epididymitis are chlamydia and gonorrhea. If caught early enough, antibiotics will cure the infection without leaving any damage. However, if the infection is left untreated, it could cause permanent scarring and blockages in the epididymal ducts.

Repairing the blockage is only possible through microsurgical resection of the epididymis under a general anesthetic. This procedure is called an *epididymovasostomy*. The blocked section is cut out and the ejaculatory duct is reconnected. The best way to explain the surgery is to compare it to reattaching a long rope or cord that was once severed. This is an open surgical procedure done on the scrotum. (See Figure 7.1 for a diagram of what the procedure involves.) Repairing blockages in the ejaculatory ducts can be done with a transurethral procedure, however. There is some risk: If the valve leading to the bladder is harmed in any way, surgery could result in retrograde ejaculation or even incontinence.

Figure 7.1 Diagram of the Epididymovasostomy Procedure

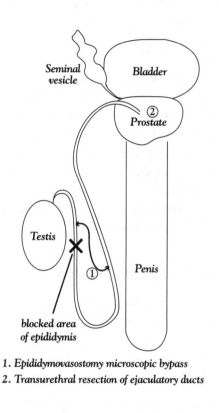

1. Epididymovasostomy microscopic bypass
2. Transurethral resection of ejaculatory ducts

Source: Keith Jarvi, M.D., F.R.C.S.(C), 1994.

Rarely, infection can cause blockages in the vas deferens. A *vasovasostomy*, similar to an epididymovasostomy, can repair the obstruction. But usually obstruction of the vas deferens is *deliberate*, caused by a vasectomy. To reverse a vasectomy, a vasovasostomy is considered highly effective, with pregnancy rates as high as 70 percent after the reversal. The best candidates for vasectomy reversals are those who had their vasectomy within the last ten years. (The Learning Channel's "The Operation" showed this procedure.)

Orchitis

Orchitis, inflammation of the testes, can be dangerous to an adult male's fertility because it can cause permanent, irreversible sterility. When orchitis occurs prior to puberty, a man's testicular function should not be affected.

Viral infections are usually the cause of orchitis, the most notorious of which are mumps. Roughly 25 percent of men with mumps get pain and swelling in one or both testicles. In this case, not only is the swelling of the testes dangerous, but the mumps virus also directly attacks the testes and can destroy their ability to make sperm. The amount of swelling, however, does not have bearing on the amount of sperm damage that occurs. In fact, some men can fully recover from mumps and go on to father children, while others remain infertile. Testicular failure is easily diagnosed through a blood test, which will show high levels of FSH and LH, signs that the testes are failing.

Mumps are certainly not the only disease that causes orchitis. Syphilis, tuberculosis, pancreatitis, hepatitis, mononucleosis, and smallpox can cause orchitis as well. However, you can have any of the above diseases, including mumps, and not suffer from orchitis.

Symptoms of orchitis include a discharge of pus or mucus from the penis, dull twinges of pain in the testicles, and lower back pain. Early diagnosis and prompt treatment of orchitis prevent further testicular damage.

Treating Common Anatomical Problems

There are some common anatomical problems that are either congenital or can result from other diseases or injury. If treatment isn't available, solutions to infertility are!

Retrograde ejaculation

As discussed in chapter 5, this is a condition where the bladder neck doesn't completely close during ejaculation, causing the semen to be propelled backward into the bladder. Men with diabetes or a history of testicular cancer can be prone to this.

There is no treatment for retrograde ejaculation, but there is a solution to infertility. Men with this problem can still father a child by having their sperm retrieved from their urine and then inseminated into their partner. The female cycle is monitored closely so that insemination can take place during ovulation. Roughly two days before "retrieval day," a man must refrain from ejaculation. The day of retrieval, he must take two sodium bicarbonate tablets with water every two hours, eight hours prior to retrieval. The sodium creates a more alkaline environment in the bladder, which allows the sperm to survive longer.

Thirty minutes before retrieval, the man empties his bladder completely. Then he ejaculates either through masturbation or regular intercourse (intercourse may not be possible if he lives far from his doctor's office). He then delivers a urine sample to his doctor's office or lab, where the sperm is washed (see chapter 5), separated from the urine (by being put into a solution), and inseminated into his partner. The average couple goes through about six of these insemination procedures and, amazingly, six out of seven will conceive.

Undescended testicles

A small percentage of all male babies are born with one or both testes still inside the abdomen. This is known as *cryptorchidism.* Out of all the babies born with cryptorchidism, the majority of the testes descend by themselves within about four months. Less than 1 percent of babies whose cryptorchidism persists may be treated with a surgical procedure known as *orchipexy.* The surgery usually is not performed until six months after birth to allow for a natural reversal of the condition. Here, the testes are manually delivered out of the abdomen during surgery (usually a laparotomy procedure) so that they will lie normally in the scrotum.

The reason why this condition can lead to sterility is because sperm cannot be produced within the warm temperatures of the abdomen. If this condition remains untreated, a male is at high risk of developing testicular cancer. Sometimes, even after treatment, a male still may have very low sperm counts. In this case, intrauterine insemination (IUI) may be an option. Up to 10 percent of men with no sperm have missing ducts. An uncommon clinical condition, affecting the lungs and pancreas, is a disease called cystic fibrosis (CF). The gene for CF is the most common cause of missing ducts. If you have missing ducts, it's crucial that you be tested for CF.

Blocked or missing ducts

Men born to women who took DES (see chapter 2) can be prone to a variety of congenital defects that include a missing or defective vas deferens or missing seminal vesicles. In these cases, the semen volume is low and may be accompanied by low or no sperm counts.

To date, there is no way to replace missing ducts, but a procedure known as *sperm aspiration* (for men who have blocked or absent vas deferens or who have had vasectomies) can allow a man to father a child. Here, immature sperm are surgically removed from the epididydmis (through an incision in the scrotum) and cultured in a laboratory, then used in an IVF procedure with the female partner's egg. (See chapter 9 for details on IVF.) Other than this option, men with these problems must seek out other parenting options, such as adoption or donor insemination, or choose a childfree lifestyle.

Hypospadias and epispadias

A common congenital problem involves an abnormal urethral opening. Here the opening of the urethra on the penis is somewhere other than at the tip: the underside (known as *hypospadias*) or upperside (known as *epispadias*). Sperm production is fine, but when ejaculated it won't be deposited directly into the cervix. This is easily corrected through plastic surgery, where a new opening at the the tip of the penis is constructed and the old opening is closed up.

Torsion

One of the reasons why the testes are ultrasensitive to pain is to protect them from serious injury. Injury to even one testicle can cause torsion, when the testicle twists inside the scrotum. Pelvic surgeries such as hernia repair or bladder surgery can also cause testicular torsion. Torsion can be surgically repaired if it's caught early enough, but if left untreated, the testicle (or both testes) shrinks and withers away (atrophy) to the point where it is the size of a pea. When atrophy occurs, there is no treatment and men with this problem will need to seek other parenting options.

Treating Immunological Infertility

As discussed in chapter 5, some male factor infertility is caused by antisperm antibodies; the sperm is coated with antibodies that harm the sperm, causing poor motility or failure for the sperm to recognize or penetrate the egg.

Women can also form antibodies to a partner's sperm, causing the sperm to clump together around the cervix or to have poor motility. Generally, though, infection or inflammation is the main trigger of male-produced antisperm antibodies, while a vasectomy procedure is also cited as a major cause. Sperm ingestion can lead to immunological infertility as well, which is discussed in chapter 3.

If there are only a few antisperm antibodies in your system, this shouldn't create a barrier to fertility. However, if the antibodies are present in large numbers, you've got a big problem.

Treatment

To date, treatment for immunological infertility is not very successful. Here, corticosteroids (anti-inflammatory drugs such as methylprednisolone, prednisone, or dexamethasone) are used to suppress the immune system. The theory is that when the immune system is suppressed, the antisperm antibodies will be less lethal on the sperm.

Unfortunately, there are some very unpleasant side effects to these drugs, which include rashes, irritability, depression, indigestion, weight gain, and fluid retention. Pregnancy rates on these drugs hover around 30 percent; however, the best way to reverse infertility is to combine the drug therapy with either IUI or IVF, both discussed in chapter 9.

Premature Testicular Failure

Men who receive chemotherapy or radiation therapy to the testes, or who are exposed to known environmental toxins in the workplace, are at high risk of suffering from testicular failure. This is when your testicles shut down and stop producing sperm. Common cancers in younger men include Hodgkin's disease, non-Hodgkin's lymphoma, leukemia, testicular cancer, and melanoma. Prior to your treatment, you should bank significant quantities of your own sperm (waiting two to four days between samples) if you do not yet have a family. Your sperm can be frozen indefinitely until you're ready for it to be inseminated into your partner.

A Word About Sexual Dysfunction

A significant portion of male factor infertility is caused by sexual disorders rather than physiological problems. Therapy is available for a variety of problems that include premature ejaculation, anejaculation, impotence, and poor libido. (See chapter 5.) Ask your urologist or family doctor to recommend you to a sex therapist or counselor if a physical cause for your dysfunction is ruled out. In many cases, sexual dysfunction is rooted in emotional trauma that can be treated through psychiatric therapy. Inappropriate emotional or physical stimulation can also result in sexual dysfunction.

Because of the way humans are built, while many women are also sexually dysfunctional (not able to climax and so on), female sexual performance does not correspond to reduced fertility the same way that male sexual performance does.

Secondary Infertility

It is possible to be infertile after having one or more biological children. This is known as *secondary infertility*. *Primary infertility* refers to couples who have never conceived. Secondary infertility carries unique frustrations because couples can't help saying, "We've reproduced once, why can't we reproduce again?" Couples experiencing secondary infertility will go through the same workups discussed in chapters 5 and 6. There are some common causes of secondary infertility that you may want to rule out first, though, before proceeding with a battery of tests.

- *Varicoceles*. As men get into their late thirties and early forties, varicoceles can develop. Get this checked out early.
- *Prostate health*. In addition to prostatitis, overall prostate health tends to deteriorate as men age. Make sure you don't neglect this aspect of your yearly physical exam.
- *Endometriosis*. This is cited as the most frequent cause of secondary infertility in women.
- *PID*. This can worsen with time if the original bacteria causing PID was never treated.

Other Factors to Consider

Age

Even five years can make a big difference in a woman's fertility cycle and a man's sperm count. Many couples have one child and then space out the next one to coincide with their first child's school schedule. For busy career couples, this spacing helps make two children more manageable.

If you've started your family later in life (after thirty-five) and are considering more children, you might look into banking your sperm and freezing previously retrieved eggs to be used in an ART procedure just in case you run into problems.

Scarring after childbirth

If you had a difficult first labor and childbirth experience and suffered from a bacterial infection after childbirth, scarring may be the culprit behind your infertility now. A laparoscopy would confirm whether this is the problem.

Stress

Stress increases enormously after one child, which can affect ovulation and sperm production. See chapter 3 for more information.

Strenuous exercise and weight loss

Many women will overdo it in the gym in a mad scramble to reclaim their slim figures after childbirth. This can affect ovulation for future pregnancies.

Whether your fertility problem is female factor or male factor in origin, if treatment of your health problem hasn't resulted in pregnancy (including the use of fertility drugs to *induce* ovulation), fertility drugs may be used to enhance ovulation in cases where ART procedures are being used. The next chapter is all about the uses and the risks of these drugs.

If fertility drugs are not an option, you may need to consider other options, such as surrogacy, adoption, or childfree living. Surrogacy is discussed in chapter 9; options to biological parenting are discussed in chapter 12.

The 24-Month Pregnancy

In an ideal infertility workup and treatment program, it takes up to 24 months for a pregnancy to be achieved. Here is a rough timeline to help you plan.

Diagnostic Testing: 3 to 6 months

This period involves everything discussed in chapters 4, 5, and 6:

- Blood tests
- Semen analysis
- Charting
- Postcoital test
- Invasive tests for checking female structure

Evaluation and Initial Treatment: 6 months

This involves finding and treating problems discussed in chapter 7.

Aggressive Therapy: 6 cycles (or roughly 6 months)

This involves using a combination of fertility drugs and insemination procedures discussed in chapter 8.

In Vitro Fertilization (IVF) Procedures: 3 to 6 cycles

This stage involves graduating to some of the IVF-like procedures discussed in chapter 9, and/or incorporating intracytoplasmic sperm injection (ICSI) procedures, where the sperm is injected directly into the egg.

Source: Adapted from *Infertility Helper* September 1995.

8

All About Fertility Drugs

As WE'VE SEEN in chapters 5, 6, and 7, fertility drugs may be prescribed to many women and to *some* men for a variety of hormonal problems and unexplained infertility. Even women who ovulate regularly may start using fertility drugs if they're undergoing any sort of assisted reproductive technology (ART) procedure, such as in vitro fertilization (IVF) or gamete intrafallopian transfer (GIFT).

In the majority of cases, fertility drugs are used to induce ovulation in anovulatory women (see chapters 4 and 6) or to increase follicle stimulation in women undergoing ART (see chapter 9) procedures. Only a tiny segment of fertility drug users are male (see chapter 5). Therefore, this chapter is directed primarily at the female reader; the last section of the chapter discusses the use of fertility drugs in men.

Some women's organizations would argue that fertility drugs would not be as widely used if the majority of patients using the drugs were male. They compare the widespread DES (diethylstilbestrol) and other disastrous women's health products such as the Dalkon Shield or thalidomide (not available in the United States). All of these products were introduced onto the market without adequately researching the long-term consequences. A large portion of this chapter focuses on the known risks of fertility drugs and explores some of the unknown potential risks.

Fertility Drugspeak

It's a little difficult to make an informed decision about fertility drugs unless you understand what you're really taking. Unfortunately, many specialists will give you a prescription with only a brief explanation of side effects and when to take your medication. Worse, even if your doctor explains what the drugs are, distinguishing between the generic drug names and brand names of all these products can be pretty overwhelming. Here's an explanation in plain English, using the generic names of these drugs only. See Table 8.1 for a list of brand names for each drug.

For most women, ovulation induction will involve the drug *clomiphene citrate*. This is also referred to as an antiestrogen. High levels of estrogen prevent ovulation from occurring, and when the estrogen is blocked out *completely*, your ovaries respond by making more follicles than they normally would, in an effort to make the estrogen it thinks is missing. (Follicles secrete estrogen, as explained in chapter 4.) Clomiphene is discussed in detail further below.

Some women will be offered more potent drugs, known as *gonadotropins*, which are administered by injection. Gonadotropins are sex hormones secreted by the pituitary gland; follicle stimulating hormone (FSH), luteinizing hormone (LH), or human chorionic gonadotropin (hCG) are all gonadotropins.

Until recently, the only way to extract FSH and LH was from one source: the urine of menopausal women. (In menopause, FSH and LH levels are naturally high to compensate for retiring ovaries.) That urine was then refined and turned into human menopausal gonadotropin (hMG). There were initially two kinds of hMG on the market, and both contained FSH and LH; one brand contained half of each hormone, known as menotropin; another kind contained mostly FSH, which was usually prescribed to women with polycystic ovarian syndrome (see previous chapter), known as urofollitropin.

But there is now a new generation of gonadotropin drugs, which are not made from anyone's urine, but instead, through recombinant DNA technology. This technology is able to isolate from a human cell the genetic code that controls the production of FSH. So in a laboratory, these cells can turn into a whole FSH factory. The result is a much purer form of FSH (about 99 percent pure) with no urine or LH to "process out."

Most women will be prescribed one of the newer gonadotropin drugs produced through recombinant DNA technology, although the older drugs made from menopausal urine are still around in a "new and improved" version, known as "purified" or "highly purified." What you're prescribed depends entirely on your doctor, but you should definitely ask whether your drug is a first generation drug. If the answer is yes, you might want to ask why your doctor has chosen to prescribe the older drug versus a newer, purer drug.

When you're on hMG (whether it's menotropin or urofollitropin), you'll also receive injections of hCG. Human chorionic gonadotropin (hCG) is a hormone secreted by the developing placenta during a pregnancy (hCG secretion is what a home pregnancy test looks for in your urine). When you're not yet pregnant, however, hCG will cause your developing follicle (at this point known as the corpus luteum) to secrete enough estrogen and progesterone to maintain a pregnancy.

Table 8.1 Getting to Know Your Fertility Drugs

Brand Name	Generic Drug	Form
Clomid	(clomiphene citrate)	tablet
Serophene	(clomiphene citrate)	tablet
Follistim*	(recombinant FSH)	subcutaneous injection
Gonal-F*	(recombinant FSH)	subcutaneous injection
Puregon*†	(recombinant FSH)	subcutaneous injection
Fertinex	(purified urofollitropin)	subcutaneous injection
Fertinorm†	(purified urofollitropin)	subcutaneous injection
Profasi HP	(pure hCG)	subcutaneous injection
Pregnyl	(hCG)	intramuscular injection
A.P.L.	(hCG)	intramuscular injection
Novarel	(hCG)	intramuscular injection
Pergonal**	(hMG-menotropins)	intramuscular injection
Humegon**	(hMG-menotropins)	intramuscular injection
Repronex**	(hMG-menotropins)	intramuscular injection
Metrodin**	(hMG-urofollitropin)	intramuscular injection
Lupron	(Leuprolide Acetate-GnRH analogue)	subcutaneous injection
Lupron Depot	(Leuprolide Acetate-GnRH analogue)	intramuscular injection
Synarel	(Nafarelin Acetate-GnRH analogue)	nasal spray
Zoladex	(Gosereline Acetate-GnRH analogue)	subcutaneous injection
Parlodel	(bromocriptine)	capsules or tablets
Dostinet	(cabergoline)	oral tablets
Factrel	(GnRH)	subcutaneous injection
Lutrepulse	(GnRH)	subcutaneous injection
Crinore	(Progesterone)	oral tablets or intramuscular injection
Prometrium	(Progesterone)	capsule

* Produced through recombinant DNA technology.
**First generation of gonadotropins made from urine.
† Brand names outside the U.S. (Canada, U.K., and so on).

Note: For information about any of these fertility drugs, contact the FDA at 1-888-INFO-FDA (1-888-463-6332), or visit the FDA Web site at http://www.fda.gov/.

Your doctor may want to put you on a *gonadotropin-releasing hormone (GnRH)* analogue prior to starting you on clomiphene or hMG. These drugs block your *entire* natural cycle by blocking out GnRH, secreted by your hypothalamus gland to kick-start the pituitary gland into secreting FSH and LH. By giving the analogue, the drug removes the control of GnRH from your hypothalamus and takes over that function instead. GnRH analogues are rather complicated drugs. Some doctors feel that controlling the cycle completely through artificial means is more effective than mixing artificial hormones with natural hormones.

Finally, there are some very specific hormonal disorders that can interfere with a normal ovulation cycle, such as hyperprolactinemia (see chapter 6) or a GnRH deficiency. In these cases, you'll be offered an exact replacement of the hormone you're not producing. These drugs are discussed further in the section, "Drugs to Correct Hormonal Imbalances."

Who Needs Treatment?

People who are offered fertility drugs fall into the following groups:

- Women who are anovulatory. This includes all the hormonal disorders discussed in chapter 6, as well as women with polycystic ovarian syndrome (PCO) (see chapters 6 and 7).
- Women who have complete ovulatory failure, a condition known as *hypogonadotrophic hypogonadism.* Surgery or radiotherapy for a pituitary tumor can cause this condition.
- Women who are in an ART program such as IVF or GIFT. In this case, while you may be ovulating regularly, in order for IVF or GIFT to succeed, you need to have *several* mature follicles in each cycle. This gives your doctor better "pickings" for the petri dishes. Your ovaries will be stimulated with fertility drugs for these procedures.
- Couples with unexplained infertility.
- Men who have certain hormonal disorders that respond to fertility drugs. See the section on "Drugs Used in Male Fertility Therapy" later in this chapter.

Operation Ovulation Induction

If you're not ovulating regularly, at least one or more of the drugs discussed in this section will be offered to you in the hope that your ovulation will be restored long enough for you to conceive. None of the medications described in this chapter is intended to be used as a long-term therapy, however. The dosages, side effects, and risks of each of these drugs are thoroughly covered in the following section. I also discuss the diagnostic tests you'll need prior to beginning treatment, as well as the tests you'll need while you're on the drugs. Finally, I identify those women who should not be taking these medications. If you're taking the drugs as part of an ART program, please refer to the section "Operation Egg Retrieval" later in this chapter. In general, your treatment will differ only at ovulation, where your eggs will be retrieved and then either put back inside you or inside a host uterus (done in the case of oocyte donation, discussed in chapter 9.)

Clomiphene Citrate

Clomiphene citrate is the most common drug used for ovulation induction (see Table 8.1 on page 173). Clomiphene comes in the form of an oral tablet and is taken for five days starting from the fifth day of your period (whether it's natural or induced). When you stop the drug, you'll get your LH surge, which stimulates ovulation and provides you with a high-quality luteal phase. Using a twenty-eight-day cycle as an example, you'd start on 50 milligrams of clomiphene on day five of your cycle. You'd take it until about day nine and then go off it. This will induce ovulation about six to ten days later (or roughly day fifteen to nineteen of the cycle). You'll need to keep track of your basal body temperature throughout this process and will probably have your serum progesterone levels taken around this time to monitor whether the drug is working. If you don't menstruate at all, you'll first have your period induced by a progesterone supplement before starting clomiphene. If 50 milligrams doesn't do the trick, the dosage will be gradually increased to roughly 100 milligrams. (Women have been known to go as high as 250 milligrams per day for five or more days per cycle, but this really isn't advised.)

It's absolutely crucial that your doctor puts you on 50 milligrams, the *lowest possible dosage*. If ovulation isn't taking place, your dosage will increase to 100 milligrams. If ovulation still isn't occurring, you should be taken off clomiphene. Going to a higher dosage is not recommended because there may be adverse reactions. Instead, you may be offered hMG, a more powerful drug. More than half the clomiphene pregnancies occur during the first three cycles and more than three-quarters occur at the 50-milligram dose. At this dose, there's a 20 percent chance of conception each cycle. Rarely will pregnancy occur when more than 100 milligrams per day (two tablets) are necessary. If you have not conceived after three cycles, intrauterine insemination will be recommended to improve your chances of conceiving. If you have not conceived after four to six cycles, more aggressive therapy may be offered.

It can take a few months to establish the right dose, but once you're on an effective dose (be it 50, 75, or 100 milligrams), you'll be on clomiphene for roughly six months. If the drug doesn't work in six months, it most likely *won't*. You see, the likelihood of conception *diminishes* with each clomiphene cycle you do. The six-month cycle takes into account the fact that you need a couple of cycles to establish the right dosage. Once that happens, three cycles of clomiphene is about the maximum most doctors will allow.

Clomiphene can also cause your cervical mucus to thicken, which can create another fertility barrier. As discussed in chapters 4, 5, and 6, high-quality cervical mucus is necessary for the sperm to reach the egg. To make sure the sperm are surviving in the cervix, a postcoital test (see chapter 6) should be done after you begin clomiphene.

It's important that the cause for your anovulatory disorder is found first and that you've completed both a male and female workup (see chapters 5 and 6). In other words, you must not take the drug unless you and your partner have been seen by a fertility specialist. Helping yourself to your sister's supply of clomiphene, for example, is a *really* bad idea!

Clomiphene works well for women who ovulate *occasionally* rather than never. It is useless in improving ovulation for women who ovulate regularly, or in inducing ovulation in women who have primary ovarian failure, which would be indicated by high levels of FSH in your blood—the result of premature or natural menopause, for example.

Costs

Clomiphene is the cheapest of the fertility drugs, costing at rock-bottom, as of this writing, about $3.50 to $4.50 per 50-milligram tablet. Prices vary from brand to brand, pharmacy to pharmacy, state to state, and country to country. Taxes, dispensing fees, delivery charges (if you're "ordering in") are not included. See "The Cost of Success" later in this chapter. Most insurance plans will be forced to cover the costs of these drugs under the proposed Equity in Fertility Coverage Act of 2001 and The Family Building Act of 2001, while others may consider these drugs "experimental." You can try to get your doctor to write a letter, which in some cases facilitates more coverage. In other cases, some drug companies have limited funds that they make available to patients to help them pay for one or two cycles' worth of clomiphene. In general, most clomiphene patients (even Canadians) should not count on getting these funds.

A word about storage

Light or moisture may affect their potency. If the drugs are not working in the first two cycles, explore the possibility that storage, rather than dosage, may be the problem. For example, bathrooms are typically the worst place to store them, yet most people will choose this area.

What are the odds?

About 60 percent of all women on clomiphene ovulate, while about 30 percent get pregnant within the first three months of treatment. There is also about a 10 percent chance of conceiving twins if you take the drug and, in fact, the risk of miscarriage *drops* (because the drug also improves the luteal phase, there is a greater chance that the pregnancy "sticks").

Who's not a clomiphene citrate candidate?

You cannot take clomiphene citrate if you have any of the following conditions:

- *Suspected pregnancy.* To avoid taking clomiphene during a pregnancy, make sure you keep a basal body temperature chart or another chart (see chapter 4) so you can keep track of your cycles. Then, you should not restart clomiphene citrate if your period is late and rule out or confirm the pregnancy before you start your next clomiphene cycle.
- *Uncontrolled thyroid disorder or adrenal disorder.* If you've been successfully treated for one of these conditions, then it's fine to take clomiphene.
- *Pituitary tumor or another organic intracranial lesion.*
- *Liver disease or a history of liver disease.* Women with liver problems won't absorb and break down the drug properly, nor should they risk pregnancy without discussing the risks with an internist.
- *Abnormal uterine bleeding* that hasn't yet been investigated or has no known cause. This suggests that you have too much estrogen in your system already, so the last thing you need is *more*!
- *Ovarian cysts or enlargement of one or both ovaries that is* not *due to polycystic ovarian syndrome.* Because the drug causes more follicles to ripen, there's a higher risk of developing ovarian cysts or enlarged ovaries. This is discussed more below.
- *Depression or a history of depression.* These drugs can cause symptoms of depression that can aggravate a preexisting history. Depression is discussed later.
- *Fibroids.* The increase in estrogen can stimulate the fibroids to grow, which is not dangerous to your general health but could interefere with a pregnancy. Discuss further the risks with your doctor so you can make an informed decision.

When should you take clomiphene citrate?

You can consider taking clomiphene citrate only if

- your partner has a clean bill of health from his workup (see chapter 5);
- you have been charting your cycles and have a clear understanding of how your own menstrual cycle works (see chapter 4);
- you have had a full workup yourself, including a full physical, pelvic exam, negative Pap smear, blood tests that check your estrogen and progesterone levels at key phases in the cycle, a clean hysterosalpingogram (meaning your tubes are open), and an endometrial biopsy that determines whether or not you have a luteal phase deficiency. (All these are discussed in chapter 6.)

If you're over forty . . .

As you age, your risk of endometrial cancer (which is an estrogen-dependent cancer) goes up, so high levels of estrogen can put you at further risk. Discuss your risk profile with your doctor *before* you go on clomiphene citrate. Depending on your doctor, you may need to have additional tests to rule out conditions that may prevent you from taking fertility drugs.

Side effects

Overall, between 10 and 20 percent of women taking clomiphene will experience side effects, while anyone taking clomiphene for more than twelve cycles may be at an increased risk of developing ovarian cancer (discussed later in this chapter).

You may recognize many of the clomiphene citrate side effects from your days on oral contraceptives. Most of these side effects have to do with increased levels of estrogen in your system. You may even confuse the side effects of clomiphene with premenstrual symptoms or even pregnancy symptoms. The most serious side effect is ovarian enlargement. This occurs in approximately one in seven women on clomiphene. Careful monitoring through ultrasound will help to isolate this symptom before it becomes dangerous. (Severe ovarian enlargement that comes on suddenly rather than gradually is called *hyperstimulation syndrome* and is discussed separately later.) Hot flashes resembling menopausal symptoms occur in roughly one in ten women, while roughly one in fifteen women will experience diarrhea, constipation, or bloating.

About one in fifty women on clomiphene will experience stomach upset, breast tenderness, nausea and vomiting, nervousness, insomnia, and vision problems, while about one in a hundred will experience headaches, dizziness and light-headedness, increased urination, depression, fatigue, skin changes, abnormal uterine bleeding, weight gain, ovarian cysts, and reversible hair loss. Some of these women may also experience cramping during ovulation (known as *mittelschmerz*). *Warning: The higher the dose, the greater the risk of ovarian enlargement and vision problems.*

It should also be noted that clomiphene can interfere with the production of high-quality mid-cycle cervical mucus; solving one barrier to fertility while creating another.

A word about visual problems

In about one in fifty women on clomiphene, visual problems may develop shortly after beginning treatment. The symptoms usually involve blurring or seeing spots or flashes (scintillating scotomata), and the problem seems to be directly linked to dosage; the greater your dosage, the worse your vision symptoms may be. On the more severe side, vision symptoms can include double vision (diplopia), seeing rings of light (phosphenes), over-sensitivity to light (photophobia), decreased visual acuity, loss of peripheral vision, and spatial distortion. If you experience these symptoms, discontinue clomiphene immediately. Your vision should return to normal within a few days. Often symptoms will first appear or will be exacerbated by a brightly lit environment. Ophthalmologists have reported noticeable changes in the eyes of patients on clomiphene. *In other words, these vision symptoms are real and not imagined.*

If you operate machinery, work under conditions where the lighting is poor, or are doing any significant amounts of driving, be on the alert for these symptoms. If you must discontinue clomiphene because of these symptoms, you must follow up with a visit to an ophthalmologist.

A word about periods

While you're on clomiphene, your periods may become lighter or heavier than usual. There may also be a two to three day delay in your period, which may make you suspect pregnancy. You may also have heavier cramping.

Don't confuse side effects with pregnancy symptoms

Obviously, many of the clomiphene side effects mimic some of the symptoms of pregnancy: nausea and vomiting, delayed period, breast tenderness, dizziness, and so on. Whenever you experience any of these symptoms or side effects, report them to your doctor and have a pregnancy test done.

Risks

To date, no increase in birth defects has been reported with clomiphene; your risk is comparable to that of the general population. However, there is the risk of a *multiple preg-*

nancy, which carries greater risks, such as premature delivery and increased complications. In unassisted conceptions, the risk of a multiple pregnancy is about one in eighty; with pregnancies conceived on clomiphene, the risk is about one in twenty, a *significant* increase! Out of all the pregnancies reported on clomiphene, 90 percent were single fetuses and 10 percent were twins. Less than 1 percent were triplets or more. See the separate section on multiple pregnancies for more details.

Clomiphene carries some severe risks, which include an ovarian disorder known as *hyperstimulation syndrome*. This is discussed in a separate section later, since hMG carries the same risks.

Finally, there have also been ectopic pregnancies reported in clomiphene pregnancies, but this risk is not any greater than in the general, fertile population. Technically though, some literature lists ectopic pregnancy as a "risk" because clomiphene cannot *prevent* an ectopic pregnancy from occurring.

If you need to discontinue treatment . . .

You may be able to resume treatment with clomiphene after taking a break from it for three months or so. Discuss this possibility with your doctor. Reestablishing treatment with clomiphene depends on the severity of your side effects, your overall health, and the dosage. Keep in mind, though, that long-term use of clomiphene is *not* recommended.

A word about monitoring

Since the point of clomiphene is to induce ovulation just long enough for a conception to occur, it's crucial that you keep track of your basal body temperature throughout the cycle. Once you start clomiphene, your doctor should take your FSH levels around day two or three of the cycle via a blood test, and retake your FSH levels around days ten to twelve to see if the levels have doubled. If they have, then all is going well, and you may continue your clomiphene cycle. On day ten or eleven of the cycle, a transvaginal ultrasound (see chapter 6) should also be done to monitor the maturation of your follicles. This monitoring is essential in order to keep watch for any adverse enlargement of your ovaries. Monitoring the cycle will also help you time your intercourse more exactly so you can conceive.

If your doctor gives you a clomiphene prescription and tells you not to come back for a month, *go elsewhere. This is a sign that he or she doesn't understand how to administer the drug.* Clomiphene, again, must be given only to women whose partners had a full workup, and who themselves have been screened for other possible causes of female infertility, such as blocked or scarred fallopian tubes. See the separate section on monitoring for more details.

Human Menopausal Gonadotropin (hMG)

As discussed in the Drugspeak section, hMG comes under the generic drug names *uro-follitropin*, which is pure FSH and is reserved for PCO women, or *menotropin*, which is pure FSH and LH in equal parts. Women will only require hMG treatment to induce ovulation if they're *not* responding to clomiphene citrate. Women who are more likely to be offered hMG are those who have very low estrogen levels to begin with, those who have PCO (these women will get urofollitropin), and those who are undergoing an ART procedure (see the section "Operation Egg Retrieval"). If you're offered hMG without first being put on clomiphene citrate, *question it*! This is not a standard or recommended approach. The general scenario is to do about three cycles of clomiphene and then graduate to hMG if you're not responding.

Getting Under Your Skin

Gonadotropin drugs cannot be ingested because your stomach digests the drug before it has a chance to work. Therefore, it has to be injected. The purer gonadotropin drugs, produced through recombinant DNA technology, can be injected just under the skin (known as *subcutaneous injection*), similar to how diabetics inject insulin. Here, a very fine needle (so that it feels like a pinprick) is used. This makes it possible for you to self-administer the drug, which allows a lot more independence and convenience.

The cruder versions of these drugs, which contained urine, could only be injected into the muscle (known as *intramuscular injection*), which meant that only a professional could administer the injections, although a partner was often taught how to give an intramuscular injection. Intramuscular injections also use needles that are five times the size, which need to go deeply into the muscle (usually the buttocks).

Your doctor or health care provider will show you how to self-administer a subcutaneous injection, and discuss issues such as where to inject, skin irritations to watch for, and so on. Each injectable drug also comes with a kit and detailed instructions. Do not attempt to do this without a "learning session." (See Figure 8.1.)

How a Typical hMG Cycle Works

A few days after your period or day two or three of your cycle, you'll go for your first baseline ultrasound, and then have your estradiol, FSH, and LH levels checked. Then, if all is well, you'll go for your first hMG injection. (All women will have these injections daily.) Assuming a twenty-eight-day cycle, you'll begin to take two ampules of hMG until day five or six. At that point, you'll return to your doctor's office for an ultrasound and a check of your estradiol (one type of estrogen) levels. Your doctor will then carefully monitor your cycle by taking daily blood samples to check hormone levels and doing daily transvaginal ultrasounds to determine the quality, quantity, and maturity of your follicles. If too many follicles develop, the doctor will stop the treatment until the next cycle to avoid a grossly multiple birth (discussed later). Basically, the hMG dosage is adjusted to the number of follicles developing, your estrogen levels, and so on. When the ultrasound reveals mature eggs of 1.8 centimeters, you'll be injected with *human chorionic gonadotropin* (hCG), which stimulates LH, creating your LH surge. Ovulation should occur twenty-four to thirty-six hours later. From a pharmacological standpoint, hCG is actually the same thing as "pituitary LH," and it's given to you because it keeps your corpus luteum working longer secreting progesterone and estrogen. A typical cycle involves anywhere from seven to twelve hMG injections.

Who Isn't an hMG Candidate?

For the most part, if you can't take clomiphene citrate, then you *definitely* can't take hMG. The only exceptions are women with liver disorders. Because hMG is *not* digested but injected, your liver doesn't need to break down the drug, so there's no reason you can't take hMG. You also cannot be on hMG if you have primary or premature ovarian failure or have had bad reactions to hMG or clomiphene citrate in the past. If you have a history of pulmonary or vascular disorders, you should be aware that hMG can cause both pulmonary and vascular complications, but you are not considered at higher risk for these symptoms than are those in the general population. If you're over forty, the drug can

Figure 8.1 Tips for Injecting Drugs Under the Skin

1. The best place to inject is tummy flab. Squeeze the flab together about 2 inches from your belly button and inject. If you have no such flab, thighs or buttocks are fine, too.

2. Rotate your injection sites. Never inject in the same place twice in a row, or in any bruised area. (See below.)

3. Expect some bruising at the site of your injection, which is normally about the size of a quarter. A little ice before you clean the area for injection and/or after you have given yourself the injection will help.

increase the risk of endometrial cancer. You may need to rule out endometrial cancer risks before you begin hMG, depending on your doctor's advice.

Finally, you shouldn't be on hMG unless you and your partner have already been screened for other fertility problems, you've had a diagnostic laparoscopy, and you've already had an unsuccessful bout with clomiphene. hMG should be the last resort for ovulation induction.

Side Effects

The most serious side effects of hMG are enlarged ovaries, which can range from moderate to severe. When severe ovarian enlargement comes on suddenly, this is known as hyperstimulation syndrome, a side effect of clomiphene citrate. *Enlarged ovaries occur in about 20 percent of all women on hMG, accompanied by abdominal distension and pain.* You should stop treatment immediately. Other side effects are abdominal pain; rash or swelling at the injection site; headache; gastrointestinal complaints; fever or flulike symptoms (fever, chills, nausea, and vomiting); breast tenderness; skin reactions; rapid heart rate (tachycardia); and rapid breathing.

As mentioned above, pulmonary disorders such as lung collapse or acute respiratory distress syndrome, in which the fluid builds up into the lung tissue, can occur. Bleeding in the abdominal region (hemoperitoneum) can also develop because hMG causes your blood vessel walls to become porous.

Periods may also be heavier, with heavier cramping, and you may feel cramping during ovulation. If your periods are delayed, you must rule out a pregnancy before you continue. As with clomiphene, some of these side effects can be confused with pregnancy symptoms; don't conclude you are pregnant until you check it out.

Side Effects of hCG

When you stop your hMG injections and begin your hCG injections, you may experience headache, irritability, restlessness, fatigue, depression, or a swelling or rash at the injection site. Some women may continue to experience side effects from hMG, too, but the above list refers exclusively to side effects of hCG. If you've demonstrated a past allergy or adverse reaction to hCG, you shouldn't be on the drug a second time.

hMG Storage

If you're self-injecting at home (your doctor will show you how), the drug should be stored in the refrigerator. hMG comes in a freeze-dried form with a separate liquid that's added just before injection. Once you mix the two substances together, you must take the drug *immediately*. You can't mix them up an hour before you plan to take it, and you can't put the leftover drug in the refrigerator to take the next day.

The Costs

This is an expensive drug. Average pricing (as of this writing) for the newer generation FSH is roughly $40 to $50 per 75-milligram vial or about $95 per 150-milligram vial. The average cost for older generation hMG is roughly $40 to $52 per one 75-unit vial. That doesn't include the cost of hCG, which runs roughly $45 for each 10,000-unit vial, which usually accompanies FSH therapy. Again, prices vary from brand to brand, pharmacy to pharmacy, state to state, and country to country. Taxes, dispensing fees, delivery charges (if you're "ordering in") are not included.

Fewer drug plans cover hMG than clomiphene citrate. You may be able to obtain coverage if your doctor writes a letter to your drug plan or health insurer. As with clomiphene, some drug companies make limited funding available to patients to help cover the costs of one or two cycles. But for the majority of patients on hMG, you're on your own. Again because of the expense, inconvenience, and side effects of this drug, hMG should be used as a last resort.

The Odds

In the end, while 75 percent of women will ovulate with hMG, the pregnancy rate on the drug drastically varies: 20 to 80 percent of all hMG cycles will end in pregnancy. Twins occur in 20 to 40 percent of all pregnancies that result from hMG (see page 186).

The Risks

The risks of hMG are similar to those of clomiphene: multiple pregnancies (occurring in 20 to 40 percent of all hMG pregnancies), ovarian hyperstimulation syndrome (discussed on page 185), and an increased risk of ovarian cancer. Ectopic pregnancies have been reported but, again, this risk is not any greater than it is for the general, fertile population.

GnRH Analogues

Some doctors will want to put you on a *GnRH analogue*—a GnRH "copycat" that takes over GnRH production for your hypothalamus, blocking its communication link to the pituitary gland. The result is that your entire hormonal axis is shut down. The shutdown occurs because your hypothalamus thinks: "Oh, I don't need to release GnRH; it's already here." The pituitary gland therefore has its "hands tied"; it cannot release FSH or LH until it receives GnRH. Your body goes into a kind of postmenopausal or prepubertal state, enabling your doctor to control your entire cycle with drugs.

These drugs are often used to treat other problems, including fibroids and endometriosis.

Costs

GnRH therapy is also expensive. Average costs as of this writing are about $150 per 5-milligram dosage (that includes the initial purchase of a kit). If you're on GnRH therapy, you're often taking it in conjunction with FSH therapy and hCG, so you need to factor in those costs as well. Sing along this time: Prices vary from brand to brand, pharmacy to pharmacy, state to state, and country to country. Taxes, dispensing fees, delivery charges (if you're "ordering in") are not included.

The Trouble with Fertility Drugs

As you've probably heard, a number of experts, ethicists, and past fertility patients have voiced their concerns about long-term or unknown risks of fertility drugs and the risks of multiple pregnancies. This section discusses in detail all the potential problems fertility drugs may cause.

Ovarian Hyperstimulation Syndrome (OHSS)

This is a condition that develops when the ovaries are overstimulated by either clomiphene or hMG and, therefore, enlarge suddenly and overproduce follicles. The condition is rarely seen with clomiphene and is more common with hMG. The symptoms of OHSS are abdominal bloating or distension, discomfort, nausea (which may be mistaken for morning sickness), and sometimes difficulty breathing (which can be confused with dyspnea).

This condition is thankfully quite rare when the dose is low and the drug is used correctly, but the higher the dose and the longer you're on the drug, the higher the risk of OHSS. Women with PCO are more prone to OHSS than other women on the drugs. In general, roughly 6 percent of all PCO women on urofollitropin will develop OHSS, but only about 1.3 percent of women on menotropin will develop the condition.

If this condition is left undetected, hospitalization may be necessary. Keep in mind that virtually no specialist will put you on fertility drugs without monitoring your cycle via ultrasounds and blood samples throughout. One of the key reasons why monitoring is done is to prevent this condition from developing.

Monitoring an Induced Cycle

Whether you're taking clomiphene or hMG, you must be monitored (on a daily basis for hMG). This means taking blood samples to monitor your serum hormone levels; performing transvaginal ultrasounds (which are clearer than abdominal) to monitor the growth of the follicles, the quantity of follicles, and the size of your ovaries (see chapter 6 for ultrasound details); and taking vaginal smears to detect the quality of cervical mucus, also a marker for hormone levels. On your own, you should also be tracking your basal body temperature and the changes in your cervical mucus. The purpose of all this monitoring is to make sure that your ovaries are not enlarging, that your cervical mucus is the right consistency (clomiphene can alter it), that intercourse is timed to coincide with ovulation, and that your ovaries are not forming cysts. You should not be on either clomiphene or hMG unless you're being monitored.

What You Should Know About Multiple Pregnancies

In the 1950s, twins naturally occurred in 1 out of every 80 pregnancies. By the 1970s, that number dropped to 1 out of every 100 pregnancies. Today, however, fertility drugs such as clomiphene and hMG have caused the incidence of multiple births to skyrocket: over the last decade, twin births have increased by 33 percent, while births of triplets or more have increased by 178 percent.

During 1980 to 1994, the number of twin births in the United States increased by 42 percent, while the number of U.S. triplet births has, ironically, tripled. Twin births are also more common in Connecticut, Massachusetts, and throughout the northeastern United States. That's because new reproductive technologies such as IVF are more common in the Northeast and because these are the states that have mandated insurance benefits for fertility treatments. In addition, the chances of a multiple birth are thought to increase as women age, but probably more to the point, the older women are when they plan pregnancy, the more likely they are to have taken fertility drugs or conceived through fertility treatment.

Fertility drugs and multiple births made the cover of *Time* and *Newsweek* in 1997 with the birth of the McCaughey septuplets. The McCaughey story is considered wonderful by some and frightening by many. Most multiple births with more than three fetuses end in disaster. Just a year before the McCaughey story, Mandy Allwood, in England, sold her eight-fetus story to the *News of the World*. Her fee depended on how many survived. All of them died; she miscarried them one by one.

Multiple births now account for more than 2 percent of all births, but take up a wealth of hospital resources ($4,600 U.S. per day for twins) because they require so much care. Twins and triplets are usually born before thirty-four weeks. Over 50 percent of twins and more than 90 percent of triplets are born premature. According to the Centers for Disease Control, the risk for low birth weight among twins is seven times greater than that among *singletons*, while twins account for 12 percent of all infant deaths, even though twins make up only 2 percent of the annual infant population. The problems increase when triplets are involved. But quadruplets and quintuplets have a 10 to 15 percent mortality rate, even with top neonatal facilities. In the McCaughey's case, it took a sixty-person medical team to bring the seven babies into this world.

A generation ago, a local obstetrician from my own neck of the woods says that he may have seen only one or two pairs of triplets in his lifetime, but over the past five years, he has seen eighty-five sets, not to mention a few quadruplets. Most fertility specialists will limit embryo implantation (see next chapter) to three or four; in Britain the legal limit is three, and may be reduced to two. The American Society of Reproductive Medicine (ASRM) guidelines limit embryos transferred to two to three.

The problem is that because fertility treatment is so expensive and fertility clinics want to boast high success rates to get patients, aggressive therapy seems to be a disturbing trend. Typical of the fierce competition between fertility clinics, a recent ad to recruit patients to a New York clinic shouts the headline: "Other doctors said they couldn't have a baby. Dr. [John Doe] gave them two." A picture of darling twin infants appears beside the headline, and the last line of copy reads: "We consistently have one of the highest success rates in the world."

Early detection is important because the gestation period for a multiple birth is shorter than with a singleton. A single pregnancy is about forty weeks long, but for twins the pregnancy tends to last only thirty-seven weeks, while triplets are born at about thirty-five weeks. The more fetuses you're carrying, the shorter the gestation period. While gestation is shorter, the chance of premature labor is higher.

Carrying more than one child also means that your risks of low birth weights and cord problems are especially high. Some unique complications include *twin-to-twin transfusion syndrome* (TTTS). TTTS is a placenta disease that occurs when you're carrying completely normal, chromosomally intact identical twins (or more) who are sharing one placenta in either separate amniotic sacs (a monochorionic-diamniotic pregnancy) or sometimes a shared amniotic sac (a monochorionic-monoamniotic pregnancy). What happens is that blood passes unevenly between the shared placenta and the developing twins. (For more information, I encourage you to call the TTTS Foundation at (216) 889-TTTS.) Pregnancy loss also increases, as well as the risks of developing all the other pregnancy problems such as *toxemia* (hypertension plus water retention plus protein in urine), gestational diabetes, and so on. Finally, if you have an existing red-flag condition (such as Rh factor) that marks you as "high risk" from the outset, that condition can be exacerbated by multiple pregnancy, and you will go from a high-risk pregnancy to a very high-risk pregnancy.

To manage a multiple pregnancy, you'll need to be under the care of an obstetrician and possibly a perinatologist (an obstetrician trained in high-risk pregnancies) if you have complications. In addition, you'll need to have a pediatrician who subspecializes in neonatal medicine waiting in the wings for your first twin to be born. Your doctor should refer you to a pediatrician/neonatal specialist sometime in the second trimester, since you're likely to deliver prematurely. You will probably need several ultrasounds throughout the pregnancy. If you're over thirty-five, you will also need to have an amniocentesis.

For more information on high-risk or multiple pregnancies, consult my book, *The Pregnancy Sourcebook*, 3rd edition.

A Question of Cancer: Déjà Vu?

As discussed in the beginning of this chapter, many women's groups are questioning the long-term effects of "ovulation inducers" such as clomiphene and hMG, claiming that the pharmaceutical and medical communities may be conducting an encore performance of DES, the Dalkon Shield (an IUD that caused pelvic inflammatory disease in users), and thalidomide (a drug widely distributed in the United Kingdom and Canada that caused horrific birth defects in the infants of users).

In January 1993, a study published in the *American Journal of Epidemiology* concluded that there was indeed an "associaton" between fertility drugs and ovarian cancer. This link was discovered accidentally during an investigation of something else: whether oral contraceptive use and pregnancy *protected* women from ovarian cancer. The study found that women who ovulated less often were less likely to get ovarian cancer. Hence, women on hormonal contraceptives, women who were pregnant (you don't ovulate when you're pregnant), and women who breast-fed (your cycle returns later when you breast-feed than if you were to bottle-feed) were more protected from ovarian cancer than women who were never pregnant or were never on hormonal contraceptives.

It was then found that infertile women who were never on hormonal contraceptives but who had been on fertility drugs *without success* were at least three times more likely to develop ovarian cancer compared to the general female population. The study concluded that while the link was certainly alarming, much more research into the *long-term* effects of the drugs was needed before *any* kind of absolute conclusion could be drawn.

The media went crazy when this study came out. Numerous articles on the dangers of fertility drugs were published, while pharmaceutical companies sent out press releases documenting that the risks of fertility drugs and cancer were not proven and that fertility drugs were perfectly safe and effective.

A second study, published in 1994, compared the number of women developing ovarian cancer, registered in fertility clinics, to the number of women expected to get cancer given the risk in the general population. The study found that the risk was at least double compared to the general population and more than ten times greater in women who had taken more than twelve cycles of clomiphene citrate. For the record, no doctor should allow more than six cycles of clomiphene citrate.

When you're on these drugs, the amount of follicles you would normally produce in a year or even two years are being produced in a *couple of months*. Your ovaries are being worked overtime.

And, because it's an *undisputed* fact that women who give their ovaries a "break" from ovulation are less likely to develop ovarian cancer, it stands to reason that women who are overworking their ovaries are more *likely* to develop ovarian cancer. It's also an undisputed fact that women in the general population who never had children and were never on hormonal contraceptives are more at risk for ovarian cancer, too.

What this cancer risk means to you

In the general population, the risk of ovarian cancer is about two per hundred thousand women at age twenty; fifty-five per hundred thousand women at age seventy. That's pretty small. If you have the genetic mutation BRCA1 or BRCA2, you have a much greater risk of familial ovarian cancer. Without the genetic mutation and without any fertility drugs, women who have never been pregnant double their risk of ovarian cancer. Being infertile increases this risk by an additional 50 to 100 percent simply because some conditions causing infertility can predispose you to ovarian cysts or tumors.

The January 1993 study concluded that there were all kinds of data that needed to be computed into the ovarian cancer "risk profile" for fertility drug users. Without this data, conclusions about the absolute risks of these drugs cannot be drawn. The study noted, for example, that

- fertility drug users who conceived (regardless of length of pregnancy) were not at increased risk;
- fertility drug users who had a history of past pregnancies (regardless of outcome) were not at increased risk;
- fertility drug users who had a history of hormonal contraceptive use were not at increased risk.

The study also noted that none of the following factors was taken into account:

- Length of treatment
- Reason for treatment
- Strength of dosage
- Drugs or combination of drugs involved

It should also be noted that the study did not investigate how the following "known risk factors" affect fertility drug users.

- Family history of ovarian, breast, colon, or endometrial cancer (those with a family history of these cancers are more at risk)
- Obesity (obese women are more at risk)
- Diet (those consuming high fats are more at risk)
- Smoking (smokers are more at risk)
- Age (women ages fifty-five to sixty-four are more at risk)
- Exposure to toxins (this plays a role in risk)
- Menstrual history (women who are anovulatory to begin with have a greater risk)
- History of diabetes or hypertension (women with these histories are more at risk)
- Race (Caucasians and Northern Europeans are more at risk)
- Geographics (women living in urban centers are more at risk)

The bottom line is that without studying how the above data affect women taking fertility drugs, the cancer risk is, as the study concludes, "very tenuous."

For the moment, studies suggest an association between fertility drugs and ovarian cancer, but no study to date has proven a conclusive link. A large Australian study found no increased risk of ovarian cancer with fertility drugs. But this isn't as comforting as it sounds: Keep in mind that very few substances associated with cancer are ever proven conclusively to cause cancer. Until very recently, even tobacco was only "associated" with lung cancer, which is why tobacco companies were able to say to the U.S. Congress that cigarettes do not cause cancer.

What you should be concerned about

We didn't know the risks of DES, for example, until the children of DES users were old enough to reproduce. The children of DES users face the most profound risks of these drugs, not the DES mothers. So how will the *children* of fertility drug users be affected by the drugs when *they* want to reproduce? We have no idea. We suspect that they will be more at risk for reproductive abnormalities (which won't be known until puberty in most cases); certain kinds of reproductive cancers; pregnancy complications; and birth defects.

To date, no increased risk of birth defects has been found among children born to fertility drug users. We won't know anything else until the babies born in the 1980s begin having enough children that can be tracked and studied.

Depression and Fertility Drugs

Depression and fertility treatment go hand in hand. A study done by Harvard professor Dr. Alice Domar, found that women who were undergoing fertility treatment experienced levels of depression that equaled those of women facing cancer or AIDS.

First, the circumstance of infertility, by itself, can trigger all the feelings and symptoms associated with biological depression. Meanwhile, the hormonal changes created by fertility drugs can also trigger biological depression. Estrogen functions as a weak antidepressant, and when analogues are introduced, your mood can head south. Finally, the cost of treatment can place such a strain on your finances, it's, well, depressing.

The symptoms of depression can vary from person to person but can include some or all of the following:

- Feelings of sadness and/or "empty mood"
- Difficulty sleeping (usually waking up frequently in the middle of the night)
- Loss of energy and feelings of fatigue and lethargy
- Change in appetite (usually a loss of appetite)
- Difficulty thinking, concentrating, or making decisions
- Loss of interest in formerly pleasurable activities, including sex
- Anxiety
- Feeling guilty, worthless, hopeless, or helpless
- Feeling restless and irritable

Women who suffer from depression also report feelings of self-blame, self-hatred, as well as headaches, gastrointestinal problems, and other physical symptoms. Thoughts of suicide are on the more extreme end of the spectrum and are really along the same continuum as self-blame and self-hatred.

If you're experiencing any of these symptoms, your health should come first. And it may be one of the stop signs I discuss in chapter 9. Refer as well to the next chapter's section "Addicted to Hope," which discusses how easy it is to get trapped into an endless cycle of fertility treatment. For more information on depression, consult my book *Women and Depression*.

Treating depression

Drug-free ways of coping with and treating depression are various forms of counseling or talk therapy. However, the "sharing" approach has been shown to be highly beneficial—particularly in cases where women share difficult circumstances or have difficulties in common. For example, several studies have shown the value of support groups and support systems in coping with many conditions, such as infertility.

The Cost of Success

The bad news about fertility drugs is that most couples have to pay for them. In the United States, very few health insurers or health plans cover fertility drugs, although many of the diagnostic tests involved in an infertility workup may be covered, and new laws are being proposed to ensure fair access to coverage (see chapter 9). Table 8.2 shows what is covered by some states.

To make matters worse, most fertility clinics in the United States will not even see you unless they have a contract with your insurer or your health insurer's written authorization or referral for your appointment.

You're expected to pay for everything at your clinic up-front, which includes any of the drugs or kits you may be purchasing from the clinic. Most clinics take all major credit cards.

Thinking of sneaking into Canada? Canadian couples don't fare much better. Their diagnostic workups will be covered by their province, while usually up to three cycles of fertility drugs will be covered at a minimum. (The winner is British Columbia, which covers 80 percent of all drug costs; Ontario covers no fertility drugs at all.)

On an international scale, the best infertility treatment coverage is in Belgium and France, where couples can expect 100 percent coverage.

A word about the illegal drug trade

Because some Western European countries fund fertility treatment, the demand for fertility drugs is high, which keeps the costs down (the old story of it being cheaper to buy something in mass quantity than in a single serving). Drug pricing is also adjusted according to the standard of living, making North America the most expensive place to buy fertility drugs.

As a result, there is currently a black market in fertility drugs. Thanks to the Internet, North American couples can purchase fertility drugs from European countries such as Belgium or France at half the cost. Mexico is also a popular spot. The drugs are usually sent right to your door within a couple of days. Of course, both Canada and the United States have strict guidelines about importing drugs, which makes this cross-border shopping adventure 100 percent illegal. But unless the price of fertility drugs drops, many couples will find the black market prices very tempting.

American couples under the impression that they can import drugs for personal use are under the wrong impression. The FDA only approves this if the drug being imported is (1) to treat a serious condition, and (2) not available in the United States. Fertility drugs meet neither condition.

Drugs That Correct Hormonal Problems

Some women who are anovulatory will be given neither clomiphene nor hMG. Instead, they may be offered one of the following drugs to compensate for a specific hormonal

Table 8.2 State Infertility Coverage as of 2001

Arkansas (coverage since 1987)	State covers up to a maximum lifetime benefit of $15,000.
California (coverage since 1989)	Coverage excludes IVF, but covers gamete intrafallopian transfer (GIFT).
Connecticut (coverage since 1989)	No specific limitations published.
Hawaii (coverage since 1987)	Coverage provides a one-time only benefit covering all outpatient expenses arising from IVF.
Illinois (coverage since 1991)	Limits first-time attempts to four oocyte retrievals. If a child is born, two complete oocyte retrievals for a second birth are covered. Businesses with twenty-five or fewer employees are exempt from having to provide the coverage specified by the law.
Maryland (coverage since 1985)	Businesses with fifty or fewer employees do not have to provide coverage specified by law.
Massachusetts (coverage since 1987)	No specific limitations published.
Montana (coverage since 1987)	Coverage applies to HMOs only; other insurers specifically are exempt from having to provide the coverage.
New Jersey (coverage since 2001)	No specific limitations published.
New York (coverage since 1990)	Provides coverage for the "diagnosis and treatment of correctable medical conditions." Does not consider IVF a corrective treatment.
Ohio (coverage since 1991)	Coverage applies to HMOs only.
Rhode Island (coverage since 1989)	No specific limitations published.
Texas (coverage since 1987)	No specific limitations published.
West Virginia (coverage since 1977)	Coverage applies to HMOs only.

Source: American Society for Reproductive Medicine (formerly The American Fertility Society), 2001.

imbalance. In these cases, they will not be taking an "ovulation inducer" but a hormone replacement. Therefore, risks such as hyperstimulation syndrome, ovarian enlargement, or cancer are not an issue.

Bromocriptine

Bromocriptine is the drug prescribed for *hyperprolactinemia*, which is discussed in chapter 6. Hyperprolactinemia means that you're producing too much prolactin, which inhibits estrogen production. High levels of prolactin are normal in pregnant and lactating women. For those who are not pregnant, alcohol consumption and antidepressant use can cause you to overproduce prolactin (see chapter 3).

Bromocriptine suppresses your hypothalamus, and hence suppresses prolactin. The most popular brand name of bromocriptine is Parlodel. This won't *cure* your hyperprolactinemia, but it will *control* it. The dosage is pretty low because bromocriptine is extremely potent. You'll start with about 2.5 milligrams per day and eventually graduate to the same dose three times a day. Once you get pregnant, you'll be taken off the drug immediately.

Risks and side effects

The side effects can be nasty: dizziness, nausea, nasal congestion, low blood pressure, and headaches. You'll usually experience the side effects at the beginning of your treatment, then find that they subside with time. This drug is considered safe, but it has only been in use for about a decade. So far, it hasn't been known to cause any birth defects, but it's still too new to yield any long-term statistics.

Before you start bromocriptine, you'll need a CAT (computerized axial tomography) scan to rule out the possibility of a benign pituitary tumor, which could be the source of your high prolactin levels. Other than that, there are no other conditions that prevent you from taking bromocriptine.

The odds

About 90 percent of women on bromocriptine will ovulate as long as they take it correctly; 65 to 85 percent of these women get pregnant. Multiple births and ectopic pregnancies do not occur with any more frequency than they do in the general population.

GnRH

In some cases, women have specific GnRH *deficiencies*, where their hypothalamus glands are not producing GnRH, which results in anovulation. Under these circumstances, you'll be put on clomiphene citrate first and then move on to GnRH only if you don't respond to clomiphene citrate.

Operation Egg Retrieval

If you're undergoing IVF or GIFT or another ART procedure, and if you're ovulating regularly, you'll be prescribed hMG, not so much to induce ovulation but to stimulate the ovaries to produce several mature follicles. If you're not undergoing IVF, clomiphene and hMG may be used together. This is not a standard practice, but it is not necessarily more risky than hMG used alone. If your doctor suggests this combination, ask why it's being suggested over using hMG or clomiphene alone. Almost all IVF programs place you on a GnRH analogue such as Lupron prior to the administration of clomiphene or hMG.

In general, the side effects and risks of these drugs are the same for you as for an anovulatory woman. You must also make sure that the cause for your infertility (whether male factor or female factor) is investigated before you undergo any kind of ART procedure. When you're on these drugs, you will also require the same level of monitoring as an anovulatory woman, but you will not ovulate. Instead, your eggs will be *retrieved* through an egg retrieval procedure. The surgical procedures that follow greatly depend on the ART procedure you've chosen and are therefore discussed in the next chapter.

Drugs After Retrieval

If you're undergoing IVF-like procedures, you will begin hCG injections thirty-five hours before egg retrieval to keep your uterus primed and receptive for an embryo. After the embryo is put back inside you, you will either begin displaying the signs of early pregnancy, or you will begin to menstruate. The hMG cycle can begin immediately after your period is over, if you haven't conceived.

If you're not having an IVF-like procedure but are having your eggs retrieved so they can be put into a host uterus (because you are donating oocytes or cannot sustain a pregnancy for some reason), then you will also receive hCG prior to your retrieval surgery. You will either have your period induced by a progesterone suppository or you will just stop all medication and shed your lining naturally. If the pregnancy hasn't established in the host uterus, you'll begin your treatment again after your period is finished.

Drugs Used in Male Fertility Therapy

When a man's levels of either FSH or LH are too low (and consequently, testosterone is low), it's a sign of a pituitary gland problem. This can be remedied with hMG, which is used to stimulate the seminiferous tubules and the Leydig cells (see chapter 5 for details).

For the majority of males taking fertility drugs, hMG (menotropins such as Pergonal) will be prescribed over clomiphene citrate, since clomiphene citrate has not been proven to be helpful for men. When menotropins are prescribed to men, they should only be taken if a man has undergone a full workup and has been diagnosed with a sperm-producing deficiency that is caused by *pituitary gland* failure. For example, if your sperm-producing problem is being caused by testicular failure (indicated through very high levels of FSH and LH), hMG is not an appropriate therapy.

hCG will also be taken in conjunction with hMG at an interval determined by your doctor. Generally, sperm production can be achieved only if hCG and hMG are used together rather than separately.

Side Effects

The only specific side effect reported with men on hMG is the development of enlarged breasts, known as *gynomastia*. This condition goes away once you stop treatment. As for headaches and nausea and the long list of side effects reported by women, there is no specific literature that cites whether these side effects are experienced only by women. No studies on cancer risks or other long-term risks have been done regarding male usage of hMG.

If you're taking hMG and hCG because of hypogonadotrophic hypogonadism (which may be caused by Kallmann's syndrome, discussed in chapter 5), hMG/hCG will be used to stimulate the onset of a puberty you never experienced. In this case, the drugs may cause what's known as "precocious puberty." This can be a dangerous situation in which your body suddenly goes into a wild, uncontrolled puberty, causing hormonal overload: huge increases in body hair, overgrowth of genitals, and a huge libido. If this happens, your hMG/hCG therapy will need to be stopped as soon as possible.

Other Drugs

Hyperprolactinemia can sometimes occur in men who are taking hMG. High prolactin levels in men are caused by a benign tumor in the pituitary gland, which will interfere with testosterone levels. This tumor can be removed, or *bromocriptine* may be prescribed to block prolactin secretions.

Finally, as mentioned in chapter 5, thyroid disorders can be common hormonal culprits that reduce sperm production. You'll be placed on levothyroxine sodium (thyroid replacement hormone), which you'll need to take daily. This drug may be prescribed after you're treated for hyperthyroidism (an overactive gland) or hypothyroidism (an underactive gland).

Fertility drugs may only first enter the treatment picture if you're embarking on an assisted reproductive technology procedure such as IVF or GIFT. All these procedures are discussed in detail in the next chapter. Whatever the reason for taking these powerful drugs, it's important that you make an informed decision. For many, the short-term outcome of a possible pregnancy outweighs the side effects and questionable long-term risks of the drugs. "I'd rather have a baby now than worry about possible cancer twenty years down the road" is a common attitude of fertility drug users, but it is not necessarily the *wisest* attitude. You owe it to yourself to learn and assess all the facts and risks before you decide.

9

Out-of-Body Experiences

IF YOU'VE FOUND the cause of your infertility, and it cannot be reversed or treated successfully, you may be a candidate for assisted reproductive technology (ART), sometimes referred to as *assisted conception*. ART is also known as NRT, which stands for new reproductive technologies. However, for the purposes of this book, I will use the more familiar term ART, which is the term still used by most fertility clinics and is still the most effective "key word" for literature or Internet searches on the subject. Couples with unexplained infertility are also ideal candidates for some of these procedures. And finally, the explosion in gay/lesbian couples using ARTs has led to what many people are calling a "gayby boom," a topic discussed at great length in chapter 10. Questions and issues surrounding ART for heterosexual and homosexual couples are different in many respects, so here's what I've done: This chapter contains all the technical information for both groups, but is skewed toward the heterosexual reader when I address questions and concerns. Chapter 10, however, is designed exclusively for gay/lesbian readers and will discuss issues around doctor bias and homophobia, gay/lesbian parenting, and so on. Single women using ARTs will find useful information in this chapter as well as chapter 10.

Until 1978, couples who couldn't conceive had two choices: adoption or childfree living. In 1978, the first "test-tube" baby, Louise Brown, was born. Since then, thousands of children have been born worldwide as a result of reproductive technologies that assist couples in the conception process. We now live in an era in which the term *family planning* has taken on a futuristic dimension. However, the technology of many of these procedures is by no means a perfected science. There is a high degree of trial and error involved and a very high failure rate as a result. Many couples need to be assisted repeatedly before they have a successful pregnancy. Although ART is a wonderful option for couples who can't conceive, it is not a panacea to infertility. In fact, the ART process is difficult and stressful and requires a committed and emotionally stable couple.

Before you and your partner look into ART, it's important to examine all the other alternatives in chapter 12. Seeking the services of a good counselor or therapist is often helpful when you're making this decision; it's difficult to be objective and realistic when you want a child so badly.

Although you may successfully conceive through the techniques discussed in this chapter, the risk of miscarriage is high and the rates of successful births are low. Ultimately, you need to weigh these risks against other options. You'll have to gauge whether you're strong enough to weather not only the disappointment and pain of infertility, but also the added anxiety of a high-risk pregnancy or the grief of potentially losing a pregnancy you worked so hard to achieve (see chapter 11).

This chapter discusses the range of ART procedures available to you as of this writing. These include in vitro fertilization (IVF) and various IVF-like procedures, some of which are dying out with the success of intracytoplasmic sperm injection (ICSI), where the sperm is injected into the egg. Since the first edition of this book, another ICSI-like procedure has emerged known as assisted hatching, which is also covered in detail.

Donor procedures and "materials" (sperm, eggs, uteri) are also fully discussed, with a large section devoted to guidelines for selecting various programs and disclosure issues.

In 1992, The U.S. Congress passed the Fertility Clinic Success Rate and Certification Act, which requires the Centers for Disease Control and Prevention (CDC) to publish pregnancy success rates for ART in fertility clinics in the United States. Now the CDC publishes these statistics in partnership with The Society for Assisted Reproductive Technology (SART), an organization of ART providers affiliated with the American Society for Reproductive Medicine (ASRM). Based on the latest statistics gathered from the Centers for Disease Control (1998) the "take-home baby" rates using nondonor eggs are roughly 8 percent for women aged forty to forty-six, and only 32 percent for women under age thirty-five. Women aged thirty-five to thirty-seven have take-home baby rates of roughly 26 percent and women aged thirty-eight to forty have take-home baby rates of roughly 17 percent. But when donor eggs are used for women in all these age categories, the take-home baby rates rise to 40 percent for women over age forty, and 43 percent for women in their thirties. According to *The New York Times*, "The most reliable way to interpret success rates is to take the most conservative delivery rate as a percent of the number of the treatment cycles that a clinic initiates."

For the purposes of accuracy, success rates for these procedures are quoted in very general terms, if at all. First, these technologies are moving so fast, success rates for each procedure are moving targets, too. Second, each clinic has its own definition of "success rates," usually involving a take-home baby only after several cycles. For that reason, you may want to review the section, "Addicted to Hope," as well as the lengthy section that discusses ethics and reproductive technology.

The average cost of an IVF cycle in the United States, not including medications and fees, is $10,000. Fees paid to sperm donors range between $25 and $75; and fees paid to egg donors range between $2,500 to $5,000. States that cover IVF treatment up to a point are Massachusetts, Rhode Island, Maryland, Arkansas, and Hawaii. States that cover corrective surgery for infertility include Ohio, West Virginia, Montana, and New York.

The procedures discussed in this chapter are very complicated and involve several steps. To truly grasp the nature of each procedure, a degree in molecular biology really helps! Since most of us can't boast this credential, I've provided you with as much information as a layperson can digest. If you're considering any of these procedures, a frank discussion with your specialist is a good idea. You may also want to consult the back of this book for a list of resources you can turn to for more information.

Who Should Manage Your ART Procedure?

First, get a fertility specialist! See chapters 2, 5, and 6 for more details. Second, unless you're unhappy with your current fertility specialist, be it a reproductive end ocrinologist/gynecologist or a urologist/andrologist, whoever has handled your workups so far and has diagnosed your fertility problem should manage your ART procedure. In some cases, you may be referred to a separate clinic that specializes in the ART procedure you want done, or another doctor with other skills may be called in as a consultant. Any ART procedure usually involves embryologists who perform all the necessary lab work; however, you may never meet these specialists. Your specialist may also provide several ART services at his or her own clinic or through the hospital he or she is affiliated with.

If you've been recommended to an ART clinic and haven't yet had a workup, you *must* go through both the male and female workups first. See chapters 5, 6, and 7 for more details.

Selecting a Clinic

If you've been recommended to a clinic for any ART procedure that involves ovarian stimulation and egg retrieval, you need to ask a number of important questions before you make your selection. You should also review chapter 2.

1. *When did the clinic/program first perform the procedure I am undergoing?* The longer the facility has been in business, the better; newer clinics may have shorter waiting lists. Also keep in mind that some ART procedures are so new that "old" may not mean anything.

2. *How many babies have been born as a direct result of the facility's efforts?* Remember, pregnancy rates are not the same as the rate of live births. If you can, find out how many live multiple births resulted, too.

3. *How many ovarian stimulation/egg retrieval cycles has the facility managed successfully?* A good number to work with is roughly twenty-five cycles per month. The more cycles the facility manages, the more experience it has with dosage adjustment and surgical retrieval.

4. *How many embryo transfer procedures has the facility done?* Again, the more the better. Experience, experience, experience!

5. *How many pregnancies have resulted from the facility's efforts?* Compare pregnancy rates to the rates of live births.

6. *What is the facility's miscarriage rate?* This is important data if you can get it. (It should be made available to you.)

7. *How many doctors will be involved with my care?* What are their credentials?

8. *What are your candidate requirements?* Most programs have age limits.

9. *Is there a choice as to the number of embryos transferred?* (This is not relevant for GIFT.)

10. *Is embryo freezing available?* This will minimize the stress involved with a second attempt.

11. *How much time should I arrange to take off from work?* This is a crucial question that many couples forget to ask. You'll need to arrange for appropriate leaves of absences, arrange for proper rest, and reduce your social commitments. Unless you're rested and healthy, the procedure won't have the optimum chances of success. If a clinic tells you that you won't need to take more than a day off work, this tells you that there is very little patient consideration at that particular facility.

In Vitro Fertilization (IVF)

Comedian Rita Rudner explains IVF like this:

My mother is worried that I will delay getting pregnant until it's too late. I told her not to worry. That I will simply freeze my eggs, and when I'm ready, have them fertilized in a dish. My mother paused, and in horror said, "Oh, but I hope you won't use a good dish!"

That's just about the best IVF explanation I've heard. And what's even more hilarious is that it's true. Now for a little more detail . . . The term *in vitro* means "in glass"; yet today, "in plastic" is more accurate. This is a process that combines using the fertility drugs discussed in chapter 8 (clomiphene citrate and human menopausal gonadotropin) to induce ovulation, removing those eggs via microsurgery and/or ultrasound, and then placing them in a plastic dish and fertilizing them with sperm.

Before you make your IVF plans, please remember that this process is expensive, stressful, and drawn out. Also bear in mind that IVF usually requires at least two attempts for a successful outcome.

IVF was originally designed for couples with female factor infertility due to damaged fallopian tubes (see chapters 6 and 7). Today IVF is also used for assisting couples who have unexplained infertility, who have a variety of male factor infertility problems, such as poor sperm count or poor morphology (see chapter 5), and who are involved in various donor programs. *IVF is the "architecture" on which all ART procedures are based.*

The Stages of IVF

IVF is an involved four-step process. The first stage is ovarian stimulation via a GnRH analogue and then human menopausal gonadotropin (hMG). Even if you are ovulating regularly, you'll be placed on fertility drugs to stimulate the production of multiple follicles on your ovary. This increases your doctor's chances of obtaining a good, "fertilizable" egg. All of this is discussed in detail in chapter 8. IG, or immunoglobin therapy, may also be used in conjunction with both ICSI (discussed later) and IVF, which helps prevent losing the embryos to immunological factors. (See chapter 9.)

In the second stage, blood tests and ultrasound are performed and eggs are collected. This is known as egg retrieval, oocyte pickup, or egg pickup. You'll be monitored daily. When your eggs are ripe, you'll undergo a procedure called endovaginal egg retrieval with the aid of ultrasound, where your doctor actually *retrieves* your eggs. (See the separate section on egg retrieval next.)

The third stage involves fertilizing the eggs in a lab. After the eggs have been fertilized by sperm, stage four, *embryo transfer*, is the final step. Stage four involves transferring the embryos from the petri dish directly into the uterine cavity with the aid of a catheter.

The fertility drugs discussed in chapter 8 do tend to create chromosomally imperfect eggs, so you may need to have more than one cycle's worth of eggs retrieved before your doctor finds an acceptable one. When this happens, the egg is nurtured in the laboratory until it is mature enough to interact with the male partner's sperm. Any other good eggs retrieved might be fertilized and frozen for future embryo transfers, eliminating the need to go through ovarian stimulation and egg retrieval again. Sperm banks allow for the storage and provision of sperm for couples undergoing IVF and ICSI treatments (it would be embarrassing if, after ovarian stimulation, no sperm were available). Embryo freezing is called *cryopreservation* (discussed in a separate section toward the end of this chapter).

You'll be given some notice about the timing of your egg retrieval. If your IVF procedure involves your partner's sperm, he'll need to abstain from ejaculation for about four days prior to delivering his semen sample to the lab. The semen sample isn't requested until enough satisfactory eggs are retrieved. Once the lab receives the semen sample, the sperm are carefully washed, which simulates the natural "capacitation" process sperm go through when they swim upstream toward the egg. The sperm are also analyzed and the best sperm are selected for the dish. Then, the sperm are placed in the dish with the egg. If the sperm and egg fertilize, the embryo will be transferred to the uterus.

As discussed in chapter 8, if you're undergoing IVF, you'll not only receive injections of human chorionic gonadotropin (hCG) during the retrieval and fertilization stage, but your uterus will also be helped along by progesterone supplements after the embryo transfer to help make it as "embryo-friendly" as possible.

If the egg and sperm do not fertilize, you'll need to try again at the next cycle (if you choose to). In some cases, the failure of the sperm and egg to fertilize in the dish indicates other problems. Further tests may be necessary, but the best semen analysis is IVF.

Egg retrieval

In the past, eggs were retrieved during a laparoscopy procedure. Today, most specialists will retrieve the eggs using an ultrasound-directed *needle aspiration* procedure. Needle aspiration does not require a general anesthetic, which translates into less stress for you.

The egg retrieval procedure involves a local anesthetic. Then, you'll undergo a similar procedure to a transvaginal ultrasound, except here, a needle aspirator is attached to the transducer. Using the picture on the screen to guide the transducer and needle aspirator, your doctor can reach your ovary and aspirate several follicles at once, retrieving them for use in an IVF-like procedure.

It's now recommended that before any egg retrieval procedure, you have what's called a *Day 3 FSH*, which will measure the level of FSH in your bloodstream at the beginning of your cycle. High FSH levels at this time are a sign that your eggs are aging (and are closer to menopause), which means that you may have more difficulty conceiving using your own eggs. Some experts feel that any exploratory surgery or other tests are a waste of time before a Day 3 FSH.

Oocyte culture and fertilization: an eggs-act science

Once the eggs are retrieved, they're placed in fluid and counted and evaluated for maturity. This takes two to three hours. A semen sample, which will be collected and washed prior to egg retrieval, is incubated and then placed with the egg. The egg and sperm are then left alone for roughly forty hours. If no fertilization takes place, ICSI may be recommended (see below) or other eggs retrieved during your cycle will be put together with new sperm from new samples. If no fertilization occurs and your egg supply is exhausted, you'll need to try again the next cycle. If the egg is fertilized, you'll go on to the final IVF stage, known as the embryo transfer or embryo replacement.

Getting eggs is becoming easier every day. For example, immature egg harvest may one day eliminate the need for fertility drugs. Here, the immature eggs are harvested from the ovaries and matured and cultured in a lab, then fertilized and transferred back into the womb as an embryo. This technique, pioneered in South Korea in 1991, may become a viable option available soon.

A problem with many eggs in women thirty-nine and older is that they are often defective. But yet another ingenious technique can now solve that problem, too. It's called cytoplasm transfer, and it involves using a liquid known as ooplasm from a donor egg, a crucial ingredient that enables your eggs to mature normally. Cytoplasm is the material of a cell outside the nucleus. If your own eggs are defective, ooplasm from healthy donor eggs can be injected into your egg's cytoplasm, which will mean that the resulting embryo will have your own genetic makeup instead of a donor's. It's akin to borrowing a teaspoon of baking powder from a neighbor for a cake you're baking. The ooplasm is the "baking powder" that enables the cake to rise, but the cake in the oven is your own.

Intracytoplasmic Sperm Injection (ICSI)

When IVF-like procedures fail because of the inability of the sperm and egg to fertilize naturally, because of either immunological infertility or various male factor problems, there are now some science fictionlike procedures that can help fertilization occur. These procedures are known as micromanipulation; ICSI (pronounced ixy as in "whistlin' Dixie") is one of them.

ICSI involves injecting one single sperm directly into the egg. So far, ICSI is yielding good results, with a pregnancy rate of roughly 30 percent. ICSI is an excellent ART procedure for subfertile men with poor sperm counts, poor morphology, or poor motility. It is also used to treat unexplained infertility, and as mentioned above, many clinics will separate an IVF attempt into half the eggs fertilized by "IVF Classic" (the egg and sperm left alone in a dish) and the other half, ICSI. There are deep ethical concerns raised over ICSI, discussed in the "Ethics" section on page 229. ICSI is considered a very effective treatment for male factor infertility. First developed at the Center for Reproductive Medicine in Brussels, the lone sperm is injected directly into the cytoplasm, or "yolk," of an egg. What is amazing about ICSI is that it allows for completely immotile sperm, immature sperm (which can be obtained directly from the testicles through round spermatid nuclear injection or ROSNI), or malformed sperm to actually fertilize an egg. And it's really working! In other words, as long as a man has some sperm cells remaining in his testicle, ICSI can be done successfully.

And what about ICSI children? It seems as though there *are* some problems with ICSI children. Belgian and Australian studies following more than eight hundred ICSI babies have found that ICSI offspring are twice as likely to have a major birth defect. Heart, bladder, stomach, and kidney defects were seen, as well as cleft palates and hernias. See the "Ethics" section at the end of this chapter for more information about ICSI concerns.

The technology of ICSI has spawned some interesting new tests that can help pinpoint why some sperm fertilize better than others and, hence, help to identify ICSI candidates. Hyaluronidase testing was designed to find out if sperm lack the hyaluronidase enzyme needed to penetrate the eggs' *zona pellucida* ("the shell"). Roughly 40 percent of all infertile men and 5 to 10 percent of all infertile men undergoing IVF are deficient in this enzyme. Even men with "normal" sperm samples can have this enzyme deficiency, which may answer some questions for couples with unexplained infertility. Without hyaluronidase, a man has less than a 5 percent chance of fertilizing an egg through an IVF-like procedure. By testing for the deficiency ahead of time, couples can be spared the pain of unsuccessful IVF and perhaps try for ICSI instead.

HOST, which stands for the hypo-osmotic swelling test, can actually probe into the semen a little more effectively. It can take a seemingly dead sample and find any live sperm that have not yet been detectable. With HOST, a technician immerses the sperm in a solution that enables the live sperm to be "spotted" and rescued into another solution that "revives" them. So far, clinics doing ICSI with HOST-retrieved sperm are achieving about a 70 percent fertilization rate with totally immotile sperm.

Embryo transfer

Generally, three or four embryos may be safely transferred into your uterine cavity, which is why multiple births are so common with IVF but many countries limit transfers to two to three embryos. See the section on multiple births in the previous chapter. Your doctor will use a catheter to insert the embryo into your uterine cavity through your cervix. You will not require a local anesthetic, but you'll need to lie still for about two to four hours after the procedure. You'll then need to rest for the next forty-eight hours, getting out of bed as seldom as possible.

After the embryo transfer is done, you'll report to the clinic about two weeks later for a pregnancy test. If your test is negative, you'll need to decide whether you're going to repeat the process and *repeat the fee*! If a pregnancy doesn't occur after the embryro is transferred, you'll have to wait three to four cycles before trying another IVF cycle.

After the transfer, you'll receive hormone injections of hCG and may be placed on vaginal progesterone suppositories. As discussed in chapter 11, the progesterone supplements, many believe, will help keep the uterus receptive for the implantation and well primed for the early part of the pregnancy.

According to a 1999 study by the National Institutes of Health, researchers have found that implantation is most likely to be successful eight to ten days after you have ovulated. The later the egg is implanted after ovulation, the less likely it will implant. In other words, there is a specific implantation "window" that is beginning to influence the practices of many IVF clinics. If this window is respected more often, pregnancy rates may increase.

Assisted hatching (AH)

Until recently, only about 10 percent of all embryos survived the transfer back into the uterus; and 74 percent of all failed IVF attempts were due to implantation. Success rates were particularly dismal for women over age thirty-eight, women with high FSH levels (common prior to menopause), women with a history of failed IVF attempts, and in embryos produced from sperm injection (ICSI). But a new ICSI-like technique, using what's called micromanipulation, may help to change all that. This technique is known as assisted hatching.

When embryos are transferred into the uterus, they're covered by an outer coating known as the zona pellucida. This coating must dissolve in order for the embryo to be able to "hatch" and properly implant. So with a little help from the lab, a microscopic glass tube is used to place a minute amount of a dissolving fluid on the outer coating of the embryo. This is done on the third day after egg retrieval, where embryos are directly exposed to the uterine environment earlier. You may be placed on steroids (medication that suppresses the mother's immune system) and antibiotics (to guard against any infections) when assisted hatching is performed. The steroids and antibiotics are given for four days only, starting on egg retrieval day.

There is a risk that the embryo may be damaged through this technique, but clinics offering assisted hatching, in selected cases, feel that the benefits outweigh the risks. The American Society for Reproductive Medicine has found AH to be clinically useful.

Is there a way of minimizing the risk of genetic or chromosomal abnormalities in a developing embryo?

There is an experimental procedure known as an *embryo biopsy*. Here, one or two cells are taken from the developing embryo when it has divided into at least eight cells. The cells are examined for genetic and chromosomal abnormalities. If no abnormalities are found, the embryo is transferred. Otherwise, the embryo is discarded. Gender can also be determined with this procedure, but the sex can be withheld from the parents upon request. However, there are many ethical concerns raised over genetic testing on embryos, discussed in detail in the "Ethics" section.

What are the odds?

IVF does not carry encouraging success rates. First, bear in mind that only 55 percent of all pregnancies occurring in normal, fertile couples will result in a live birth. As for IVF, roughly 23 percent (less than 10 percent for women over age forty) of all IVF pregnancies will result in a live birth. ICSI and assisted hatching are helping to up the ante considerably.

Within eleven to fourteen days after the procedure, a blood test can tell you whether a pregnancy has established itself. Although couples do conceive with IVF and do give birth to healthy children, the rate of miscarriage with an IVF pregnancy is greater than in the general population. Twenty-five to 30 percent of all IVF pregnancies will end in a first-trimester miscarriage, compared to the miscarriage rate of 15 to 20 percent in the general fertile population. Unfortunately, a woman's age does play a huge role in miscarriage statistics, which is why IVF carries rather dismal success rates after age forty unless donor eggs are used (see earlier page 200). The miscarriage rate ranges between 45 and 60 percent. But with immunological therapy, miscarriage rates can be reduced (discussed more in the next chapter).

Review chapter 11 for more details on pregnancy loss and the signs and symptoms of a first-trimester miscarriage. It's important to be prepared for these symptoms throughout the first trimester. The rates of miscarriage drop dramatically after twelve weeks, and at that point, the risk of pregnancy loss is the same with IVF pregnancies as in the general population.

How many IVF attempts should we endure?

If you haven't conceived after four *completed* IVF attempts, it's probably time to seek out alternatives (see chapter 12). However, many women may have one or more IVF cycles interrupted for a variety of reasons.

- *Poor follicular development*. This is often due to mistiming your hormone injections. When the follicle pickings are slim, you'll need to menstruate and start IVF at the next cycle.
- *Natural ovulation occurring prior to egg retrieval*. If your blood tests show that your lutenizing hormone (LH) surge has occurred, indicating natural ovulation prior to the egg retrieval procedure, your IVF cycle will need to be discontinued and started again at the next cycle.
- *Too many follicles*. In some cases, your ovaries can become far too stimulated and produce so many follicles so early in the cycle that it's dangerous to your health. In this case, your doctor may stop the cycle and perhaps lower your fertility drug dosage during the next cycle.
- *Adverse reactions to the fertility drugs*. This is covered in chapter 8. There are a variety of adverse symptoms you may develop, such as pain and enlarged ovaries, that may necessitate stopping the IVF cycle before your eggs are retrieved.

Who's an IVF candidate?

IVF is obviously not for everyone, but there are some specific cases where it is an ideal option.

- *Women who have tubal blockages of some sort*. IVF in this case is tried *after* microsurgery, which can successfully "declog" a fallopian tube. After microsurgery, you'll try to conceive for another year or so before you seek out IVF. It's best to discuss the pitfalls and benefits of repeated microsurgery versus repeated IVF attempts. Keep in mind that many doctors will advise you to go directly to IVF instead of trying to repair badly damaged tubes. Once you've made your decision, you'll be required to go through a screening process by your selected IVF program/clinic, discussed below.
- *Women with endometriosis*. Again, your doctor will first try to treat your endometriosis through drug therapy and/or microsurgery (see chapter 7). If you don't respond and you still can't conceive after at least a year, you can seek out IVF.
- *Couples with immunological infertility.*
- *Men with low sperm counts.*
- *Men with poor morphology.*
- *Women who don't get pregnant with fertility drug treatment.*
- *Couples with unexplained infertility.*

- *Gay and lesbian couples who cannot get pregnant with artificial insemination and/or fertility drugs.*

Guidelines for making the IVF decision

1. *Are you familiar with the procedure, the costs involved, and the success rates?* If you can afford only one attempt, you might want to save your money and seek out an alternative. Most couples try once or twice. Most successes require at least a second attempt.
2. *Are you prepared to deal with the stress involved?* If you feel stressed now, wait until you begin IVF. You need to be in superb psychological "shape."
3. *Are you prepared to deal with a failed IVF attempt?* Remember, even if you're lucky enough to conceive, the miscarriage rates are high. Can you *really* handle losing this pregnancy? You might want to review chapter 11.
4. *Have you and your partner figured out how many attempts you're willing to go for?* Know your limits in advance, and know when to say "enough is enough."

Selecting an IVF program/clinic

Review IVF programs with either your reproductive endocrinologist/gynecologist or your andrologist/urologist. If this fails, refer to the resource list at the back of this book and contact some of the organizations for IVF clinic referrals. Then review the questions under the preceding section.

The screening process

Once you've made your decision on an IVF clinic, there is a screening process you'll need to undergo. For most programs, you'll need to meet these basic requirements:

1. *Can you ovulate on your own?* In order for fertility drugs to work best, you'll need to be able to ovulate on your own and just have your ovulation "augmented" by the drugs.
2. *Do you have accessible ovaries?* If you have endometriosis growing all over your ovaries, scarring as a result of PID, or numerous fibroids blocking the way, your doctor will have a harder time getting to the eggs.
3. *How old are you?* Your fertility does decline as you age. Most programs have cutoff ages of about forty but may give priority to women over thirty-five.
4. *Have you had all your prepregnancy screenings done?* You'll need to be screened for certain conditions such as rubella. Check out chapter 2 for more information.

5. *Is the male partner's semen analysis normal?* It's hard to believe that some couples haven't checked this out before seeking out IVF, but it happens. In any event, if there are sperm problems, IVF won't work! Review chapter 5.

6. *Are you willing to go for a psychological workup?* You had better, because all programs recommend pretreatment counseling first. If you're not psychologically prepared, IVF will do you no good.

7. *Can you afford it?* You may need to disclose your income and/or assets to the clinic. They won't attempt IVF if you can't pay for it.

Some Valid Questions

Q. *Is there a disproportionate number of male or female sexes with IVF babies?*

A. The boy/girl ratio is the same as in the general population.

Q. *Do the risks of birth defects increase with IVF babies?*

A. The birth-defect statistics are the same for IVF babies as in the general population. There are some concerns seen with ICSI babies, discussed further on.

Q. *Are there any special foods, herbs, or exercises I can do to increase my chances of success?*

A. Review the section on complementary and alternative therapies in chapter 12.

Q. *Can I undergo IVF with donor eggs or donor sperm?*

A. Absolutely! IVF is an ideal solution if you need to mix and match reproductive material. See the separate section on donor insemination and oocyte donation.

Cryopreservation

Whenever you produce extra embryos in an IVF procedure, you'll be asked if you'd like to freeze them for future IVF attempts. Cryopreservation will reduce much of the expense and anxiety involved with a future IVF attempt, since you will not require ovarian stimulation or egg retrieval. Instead, on your second attempt, your cycle will be monitored only to gauge when your endometrium is receptive to the embryo. Then, you'll have a frozen embryo thawed in the lab and transferred into the uterine cavity. The most successful freezing of a human embryo is when it's done at the "pronuclear" stage, which is anywhere from the first to the sixteenth cellular division. These embryos can be stored for up to three years. Sixty to 80 percent of all embryos are viable once they're thawed. Freezing eggs and ovarian tissue is discussed in detail in chapter 7.

Other Works of ART

The following procedures are some first-generation ARTs still being done by some centers, but a combination of factors are making GIFT and ZIFT (see below), in particular, obsolete. First, because these procedures require you to have healthy fallopian tubes, and a general anesthetic is necessary, it's not as practical a procedure. Second, even when no specific male factor problem has been found, ICSI is often recommended to couples who are trying IVF. Many centers suggest a half-and-half approach: Fertilizing half the eggs using ICSI to boost success rates.

Nevertheless, GIFT and ZIFT may still be available at several clinics, and because they're cheaper, some couples may want to give them a whirl.

Gamete Intrafallopian Transfer (GIFT)

This is a very similar process to IVF, but it's about half as expensive and requires about a third of the time. The entire GIFT procedure takes about forty to sixty minutes. GIFT carries slightly higher success rates than IVF, yielding a pregnancy rate of about 35 percent, but it also carries the same risks and stresses as IVF. The only differences are the following:

1. You need one good fallopian tube, normal semen, and a good postcoital test (PCT) result (see chapters 5 and 6). Usually, couples with unexplained infertility are the best candidates. (GIFT has been used on women with endometriosis or cervical mucus problems, couples with immunological infertility, or men with low sperm counts or poor motility, but without a good PCT test, the chances of success are much lower.)
2. Instead of fertilizing the eggs in a laboratory, the woman's mature eggs and her partner's washed sperm are mixed in a syringe together and inserted via laparoscopy right into her fallopian tube. A general anesthetic is necessary, which may make recovery uncomfortable. Then, you wait for nature to take its course.

What's involved?

GIFT was developed in 1984 primarily for couples with "unexplained infertility" to facilitate a formal "meeting" of the sperm and egg. Like IVF, fertility drugs are used to stimulate the ovaries to produce multiple follicles. And, like IVF, the follicles are retrieved. Unlike IVF, there is no fertilization process that is done in a laboratory. Instead, roughly two hours prior to egg retrieval, a semen sample is delivered and put inside a centrifuge (that spinning thing) where it's washed and then placed in a test tube. The active sperm swim to the top of the test tube and are then placed inside a catheter. The mature egg is placed inside a separate catheter. Each catheter is then inserted into the fallopian tube via a laparoscopy procedure under a general anesthetic. Like an IVF procedure, a woman undergoing GIFT will need to rest quietly after the procedure and report for a pregnancy test roughly two weeks later. If pregnancy doesn't occur, a maximum of four GIFT cycles is recommended.

Zygote Intrafallopian Transfer (ZIFT)

ZIFT is what you get when you cross GIFT with IVF. ZIFT eliminates that blackout period associated with GIFT. Essentially, ZIFT is exactly the same procedure as GIFT except that instead of transferring raw egg and sperm into the fallopian tube, the egg and sperm make a pit stop in a petri dish, where they are fertilized but not cultured into embryos. Instead, the fertilized egg and sperm are transferred in their "undivided" state, which is called a zygote. To refresh your memory, raw or untampered egg and sperm are gametes; fertilized egg and sperm prior to cellular division are zygotes; fertilized egg and sperm that have begun cellular division are embryos.

In a ZIFT procedure, the transfer of the sperm and egg is done eighteen to fifty-two hours after egg retrieval, so the egg and sperm can fertilize. Like IVF, either laparoscopy or an ultrasound-guided transvaginal procedure is used to transfer the zygotes into the fallopian tube.

Artificial Insemination (AI)

AI is an option for cervical mucus problems, low sperm count, poor motility, or sperm antibodies. AI is also an option for psychological problems that affect male sexual performance (such as impotence), and for physical problems such as obesity coupled with a small penis, which can also affect male sexual performance. Here, the male partner's sperm is collected semen-analysis style (see chapter 5), washed, and then injected by syringe either very high into the vagina (this carries only a 13 percent success rate) or directly into the uterus (this carries a 10 to 25 percent success rate). This is done only after you've tried to treat your infertility with other means. When a woman undergoes insemination with a stranger's sperm or sperm that is not her own partner's, AI becomes *DI—donor insemination*—discussed later. Generally, DI is an ideal option for couples with untreatable male factor infertility (resulting in azoospermia), or for single women or lesbian couples desiring children.

This is not a difficult procedure at all, but any woman undergoing AI must be able to ovulate, be clear of any luteal phase defects in order to have an "embryo-friendly" uterus, have a good set of fallopian tubes, and have no other pelvic abnormalities.

AI recipes

There are three ways to artificially inseminate. Homologous insemination (also known as "cup insemination," or "the cup") is when the male partner's semen is washed, separated to improve motility, and placed in a diaphragmlike cup at the cervix during ovulation. In order to place washed sperm in the cup, you'll need to be inseminated at your clinic or doctor's office. However, in many cases, doctors may show their patients how to insert the cup properly so that between sperm washes, couples can do the procedure with fresh, unwashed sperm.

Intracervical insemination (ICI) is a little more involved. Here, a GIFT-like spinning of the semen (via centrifuge) is done to collect the best sperm. It is then placed in a catheter, which is used to pass the semen directly into the cervical canal. For each ICI attempt, you'll need to be inseminated at your clinic or doctor's office. Many couples will combine ICI with the cup to improve the odds between ICI attempts.

Unfortunately, the success rates for both the cup and ICI are low; so far these procedures haven't proved to be any more successful than spontaneous conception for oligospermic (low-sperm count) men.

IUI (intrauterine insemination) is probably a more familiar acronym. As discussed, IUI yields far better results (10 to 25 percent) than ICI or the cup as long as the insemination is timed properly. Just before ovulation, the semen is washed and spun with a sample of the male partner's blood, which creates a pellet of sperm with no semen. The dead or immotile sperm are then separated from the good sperm, placed in a catheter, and placed directly into the uterus. Sometimes fertility drugs are combined with an IUI procedure.

Microsurgical Epididymal Sperm Aspiration (MESA)

MESA doesn't carry the same questionable morality as microinjection or zona drilling. MESA is really a rescue mission using microsurgical techniques. The money is in the bank, you can count it and see it, you just can't withdraw it. As discussed in chapter 5, when there is an absence or defect of the vas deferens, a man may have perfectly normal sperm that are obstructed. This is an entirely different problem than a testicular defect. In this case, the sperm are alive and well but are trapped inside the epididymis.

With MESA, the sperm can be rescued from the epididymis and brought together with the female partner's egg through IVF or ICSI. For a woman, the IVF procedure is the same as for any other woman undergoing these procedures. But for the male partner, instead of delivering a sperm sample, he'll undergo a microsurgical procedure under a general anesthetic in which his sperm are aspirated from his epididymis and transferred into the woman. MESA is recommended for men with a congenital (present from birth) absence of the vas deferens, failed vasectomy reversal, or other problems due to obstruction of the vas deferens.

If MESA cannot be done, an *alloplastic spermatocele* can be inserted. This is a device that can be implanted into the working part of the epididymis. This implant acts like a pouch that collects sperm, which can be aspirated by a needle and artificially inseminated into the female partner. Occasionally, the epididymis is missing or damaged. Sperm can now be extracted directly from the testes for use in an ICSI procedure.

Nonsurgical Techniques That Improve Sperm

Whenever a couple undergoes an IVF-like procedure or any of the artificial insemination procedures discussed earlier, there are several techniques designed to improve the odds by improving sperm quality.

Washing

Washing is now a standard procedure in any IVF/GIFT-like procedure, regardless of sperm count. The sperm are separated from the semen by being spun in a centrifuge. This removes the proteins and enzymes that protect the sperm's head, enabling it to enter the petri dish or fallopian tube fully capacitated, a process that would occur if the sperm were allowed to naturally swim up the reproductive tract. The technique involved in washing and separating sperm to improve motility is highly technical and is therefore too complicated for the average person to truly comprehend. However, despite the complexities involved in the lab work, the only thing a male patient needs to do is deliver a sperm sample. If you're curious about the whole sperm washing process, your doctor will be happy to draw you a diagram.

Filtering

Filtering is reserved for men undergoing ART because they've had poor semen analyses in all areas. Here, fine spun-glass fibers are put into a syringe with the sperm, where they are required to pass through the fibers. In theory, the dead sperm should stick to the filter and not make it through. This is a highly experimental procedure with unconfirmed success rates.

Improving volume

When there is more semen than sperm, getting past the cervix may be a problem, since most sperm is in the first few squirts of ejaculate. Men with poor sperm volume or viscosity are encouraged to withdraw from the vagina just after ejaculation starts. Or they may withdraw prior to ejaculation, collect their semen, and drop it off at a lab for an artificial insemination procedure.

If the problem is more sperm than semen, then the sperm will never make it to the cervix. In this case, the semen is collected and washed and artificially inseminated.

Donor Procedures

Today, both men and women donate reproductive material to help couples and singles biologically parent a child. Until fairly recently, donor insemination (DI) was the only ART procedure that came to mind when one thought of a "donor." However, surrogate mothers are also considered donors, donating either their eggs and wombs (the traditional surrogate mother), or their wombs only (known as host uterus, where the egg comes from a woman other than the host). Many women also donate just their eggs, known as oocyte donation. The bottom line is that many children are born from the reproductive materials of three people rather than two: donor sperm, donor oocytes, and donor womb. Although this makes for nightmarish family law legislation, today donor procedures are proving to be satisfying solutions for thousands of couples who desire children.

The donor procedures themselves are not in any way different from the acronym soup I've covered so far: IVF, ICSI, or AI can all be used to mix and match genetic materials. The pressing physiological issues surrounding donor procedures involve *appropriate screening*.

Donor Insemination

It's important that you have an accurate diagnosis of untreatable male infertility before you make this decision.

DI is an option for couples with untreatable male infertility, for single women desiring children, or for lesbian couples desiring children. The costs range between $250 and $500. DI usually doesn't have to involve fertility drugs unless the woman does not ovulate regularly or is undergoing a more involved procedure. For example, DI can involve any of the artificial insemination procedures discussed above, IVF or ICSI.

Safe DI

I *urge* you not to try self-insemination at home with a turkey baster! In order to have successful DI, you must have "safe DI," and make sure that you select a program that screens its donors not only for STDs such as HIV or hepatitis B, but also for a range of genetic problems that could endanger a pregnancy. Even if you select your own donor and know him well, it's not possible for a complete screening to be done unless you involve a qualified lab. Compiling your own "questionnaire," for example, just won't cut it! Of course, not all sperm banks or DI programs practice appropriate screening procedures. You'll need to assume the "buyer beware" mentality while hunting for a donor or DI clinic.

Guidelines for finding safe DI programs

1. Find out how long your DI clinic/sperm bank has been screening for HIV. Then, ask how old the "oldest" sample is. Any sample taken before 1990 still may be tainted with HIV, the AIDS virus.
2. Ask for a list of all the conditions the donor is screened for prior to delivering the sample. Again, HIV isn't the only infection you'll want to avoid. The donor should be free of all chlamydia, mycoplasma, gonorrhea, herpes, hepatitis B, and so on. The donor should also be free of genetic problems, such as Tay-Sachs disease or sickle cell anemia.
3. Ask about the screening process. First, all clinics should be using at least Red Cross guidelines for screening donors, but good clinics are even stricter. These guidelines include asking about sexual habits and histories that go back to 1977 (that is, "Have you slept with prostitutes, other men, etc., since 1977?"). Second, as of 1986, most donors should have been tested at the time of their deposits. Their semen should have been frozen, and then the donors should have been retested in 180 days for HIV. If they were still negative, their semen was used. But HIV can take up to six months to show up in an AIDS test. Select a donor program that screens in six-month intervals to be safe. Age of the donor is also important. There is a significantly higher risk of chromosomal abnormalities (like Down's syndrome) when both donor and recipient are over the age of thirty-seven.
4. Ask if the clinic keeps permanent records of donors (confidential), which can be made available to a couple or offspring if requested. Will nonidentifying information on the donor be released to adult offspring if requested? For example, if two DI adults meet from the same program, will they be able to find out if they have the same father? Nonidentifying information can include

information about the donor's education, anatomical features (which can be computer generated), personality traits, and medical/genetic makeup. However, there are many "known" donors, too.

5. Is the sperm fresh or frozen? Until 1986, most sperm banks preferred to use fresh semen over frozen, because fresh yielded higher success rates. Today only frozen semen should be used to reduce the risk of HIV infection. Fresh semen is *not* acceptable. But freezing is now used as a method to improve the quality of sperm anyway, so there is no longer a reason to use fresh sperm.

6. Does your clinic/program enforce a limit as to how many offspring one donor can father? The American Fertility Society recommends ten pregnancies per donor as a maximum. This number is based on population density, lowering the outcome/probability of two half siblings meeting and marrying.

Once you've selected your program . . .

Once you've chosen a donor clinic/program that you're comfortable with, you'll discuss with an assigned counselor what kind of physical features you require, genetic lineage, and so on. When that process is complete, you'll be able to choose the AI procedure that you're most comfortable with: IUI, ICI, or even the cup, but most clinics will do either ICI or IUI. At the time of ovulation, the insemination will take place in the clinic. Prior to insemination, it's crucial that the woman undergoes a complete physical and pelvic exam to screen for other barriers to fertility or for problems that may endanger a pregnancy. Once the insemination is done via ICI or IUI, a cervical cap or nonabsorbent sponge will be placed at the cervix to keep the sperm in place. You may require several attempts before a pregnancy establishes.

The success rates of DI are usually higher than AI because both participants are usually completely fertile. Meanwhile, couples seeking AI are doing so to compensate for an already established fertility problem. Success rates range between 40 and 80 percent. Because of the stress involved, a woman's otherwise healthy cycles may become irregular, but this will usually correct itself without the use of fertility drugs.

Surrogate Parenting

Surrogacy is DI in reverse. It is an option when the female partner cannot ovulate and cannot carry a fetus. Here, a fertile surrogate mother is artificially inseminated with the male partner's sperm. This will produce a child that has the male's and surrogate's genes. It is also an option for gay couples (usually this involves coparenting with a lesbian couple). See chapter 10 for more information.

Finding a suitable surrogate is a little more complicated than finding a suitable male donor because there is far more involvement with the surrogate, who will complete the pregnancy and give birth to the child. However, the process involves finding a program that screens surrogates for STDs, HIV, and a range of genetic problems. It also involves selecting a surrogate who has genetic features similar to those of the female partner's.

Surrogate parenting is a custom that goes back to the Old Testament. The first case of surrogacy involved Sarah and Abraham. The infertile Sarah (who probably just needed some clomiphene citrate) "offered up" her handmaid, Hagar, to her husband Abraham. With Abraham's sperm, Hagar conceived and bore him a son, Ishmael. (Unfortunately, Sarah got very jealous later on and cast out Hagar into the wilderness. Then, she herself conceived a child at the age of one hundred—that's really pushing back the biological clock!)

Surrogate mothers can be found through a donor clinic or program, or by contacting family law practitioners who specialize in adoptions (see chapter 12). Surrogacy is considered an offshoot of adoption. The lawyer will draw up a contract between the infertile couple and the surrogate mother, addressing issues such as miscarriage (will she try again?), and so on. If the surrogate changes her mind, the contract is no guarantee that the courts will take your side. You'll also need to pay a fee to the surrogate, which can vary between $10,000 and $100,000. Much debate continues to surround surrogacy fees. Some feminists argue that in theory, women should be paid well, not just compensated, for such a service. In other words, a woman should be paid for nine months of work at least, at a higher rate than average, for performing an extremely specialized service.

Fortunately, there are a few offshoots of surrogacy that enable women to biologically mother a child, by borrowing only the uterus and not the eggs. For example, women with structural or medical problems that prevent them from carrying a fetus to term. In this case, an IVF procedure is performed with the woman's own eggs and her partner's sperm. The embryo is transferred into another woman's uterus, who will than carry the baby to term. The child, therefore, is the genetic offspring of the infertile couple and does not biologically belong to the carrier in any way. In order to do this, a woman must be able to ovulate on her own, and the male partner must be fertile.

Often, a relative of the woman is selected—usually a sister or mother—who can share the pregnancy experience with her. The success rate is about the same as IVF, but might work better in this case because the gestational carrier may have a more receptive uterus.

Oocyte (Egg) Donation

Whenever a woman has her eggs retrieved for an IVF-like procedure, she will be asked about egg donation. Egg donors are also recruited through ads or fertility clinics. Because donating an egg is more invasive than donating sperm, egg donors are handsomely compensated. The average compensation can range from $5,000 to five figure amounts depending on buyers' motivation, donor costs, and so on. (Canada has banned fees to egg donors.) This attracts a number of younger women who are happy to do it for the money. As discussed in chapter 7, both mature and immature eggs can now be frozen and thawed, while earlier I discussed an offshoot of donor eggs involving ooplasm.

As in any DI procedure, anyone undergoing a procedure with donor eggs will need to make sure that the donor is screened for all the conditions previously discussed, such as HIV and other STDs. There are some unique conditions that apply to the oocyte screening process.

1. All donors should be of legal age.
2. Younger donors tend to provide better pickings. Any woman over thirty-four years old should have her age revealed to the recipient so that appropriate testing during pregnancy can be offered.
3. Previous pregnancies by the donor is an asset.
4. The donor should be screened for any X chromosome-linked genetic disorder.
5. All risk factors for HIV infection should be taken into consideration (intravenous drug use, and so on). If the donor falls into a known risk factor group but tests negative for HIV, she should still be disqualified.
6. The donor should be screened for all conditions that would create a high-risk pregnancy, such as Rh incompatibility.
7. The recipient should be offered a choice of having the donor's eggs fertilized and frozen, and then having the donor recalled for HIV testing six months later. If she still tests negative, the embryos may be used.

Who can benefit from donor eggs?

Any woman who is not ovulating properly or not at all can receive donor eggs. These women may be anovulatory and do not respond to fertility drugs, or they may be suffering from premature ovarian failure as a result of early menopause or cancer therapy. Whatever the reason for their ovarian failure, as long as they have a viable uterus and can sustain a pregnancy, they can undergo IVF or GIFT (if they have good tubes) with donor eggs and their partner's sperm. Unfortunately, women pregnant with donor eggs have a higher rate of pregnancy loss and a higher implantation failure rate. This is believed to be caused by an overall reduced capacity to maintain a pregnancy in the first place.

The most progress with oocyte donation has been made in treating women with premature ovarian failure, which occurs in 1 to 3 percent of the female population. In this group, ART with egg donation is the most successful treatment for infertility, with success rates as high as 50 percent. The pregnancies that result are usually normal, allowing the mothers to breast-feed after birth. The price of a donor egg cycle is equal to the price of adoption: $14,000 to $20,000. Other women who can benefit from oocyte donation are those who carry X-linked genetic diseases; those whose eggs cannot be fertilized despite several IVF attempts; those who have inaccessible ovaries as a result of endometriosis or PID, for example; and those who suffer from repeated miscarriages (see next chapter).

Pregnancy after fifty

Women over forty are classic candidates for donor eggs. Generally, the rate of infertility in women over forty is 30 percent greater than in younger women, while the miscarriage rate in women over forty is about 50 percent using ART. Therefore, success rates using traditional ART methods are less than 10 percent. Because of egg donation, these dismal ART statistics are changing. It's found that eggs from younger women have an equal rate of success in ART procedures as the ART statistics in the under-forty age groups.

As a result of egg donation, a whole new group of women can now become pregnant: women over fifty. A combination of second marriages, second chances, and disposable incomes is making pregnancy after fifty a new option for women who thought it was too late.

Actress Adrienne Barbeau gave birth to twins at age fifty-one. In fact, if so inclined, women well into their sixties can become pregnant through egg donation. A few have already made headlines by doing just that, including Arceli Keh, a sixty-three-year-old California woman who told her fertility clinic she was fifty-three. In Italy, a sixty-two-year-old woman conceived through ART.

Many clinics refuse ART to women over forty-something. Most clinics have a cutoff age of forty-five, but this is changing as donor eggs make it possible for any postmenopausal woman to carry a child to term. The prevailing guidelines are that the line should be drawn where nature draws it. See the "Ethics" section for more on this issue.

Yes, egg donation is a wonderful option for women over forty. But it's important to note that in almost all cases of egg donation pregnancies in women over forty-five, the pregnancies are high-risk, meaning that health problems such as gestational diabetes, high blood pressure, prematurity, and placental problems—coupled with a C-section delivery—are part of the package.

What does oocyte donation involve?

Egg donation requires that both the donor's and the recipient's cycles be synchronized, which means both donor and recipient must go on fertility drugs and have frequent blood tests and ultrasounds. Any woman who decides to donate her eggs will be placed on fertility drugs to stimulate multiple follicles on her ovaries. The eggs are then retrieved using the same procedure discussed in the IVF section. Meanwhile, the recipient of the eggs will have her uterus prepped with appropriate hormonal therapy so that she can sustain the pregnancy. If the recipient ovulates naturally, she will have her cycle controlled by artificial hormones that will interrupt the natural cycle. An endometrial biopsy will be done on the recipient prior to embryo transfer to make sure that the endometrium is the right thickness to sustain an implantation.

When the oocytes are retrieved, they will be mixed with the male partner's sperm and transferred into the recipient in an IVF-like procedure.

Egg donors are limited to ten donations to limit the chance of their offspring meeting and marrying in the future.

Who is an appropriate donor?

In the past, the donors were usually infertility patients who agreed to donation. But today, young women who need money for college tuition are among the largest pools of donors. As discussed in chapter 9, while there are no egg banks available yet, more people are using anonymous donors. Some use classified ads, and there are also anonymous donor programs, but the waiting lists are up to five years. In California, there are even egg donor brokers who charge a finder's fee for locating a good egg. Often, donors are close relatives or friends of the recipient. Many couples specify that the donor must be a certain religion. For Jews who accept non-Jewish eggs, rabbis say the child is Jewish if born from a Jewish womb. Essentially, any premenopausal woman is an appropriate candidate. Once she is selected (or has agreed to donate), a full physical, STD screening, and psychiatric workup are required. The donor also needs to provide her full medical history and a family medical history. Oocyte donors can be a sister or other relative of the recipient. Some centers advise against asking a relative or friend to donate because the decision is often made out of debt or out of guilt. Egg donors are from all walks of life, including students, nannies, and professionals.

Reasons egg donors give for donating:

- Compensation for a phantom child lost to abortion
- Empathy for the infertile couple
- Altruism

However, cold hard cash is usually the best incentive, studies show, for attracting a donor.

A Word About Disclosure

If you give birth to a child who results from one or more donors, you and your partner will need to discuss whether you will disclose your child's true identity to family members, friends, and, most important, to the child. This is a highly individual choice. Whatever you do, don't make the decision without weighing all the pros and cons. For instance, would telling unreceptive family members damage the child's relationship with them, or your relationship with them? Seek out other couples who have children of donors and see what their disclosure process involved. Ultimately, there is no right or wrong answer regarding disclosure, just open- and closed-minded people. There are numerous books that can help a child accept his or her beginnings. One can compare this new controversy over disclosure to issues concerning adoption disclosure. Twenty years ago, many people thought it was wrong to tell an adopted child that he or she was in fact adopted. Today, almost all children who are adopted are informed that their parents are not their biological parents. You might want to take the Pennsylvania Reproductive Associates Infertility Survey (PRAIS) in Table 9.1. A low score indicates that you have a preference for disclosure.

The concerns over DI disclosure have become more complex as ethical issues surrounding DI have gained more attention. There are concerns for the donors and concerns for the offspring.

There is a fear that by disclosing information on the donor, it will dry up the supply of donations. But not disclosing information on the donor could result in damage to the offspring. The secrecy over DI also stigmatizes the offspring, but the age of the donor has much to do with how open he or she wants to be.

A U.K. study carried out in 1996 demonstrated that 53 percent of mature donors with families of their own tended to have fewer problems with their identities being known at some point in the future, compared to only 9 percent of younger donors. Younger donors are willing to donate for financial reasons, while mature donors seem to be more altruistic.

Some experts muse whether two sets of donors be made available to a couple looking at DI: One "known" and one "anonymous," letting the couple make the final decision, using the same risk/benefit or "best interests" criteria reserved for other forms of medical research or procedures.

The problem is, no matter what the couple decides about disclosure prior to conception, many or even new disclosure issues resurface once the child arrives or matures. First, you cannot predict how you will feel once the child is born. Counselors and past infertility patients advise waiting six months before making your final DI decision. This will allow you some time to grieve for the loss of your never-to-be-born genetic offspring and work out some of the DI issues and questions listed above.

Table 9.1 Pennsylvania Reproductive Associates Infertility Survey (PRAIS)

Author's note: A low score indicates a preference for disclosure

Name _____

Gender: _____ male _____ female

Age _____ Occupation _____

Religion: _____ Catholic _____ Protestant _____ Jewish _____ other

Marital Status: _____ married _____ single _____ divorced _____ separated _____ widowed

Experience with infertility: _____ myself _____ friend _____ family _____ none

This survey looks at people's opinions about different kinds of infertility treatments for married couples. Please take a few minutes to answer as openly as possible. Circle the number of the response that most closely represents your opinion. It is important that you answer each question and leave no blanks. Listed below are brief explanations of less familiar medical terminology:

Donor sperm: The sperm of another man is used to fertilize the egg of a woman whose husband is infertile.

Donor egg: Another woman's egg is fertilized with the sperm of the husband whose wife is infertile and wife carries the pregnancy.

In Vitro Fertilization (IVF): When the couple's egg and sperm are collected medically and allowed to fertilize in a laboratory; the fertilized egg (embryo) is then placed in the wife's body.

Gestational Carrier: When a woman is medically unable to carry a baby in her womb, her egg is collected and fertilized with her husband's sperm in a laboratory. The fertilized egg (embryo) is carried by another woman (gestational carrier), and at birth the baby is given to its biological parents.

	Strongly Agree	Agree	Disagree	Strongly Disagree
1. Parents should tell their child that they used donor sperm to conceive that child	1	2	3	4
2. Men who permit their wives to be artificially inseminated will have mixed feelings about their children	1	2	3	4
3. I believe that gestational carrier programs should be illegal	1	2	3	4
4. I do not consider egg donation a sin	1	2	3	4
5. No matter how much a woman will love a child born to her using a donor egg, she will never feel it is truly hers	1	2	3	4
6. If I used donor sperm, I would tell my friends	1	2	3	4
7. I would feel dirty having an unknown man's sperm in my body (males: answer as if you were a female)	1	2	3	4
8. If a man is sterile, he is less virile	1	2	3	4
9. I would be willing to be a sperm/egg donor	1	2	3	4
10. Children born of donor sperm or eggs are the same as any other children	1	2	3	4
11. The woman who conceived a child through donor insemination will love him/her more than her husband will	1	2	3	4
12. Legally, the man who donated the sperm is the father	1	2	3	4

13.	Parents should tell their children they were conceived through in vitro fertilization	1	2	3	4
14.	Men who donate sperm have a moral responsibility toward that child	1	2	3	4
15.	I would feel OK about my husband donating sperm (males: answer as if you were a female)	1	2	3	4
16.	Parenthood is given to those who are truly deserving	1	2	3	4
17.	Couples who use donor egg or sperm to have a baby are asking for trouble	1	2	3	4
18.	If I used donor eggs or sperm, I would tell my family	1	2	3	4
19.	Parents should tell their child that they used a donor egg to conceive the child	1	2	3	4
20.	I would feel OK about my wife donating eggs (females: answer as if you were a male)	1	2	3	4
21.	The man or woman who donates sperm or eggs should have legal rights as the child's genetic parent	1	2	3	4
22.	I would choose adoption before I would choose to use a donor	1	2	3	4
23.	A woman who uses donor sperm is hurting her husband, even though he agrees	1	2	3	4
24.	No one should know that the child was conceived by use of a donor except the involved couple and the medical personnel	1	2	3	4
25.	Couples who use IVF are being selfish	1	2	3	4
26.	Feelings about having a child conceived by use of a donor will always bother the couple	1	2	3	4
27.	I do not consider donor insemination a sin	1	2	3	4
28.	No matter how much a man will love a child born to his wife through donor sperm, he will never feel that it is truly his	1	2	3	4
29.	If I used donor eggs, I would tell my friends	1	2	3	4
30.	Couples who use donors are being selfish	1	2	3	4
31.	Using a gestational carrier is like playing with fire	1	2	3	4
32.	Making a child belongs to a married couple—not to medical science	1	2	3	4
33.	Parents should tell their children they used a gestational carrier	1	2	3	4
34.	Women who use donor eggs will have mixed feelings about their children	1	2	3	4
35.	Being a gestational carrier places tremendous stress on the carrier's marriage	1	2	3	4
36.	I believe gestational carrier programs are unethical	1	2	3	4
37.	Using a donor egg or sperm is committing adultery	1	2	3	4

PRAIS © is reprinted with permission of Pennsylvania Reproductive Associates, 1994.

The following list raises the questions that many experts and ethicists are discussing worldwide with respect to gamete (sperm or egg) donation. Use this list to examine your own wishes or feelings on the subject.

1. Is there a gender difference when looking at psychosocial issues of DI offspring? In other words, does the child bond more with the mother because of the biological or childbirth connection?
2. Should we be worried about a mother's possible repression of (or disinterest in) traits foreign to her in the child?
3. Are there cultural/ethnic differences between the donor and recipient that could affect one's ability to love and connect to a child?
4. What should potential parents know about the donor?
5. Is it acceptable to use a known donor (relative)?
6. Should the child be told about the donor?
7. Will the means of conception stigmatize the child? In other words, will the child be accepted by the extended family? Will the nongenetic parent accept the child fully? Will the child be socially stigmatized in peer group settings?
8. What will the child want to know about the donor?
9. What situations will arise where parents will have to pretend the child is not a DI offspring?
10. What if one parent changes his or her mind about disclosure?

What are the long-term consequences of secrecy?

This all depends on you, your friends, your family, your child, and your child's future friends. Much depends on fate and "the gods" as well. But here are some common fears and unanswerable questions:

- Family or friend's won't accept the child.
- The child's self-esteem will suffer.
- The child's relationship with the nongenetic parent will be affected.
- The child won't have a family tree.
- One or both parent(s) won't be able to love the child.
- Will the burden of secrecy affect the couple's relationship to one another, or as a family unit? In other words, will DI become the "dirty secret" or the "skeleton in the closet"?
- What if the child becomes ill and medical information is needed?
- What if the nongenetic parent becomes ill and wants to disclose DI to the child prior to death?

- What about divorce, death of a spouse, and so on?
- What about possibility of accidental revelation? Will the child be "outed" in public?

Gay and lesbian couples who plan DI offspring will not have to face as many of these questions; the child's means of conception will be fully disclosed (to the child and family anyway) because of the nature of his or her family unit. In fact, heterosexual couples may be able to follow the lead of the gay/lesbian community with respect to DI disclosure issues. On the other hand, with the number of DI children being conceived by gay/lesbian couples, this, in itself, may pave the way for one more group to come out of the closet: DI children from all kinds of families. See the next chapter for more details.

Addicted to Hope

The issue of stopping treatment is a concern for couples who are taking fertility drugs alone or in combination with an ART procedure. These treatments can become addictive unless you define when "enough is enough" *before* you start. Many couples report that the addiction lies in the hopefulness at the beginning of each new cycle. However, as each menstrual flow arrives, the despair gets deeper and deeper until you can't dig yourself out. Treatment is like being addicted to a miracle. "Just one more cycle and then we'll stop" can go on for longer than the recommended cycle-length of the fertility drugs, and in some cases, for longer than two years—an eternity for fertility treatments.

Before you begin your treatment, you should set down your own *financial* and *time* limits. For example, some couples plan for three in vitro fertilization (IVF) cycles and one gamete intrafallopian transfer (GIFT) cycle. Some couples plan for three clomiphene citrate cycles and one IVF cycle. You should then discuss a fallback plan in case treatments don't work. This may include adoption, childfree living, or plans to continue to try to conceive naturally (as may be the case for unexplained infertility, irregular cycles, or borderline low sperm count).

One couple with unexplained infertility actually went on oral contraception after their treatment cycle because the hopefulness/despair merry-go-round at the beginning of each natural cycle, and the beginning of each *period*, was just too much for them to handle emotionally. For this couple, oral contraception was the only way they could get on with their lives.

The Issue of Failure

For some, stopping treatment is admitting defeat or failure. Yet, in the general fertile population, few will sacrifice what you have to reproduce. Issues like child abuse, deadbeat parents, and unwanted children infuriate those of us who cannot conceive. Where's the fairness in denying so many committed parents-to-be of biological reproduction when, clearly, so many people who *don't* deserve to be parents can reproduce at the drop of a hat? There is no fairness.

For philosophers, the "problem of evil" is what has kept the question of deity in a fiery debate over the centuries (that is, "If there is a God, why is there so much evil in the world?"). For infertile couples, the justice in who gets to reproduce and who doesn't is a philosophical and spiritual quandary. For many, it is the spiritual straw that may turn us away from religion, or draw us into it.

Stop signs

For every person in treatment, there are different stop signs that tell him or her that "enough is enough." The following is a list of signs compiled from other couples' experiences. If you're currently in treatment and you've seen one of the emotional and/or physical signs below, it may be time for *you* to stop.

1. The fertility drugs are causing painful or adverse symptoms, ranging from physical pain to severe mood swings.
2. You're already in debt and cannot afford another cycle.
3. You cannot stand to be around anyone but your partner and your doctor. You can't remember the last time you chatted with a friend.
4. You can't remember the last time you did anything for pleasure—reading, sports, going to a movie—that did *not* revolve around infertility.
5. You and/or your partner are incapable of becoming sexually aroused just for "fun."
6. You eat, drink, and sleep infertility. You're so obsessed about your infertility that it's interfering with your job, your sex life, your social network, and your relationship with your partner.
7. You're showing signs of depression: apathy, loss of interest in formerly pleasurable activities, change in appetite (usually decreased), fatigue, guilt, self-loathing, suicidal thoughts, poor concentration and memory, sleeplessness (waking early and not going back to sleep), and anxiety.

Wait a Minute . . . Slow Down: Ethics and ART

Ethics and the reproductive technologies is the topic of not just another book, but a whole series of books. One book for every scenario, in fact. This section is an incredibly brief, "reader's digest" version of just some of the issues ethicists worldwide are discussing. There are many more questions than answers. And some questions have many possible answers. The one thing everyone can agree on is that we need to think about what we're doing more carefully in the future. It's not that the technology has to stop, but we may need to slow down and catch up to it. Many experts feel that the technology is out of control and way ahead of our ability as a human race to "wrap our heads around" what we are actually doing. Other experts disagree, however, which has produced a myriad of philosphical and ethical stalemates.

The General Ethical Quandaries

As you can see from the disclosure issues raised in the last section, even a simple procedure such as artificial insemination carries unanswerable ethical questions. But there is also a broader social issue raised with respect to donor sperm, eggs, and surrogacy.

One of the things people are worried about is the issue of distributive justice, a guiding principle for medical researchers discussed on page 35. This means that the burdens and benefits of new or experimental treatments be distributed equally to all groups of people. But when there is limited coverage for the expense of fertility drugs and IVF, only those who can afford treatment are able to access treatment, creating a situation where the infertile rich have more reproductive choices than the infertile poor. Furthermore, since we compensate sperm and egg donors with money for their donations, are we creating a situation where we are taking reproductive "materials" from the poor (who may be selling them to pay the rent) to benefit the rich?

Another troubling notion is that of informed consent, discussed on page 33, also a guiding principle for medical researchers and practitioners. Since some of these procedures are extremely technical and carry uncertain odds and many unknown risks, are people making truly informed decisions? In order for someone to make an informed decision, there must be full disclosure of all risks and benefits; that person must completely understand what's being explained; that person must be fully competent; and that person must feel free to say yes or no according to his or her own wishes, values, and "gut feeling" without any coercion or coaxing. Given the highly technical and experimental nature of these procedures, and the emotional states (see previous section) of many of the people seeking out ARTs, is it even reasonable to expect that people can make informed decisions?

A third issue that concerns people is the notion of beneficence, discussed on page 34, a guiding duty by medical practitioners to (1) do no harm and (2) minimize harm by pursuing a greater good. Which raises the questions: Is anyone being harmed by ARTs? Are more people being helped than harmed? Is the knowledge gained by these technologies worth the personal sacrifices made by many of the people involved in ARTs?

These issues, again, are just the tip of the iceberg. There are no definitive answers to these questions but plenty of heated debates. So imagine trying to weigh these issues when faced with the following cases, some representing the most wild dilemmas ever to face the human race.

Dead men's sperm

Known as posthumous reproduction, this is when sperm is retrieved from a dead man. Between 1980 and 1995, there were about forty-three requests for this procedure; half of the requests occurred between 1994 and 1995. By today, the requests have at least tripled. In order to honor these requests, sperm must be harvested within twenty-four hours of death, using one of the "rescue mission" techniques discussed earlier. Specific concerns raised by ethicists over this issue are:

1. When is it in the best interests of the offspring?
2. Who should be able to make such a request?
3. Should sperm be retrieved from boys under sixteen?
4. Can consent to this be achieved through a living will?

Similar questions are raised with the issue of frozen sperm collected from a man who then dies, but the fact that the sperm was "banked" to begin with may be evidence that some consent is present. Right now, there are no laws or regulations to fall back on with respect to posthumous reproduction.

Grandmothers getting pregnant

Sixty-three-year-old women are having babies with ART. The questions emerging from this new reality are:

1. How old is too old? When are we going to place limits?
2. Who are we to judge? Don't men have babies right up until they die? With women living longer, why isn't this okay?
3. Is it socially acceptable to allow women to be raising teenagers when they're well into their seventies?

Borrowing gametes from first degree relatives

This refers to the practice of women borrowing eggs from sisters or daughters; and men borrowing sperm from brothers, sons, or fathers. The requests are made by infertile people who want to continue their gene pool in some way. Some IVF programs allow a woman's sister to donate eggs, but do not allow a man to get sperm from a brother. The reasoning is that while there is a limited supply of donor eggs on the market, there is no shortage of donor sperm.

Gamete exchanges between siblings is considered morally allowable by many. But few people are willing to allow their morals to stretch to the point of allowing gamete exchanges between parents and children. In the case of a son borrowing some sperm from Dad, the man the offspring might call "Grandpa" would be the father; and the man the offspring might call "Dad" would be his brother. In the case of a daughter giving her mom some eggs, the woman the offspring might call "Mom" would be her grandmother; and the woman the offspring might call "Sis" would be the mother. The mother-daughter scenario could occur when a forty-something, divorced woman remarries and wants to start a family with her new husband. The daughter she approaches for eggs is the daughter she had in her late teens or early twenties. (Similarly, a remarried man could approach a son from a first marriage.) A few cases of mothers carrying embryos fertilized in a dish with the daughter's egg have been documented.

Secretly adding some donor sperm to hubby's

There has been a documented request by a woman to "sneak in" a little donor sperm into her infertile husband's sample. The request was turned down on ethical grounds. But according to Dr. Robin Baker, in his book *Sperm Wars* (discussed later), this happens all the time in natural surroundings: It's called infidelity and considered to create optimum chances for conception as two sets of sperm wage war against each other in a fight for fertilization. In fact, Dr. Baker insists that roughly 10 percent of all children born to married couples do not have their "father's" genes. Was this woman's request an expression of her inborn evolutionary will?

Genetic discrimination

A routine practice with IVF is to create multiple embryos in a lab, perform biopsies on them, and then implant only those with no indication of a genetic defect. This practice smacks of eugenics, the science of creating or breeding genetically superior humans. Eugenics was what spawned the "master race" politics that governed Germany during Hitler's reign. Discriminating against disabled embryos is awfully slippery business. And it's something the 1997 film *Gattica* calls attention to.

Frozen embryo or gamete "bank accounts"

To whom do these reproductive materials belong? There are no laws in place with respect to disposing of any unwanted embryos. What happens when donors or "owners" die, and there are claims being made on the materials? Unforeseen circumstances, such as death, divorce, or other family problems, may prevent embryos from being implanted into the natural mother; sperm or eggs going to the right recipients.

Doctor's morals versus patient's rights

Since there are no laws or precedents governing many ART scenarios or requests, a situation has been created where doctors are using their own rules of morality to accept or refuse patients. The general rule for accepting ART patients is that they must have a chance at a successful pregnancy and must not have serious psychiatric disabilities. Their ability to pay for the procedure also factors into the decision.

But what if a lesbian couple wants to have an ART procedure, but is refused by a homophobic doctor, who believes that a gay/lesbian lifestyle is deviant? What if a forty-six-year-old woman is turned away because the doctor feels that she's too old? What if a single woman is denied treatment because she is considered unfit, by virtue of the fact that she is single, to parent a child?

Who is the patient?

Who is the ART patient? Is it the couple or single woman desiring the procedure, or the child potentially created? Is it the donor of the gamete? After the transfer of a single embryo into a single uterus, the interests of several people are involved: The parents-to-be; the offspring-to-be; a possible sperm donor or egg donor; and even society at large, which is asked to accept the family that is being created.

And then matters are further complicated when more than one embryo is implanted, and selective reduction needs to be done to save the pregnancy. Which embryo gets to stay and which embryos have to go?

What Would Darwin say?

Transposed onto the moral dilemmas ARTs create is the issue of evolution itself. Are we interfering with the natural order? Since there are many things we still don't understand about our own evolution, are we introducing dangerous practices that threaten the "nature of things?"

Evolutionary biologist, Dr. Robin Baker, author of *Sperm Wars*, presents some startling facts about the natural human reproduction process. If the theories he puts forward are true, certain ARTs may be interfering with nature on a much grander scale than anyone thought, while some ARTs may be serving nature on a grander scale than anyone believed.

The nature of conception

Apparently, a woman's fertility cycle is bred to be confusing to both her partner and herself. Evolution has granted her this so that she may be able to hunt around for better genes on the sly, to optimize her own chances of conceiving and continuing her gene pool. As mentioned above, roughly 10 percent of all children really do "look like the milkman." And women are most likely to be unfaithful to a monogomous partner when they are most fertile.

The man's body knows it has a poor chance of fertilizing the egg. So the sperm has adapted to compete with the lover's sperm. According to Baker, less than 1 percent of the sperm in a healthy human ejaculate are built to actually fertilize ova. The rest are built for combat in a game of sperm warfare. Everyone since 1900 has at least one ancestor who was conceived through sperm warfare, meaning that we are here because the ejaculate of that one ancestor was competitive enough to win the sperm war. Apparently, in any given sample, you'll find the following characters:

- The "egg-getters." These are the Ivy League, cream-of-the-crop sperm that get to try for the egg prize. They are fast swimmers, beautifully shaped, with great heads.
- The "kamikaze" or "killer sperm." These are sperm that are designed to "defend" the territory, preventing another man's sperm from getting to the egg. They are the "secret service" sperm; they swim around looking for enemy sperm and when they find one, they kill it. They are well built, too, but with average-shaped heads.
- The "deviants." These are sperm "nerds" with various defects, such as two heads, funny midpieces, and oddly shaped tails. It's not uncommon to find utter monsters—with four heads—either. These sperm are designed to do the "dirty work" and are simply there to block the entrance to the cervix, preventing foreign sperm from entering. They are basically "doormen."

Is ICSI more problematic than we thought?

If we accept Dr. Baker's theories about sperm, then the notion of ICSI is a little frightening. What happens if we're injecting "deviant" or "killer" sperm into the egg instead of the rightful "egg-getters"? What is the integrity of the sperm that is being injected? Many experts have voiced concerns over ICSI, feeling that it is still experimental and should not be offered routinely until more extensive research is done.

Is DI more natural than we thought?

On the other hand, maybe DI is a much more natural process than we think. Is DI any more "unnatural" than infidelity?

Legislation, Anyone?

Australia, Canada, and Europe have been trying to carve out legislation regarding ART, but because restrictions on ART can also be viewed as running counter to patient autonomy (see page 32), legislation is slow to pass. The most sweeping legislation put forward so far is Canada's Bill C-47 (see page 235). In the United States, case law over various ART disputes are beginning to set legal precedents, which in the future may form standards. Right now, the United States is much more concerned with passing legislation that enables more couples to have fair access to ART procedures for all couples who desire it. For example, in the 2000–2001 session of Congress, one bill was introduced in the Senate and three bills were introduced in the House of Representatives that require insurance coverage of infertility services. The Senate bill was called the Fair Access to Infertility Treatment and Hope Act of 2000 (FAITH—to view it, go to http://thomas.loc.gov and enter S.2160 in the By Bill Number search field); FAITH did not pass. But The Family Building Act of 2001 (view it by going to http://thomas.loc.gov and entering HR 389 in the By Bill Number search field) and Equity in Fertility Coverage Act of 2001 (view it by going to http://thomas.loc.gov and entering H.R. 568 in the By Bill Number search field) are bills that would require health insurers in the United States, group health plans and HMOs to cover a good portion of infertility treatments. From an ethical viewpoint, this would help to correct problems with justice and infertility treatment (see page 35 under Justice).

Congress defines ART as "all treatments or procedures that involve the handling of human egg and sperm for the purpose of helping a woman become pregnant." Congress recognizes IVF, GIFT, ZIFT, embryo cryopreservation, egg or embryo donation, and surrogate births as procedures requiring insurance coverage.

As for legislating "high quality" ART procedures, there are no congressional bills on the agenda. Quality is currently regulated by professional societies in the United States Right now, American fertility clinics follow practice guidelines issued by the American Society for Reproductive Medicine (ASRM). Limiting the number of embryo transfers, or screening guidelines for donor gametes, are examples of ASRM practice standards or guidelines. The ASRM also issues guidelines regarding obtaining informed consent about the freezing or cryopreservation of unused embryos. Couples need to give consent regarding the clinic's time limit on storage of frozen embryos, and the circumstances warranting the disposal of frozen embryos. (Normally, the death of one or both partners, the dissolution of partnership, nonpayment of storage fees, or loss of contact with the gamete "owners" are all considered valid reasons for disposal). But in light of new developments with cloning, couples may not be aware of how "disposed" embryos can be used; can they be used for cloning, for example? (See page 236.)

Bill C-47

Canada introduced a precedent-setting federal bill in 1996 that bitterly divided experts. It is still being debated and still has a chance to become law as of this writing. Known as bill C-47, or the Human Reproductive and Genetic Technologies Act, this potential law would make Canada the only country in the world where it will be illegal for a donor to be paid for gametes, reflecting an international trend toward noncommercialization and altruistic donation. The reasoning is that if people don't get paid for donating a kidney, why should they be paid for donating gametes? The idea is to prevent the temptation for people to sell live body parts for profit. And many mature DI offspring, born in the late 1970s and early 1980s, find it degrading that lives were paid for with a credit card. Bill C-47 would also make the following practices illegal:

- commercial surrogacy (paying someone to be a surrogate)
- sex-selection for nonmedical purposes
- creating animal-human "hybrids" (that is, preventing some mad scientist from crossing a goat with a man to see what happens)
- using gametes or embryos for any reason without consent from the donors or owners
- altering genes
- cloning human embryos for the purposes of procreation (see next section)

Obviously, the complexity and stress involved with any ART procedure is monumental. This makes a failed attempt or even a miscarriage all the more traumatic. Options to biological parenting may become more appealing if you have a bad ART experience, and decisions about your parenting future may become clearer as you go through the ART haul. In any event, chapters 11 and 12 should be read by any ART candidate to prepare for a pregnancy loss and to prepare for other alternatives, including adoption and childfree living. Reproductive technologies are giving same-sex couples more alternatives, too. While in the past, same-sex couples were not able to have biological children because of their lifestyle, the reproductive technologies have changed all that. Family planning for same-sex couples is the next chapter.

Understanding Cloning

As the technology continues to advance faster than the ethics, we are facing another kind of "nuclear" war—a war over what to do with the human cell nucleus. Nuclear transfer technology (the "nucleus" is the cell's center) is known as cloning. What happens in cloning is that the genetic material is taken from an adult cell and placed into an egg whose own genetic material has been removed. Since the egg has a complete set of genes from the adult cell that was transferred, it begins to divide into multiple cells, turning into an embryo that is made up of the genetic material from an adult cell, which can be transferred into somebody's uterus and grow into a baby.

To illustrate what would happen with a cloned baby, let's use a real example. Let's say Oprah decided to clone herself. What Oprah would get from the adult cell used to clone her baby would be a baby. The baby would look like her, but it would be impossible for this child to be "Oprah" unless it was completely socialized the same (it would have to be born the same year as Oprah and have all the same childhood experiences of Oprah, influenced by the same people as Oprah, and so on). To be Oprah, the cloned child would have to have the same life as Oprah—which is impossible. Any change to the environment gives us a different child, even though it looks like Oprah genetically. Nature clones people in the form of twins, and we know that even with identical twins, they are often completely different people with different souls, ambitions, thoughts, and so on. Oprah is "Oprah" because of many unknown factors. Given a different education, different advantages in childhood, different parents, and she could have been as many different kinds of people as anybody's offspring can become. In essence, a cloned baby will appear to the adult that cloned the baby *as simply a baby* who will grow up to be a completely different person. We are concerned that cloning will attract an ego maniac to clone "oneself" in the hopes of achieving immortality. What will actually happen, however, is that the ego maniac will have a child and become a normal mother or father, facing the same challenges as any other parent does when a child resembles them. Given what we know about psychological relationships, the more the child resembles the parent, in fact, the more the child will probably rebel against the parent. Biology, therefore, is not destiny!

One of the most significant bills to have passed is known as the Cloning Prohibition Act of 2001. This law makes it illegal for anyone to use cloning technology to initiate a pregnancy. That said, it is difficult to police, and in the late 1990s, "mad fertility specialists" were announcing that they were ready to begin cloning technology for infertile couples. Not-so-mad fertility specialists were also convinced that many fertility clinics would "clone" in a don't ask/don't tell environment, too. It is not inconceivable (no pun intended!) given the desperation of many couples, and the financial greed demonstrated by many fertility specialists, that cloning babies is an ethical dilemma we need to think about today.

Just after the 2001 Thanksgiving holiday in the United States, scientists from the private company Advanced Cell Technology, based in Worcester, Massachusetts, announced it had created the first human embryos ever produced by cloning, although the embryos died before they had even eight cells—which is not exactly a successful cloning venture. So although creating another healthy human being using cloning technology is still considered a challenge, cloning a human embryo for the purposes of procreation was the Worcester researchers' intent; their intent is to grow human "replacement parts" for people requiring organs, new pancreas cells to combat diabetes, and so on. But now that the technology is here, it can be used for terrible things or wonderful things: it depends on who is using the technology—similar to the dilemmas faced with the first "nuclear" technology.

Cloning human embryos should not be confused with stem cell research from human embryos. The Stem Cell Research for Patient Benefit Act of 2001 allows stem cells from human embryos to be used to generate tissues, including neurons and heart, kidney, blood, and liver tissues. What couples seeking fertility treatment need to understand is that when embryos are disposed of, and they sign consent forms agreeing to disposal terms, their embryos may be used for these purposes.

10

Gay/Lesbian ART:
Same-Sex Parenting Through
Reproductive Technologies

FERTILITY ISSUES ARE different for heterosexual and same-sex couples using assisted reproductive technologies (ARTs). In the first case, ART is required because of a physical or unexplained cause of infertility. In the second case, both partners are usually fertile; it is only the gender preference that prevents pregnancy. For same-sex couples then, this is indeed the fertility, rather than the infertility, sourcebook. This chapter tells you not why you can't get pregnant, but all the ways you can get pregnant. And with whom.

Right now, the gay/lesbian community is in the midst of a full-fledged baby boom (dubbed the "gayby boom"), mostly due to lesbian couples helping themselves to sperm banks or the sperm of gay friends in coparenting arrangements. Not only does ART help gay/lesbian couples have biological children, but it is helping to "out" all gay/lesbian parents and their children.

Right now, between six and fourteen million children in the United States alone have at least one gay parent. In a *Newsweek* poll, 57 percent of adults polled felt that same-sex couples made just as good parents as heterosexual couples. Thirty-one percent of those polled did not think so. But just as many people who say they are against "racism" make racist remarks; people who say that "some of their best friends are gay/lesbian" are often homophobic in their beliefs and behavior, too. And that can prevent many same-sex couples from reproducing or adopting, denying them the right to pursue happiness.

Homophobia and Heterosexism

In order to understand the issues facing same-sex parenting, it's important to understand two of its major obstacles: homophobia and heterosexism.

The term *homophobia* literally means "irrational fear of homosexuality," but the definition also includes the fear of bisexuals (people who have same-sex as well as heterosexual relations), and transsexuals (men and women who have altered their sex). This fear fuels the hatred and harassment that target the gay and lesbian population. Homophobia tends to be expressed differently by heterosexual men and women. Homophobic behavior can include open displays of violence, which can take the form of assault, vandalism, rape, and even murder—not unlike lynching. The more subtle forms of homophobia include:

- demeaning jokes
- verbal abuse (name-calling)
- policies and legislation that deny rights or benefits
- routine housing and employment discrimination
- ostracization by heterosexual peers

Some of the worst offenders in homophobic behavior are heterosexual women, who may openly say that they "hate lesbians" or avoid places where there are "too many lesbians." In certain predominantly female professions, such as nursing, homophobia is expressed through ostracizing or downgrading lesbian colleagues in subtle ways. In the extreme, many heterosexual women will even refuse to identify themselves as "feminists" for fear of being branded "lesbian."

Heterosexism means to perceive anything other than heterosexuality as "abnormal" or "deviant." This is slowly changing, thanks in large part to Ellen Degeneres, star of the now defunct "Ellen" show, whose coming out on television was the biggest media event since the birth of little Ricky on "I Love Lucy." But some critics of Ellen Degeneres have still labeled her "Ellen Degenerate," openly stating their heterosexist beliefs.

Given these societal attitudes about gay and lesbian lifestyles, gays and lesbians routinely hide their identities by "passing" as heterosexuals. Lesbian women, in particular, often lead completely unassuming existences as heterosexual housewives and mothers; many of these women only come out as lesbian much later in life, after their own children have grown. Gay and lesbian teenagers fearing discrimination, and all the negative images about homosexuality, often commit suicide. In fact, the highest teen suicide rate is among gay and lesbian youth.

Having children therefore raises questions for many same-sex couples about whether they will be exposing their offspring to the unpleasant realities of homophobia. Many couples also wonder not just how society will accept their children, but how their own families will accept them. In fact, many similar issues raised in the "Disclosure" section in chapter 9 come up for same-sex couples. Except in this case, the disclosure is not so much about the donor gamete, but about the parents' lifestyle. How will the child's school chums react, for example, when he or she says: "I have two mommies."

But having children is also helping to curb homophobia and heterosexism. For example, what is helping to soften the "coming out" scene for parents is that their gay and lesbian children can still have a family—complete with lifetime partners and in-laws, children, a dog, and a station wagon. In other words, parents of gay and lesbian children today no longer have to accept a life without grandchildren when they accept their children's sexual orientation.

Heterosexist and Homophobic Medicine

The medical community was heterosexist until quite recently. In fact, well into the 1970s most homosexuals were considered "deviants," and homosexuality was considered to be a form of mental illness or, at best, "abnormal" behavior. During the 1940s and 1950s, for example, North American doctors attempted to "treat" gay men with testosterone injections, believing that it would cure their homosexuality. In Nazi Germany, homosexuals were slaughtered along with the mentally handicapped, Jews, Gypsies, and other "undesirables."

The low point in "homophobic medicine" is highlighted in Randy Shilts's book, *And the Band Played On*, a book that tells the tale of how the medical community took its time in dealing with AIDS (originally known, by the way, as GRID, for Gay-Related Immune Deficiency). Years of valuable time were wasted because patients dying from AIDS were (according to Shilts) not considered to be important to society anyway. But the delay in recognizing AIDS as a health crisis and attempting to contain the virus is exactly what led to its spread into the blood supply and heterosexual population. It took the deaths of thousands for the blood supply to be cleaned up. The bottom line is that we have all paid the price for the delay to contain AIDS, which was a direct result of devaluing the gay patients dying from AIDS. For lesbians, the AIDS crisis drew them from the women's movements into the gay/lesbian community. Prior to AIDS, lesbians were often not respected by gay males because they were women; while the women's movement often shunned them because they were homosexual. Lesbian women were natural caregivers for gay men dying of AIDS because lesbians, for the most part, were at extremely low risk for AIDS. They became allies, which would form the basis of a new partnership between gay men and lesbians.

Access to fertility clinics

Nondiscriminatory access to ART is a pretty recent event for the gay/lesbian community, even though without the contribution of sperm from gay men, most banks would go out of business! A true fable from down under beautifully illustrates the history of access to fertility clinics. In 1979, just prior to the widespread popularity of ART, the first publicly funded clinical artificial insemination program in Australia accepted a lesbian as a client. The program stated that it did not discriminate on the basis of age, marital status, or sexual preference. By 1981, because of controversy over its successful IVF and embryo freezing program, the clinic became far more conservative to appease public outcries. As a result, it began to reconsider its position on accepting "single" women (which, of course, also meant lesbians) into the program. Threats of lawsuits by single women postponed the clinics decision until 1984, when it finally limited services to married women only. Insemination was only available to women who could prove that their husbands were infertile. Lesbians and heterosexual single women were therefore denied access to a clinic they supported with their taxes. This story repeated itself all over North America, until recently.

Clinics that serviced single heterosexual women and lesbians often insisted they undergo a full invasive workup (see chapter 7) prior to insemination. High fees and hormone therapy to "regulate" cycles—when it wasn't necessary—was also part of the package, often accompanied by heterosexist psychological tests or profiles for eligibility. Then, after the workup, many women were still refused insemination because of a "change in policy" or because the clinic had decided that, upon reflection, the woman was not a "suitable candidate" for insemination after all. (See the "Ethics" section in chapter 9.)

Lines such as "there is no medical necessity" to inseminate you, or "we must reserve treatment for clients who really need it, lest we lose funding" were the norm. Some clinics insisted that single women (regardless of orientation) were too "psychologically unstable" to raise children. Some doctors told lesbians, in particular, that they did not want to accept them as clients because "they were afraid of being sued for paternity," and that "they've had bad experiences with 'militant women like you.' "

To combat the harassment of traditional sperm banks, women's organizations have tried to form their own sperm bank or sperm networks, but problems arose with the logistics of freezing (people with the know-how refused to divulge "trade secrets"). In some cases, even advertising for donors became difficult as newspapers would refuse to run the ad because it was "dirty" or would charge five times as much.

Good neighbors

What has helped make access to sperm easier for lesbian couples is who they know: gay males who also want children or who simply don't mind being a good neighbor. As gay men and lesbians began to organize themselves into an efficient baby-making industry on their own, a virtual explosion in same-sex parenting began. A partnership between gay men and lesbians, which began with the AIDS crisis, was now helping to end a parenting crisis for millions of gay and lesbian couples all over the world who desired genetic offspring. Ironically, many clinics who in the past had closed their doors to lesbians are now competing for their business. And business is booming. High-profile Hollywood singles and lesbians are also helping to make it easier for single heterosexual women and lesbian couples to have families. Melissa Etheridge was one of the first high-profile lesbians to announce her partner's pregnancy, while Madonna went ahead and had a child without a husband. Meanwhile, Rosie O'Donnell is helping to make it chic for a single woman to adopt children.

And grown children of gays and lesbians, who were conceived prior to one parent coming out, are helping to dispel the following myths:

- "Children of gay parents are more likely to be gay." Studies done so far report that these children are not any more likely to be gay than the kids of straight parents.
- "Kids of gay parents have more problems in school and with relationships." Psychologists agree that children of gay parents have no more psychological problems than any other kids, and do just as well in school.

How Two Mommies Can Meet Daddies

One of the most popular routes for same-sex parenting is coparenting. Here, lesbian and gay couples often meet at "mixers" arranged by organizations in their gay/lesbian community for prospective parents. Often meetings are arranged through friends or colleagues, and sometimes through personal ads in gay and lesbian newspapers and magazines.

Many scenarios can take place but here's what results for two mommies:

1. Lesbian couple approaches gay couple and together they discuss what kind of parenting arrangement best suits them. The gay couple decides whose sperm will be used; the lesbian couple decides which partner will be inseminated (see next section). One of the lesbian partners self-inseminates and gives birth while the other lesbian partner, along with the father, adopts the child. Sometimes the father's partner also adopts the child, resulting in two mothers and two fathers. (See "Legal Stuff" on page 246.)
2. Lesbian couple approaches a single gay male for a similar arrangement, or vice versa. The child in this case may have one mother and one father, or two mothers and one father.
3. Lesbian couple approaches a single gay male and asks simply for a donation, whereupon the donor gives up any legal connection to the child.

4. Lesbian couple makes a trip to a sperm bank and selects an anonymous donor.
5. If the couple desires a child that has genetic traits of both partners, sperm could be donated by a male sibling or cousin of one partner and inseminated into the other.

Who Should Get Pregnant?

In many lesbian relationships, there is one partner who is an obvious choice. She may be younger (under thirty-five) and have a less demanding job than the other partner. Sometimes the choice is not so obvious and will be based on the desire to experience pregnancy and childbirth, health benefits (or spousal health benefits), and medical history. For example, having children prior to age thirty-five and breast-feeding can reduce one's risk of developing breast cancer. (Breast cancer is diagnosed frequently in the lesbian community because women who have never been pregnant are at higher risk.) On the other hand, if one partner has a condition such as diabetes, which isn't very compatible with pregnancy, then the nondiabetic partner might be a better choice.

A fringe benefit of same-sex parenting for women is that if both partners desire pregnancy, they can simply take turns getting pregnant. (Even with the same gay couple, "switching sides" for child number two.) And child spacing "rules" need not be observed, either. The usual advice is to space out children so that the body can recover. But while one partner is breast-feeding baby number one and enjoying motherhood, the other partner can begin conceiving with baby number two. The result is more children closer together, with less stress on the body.

Insemination Arrangements

As discussed in chapter 9, it's important to practice safe insemination. If your coparent is HIV-negative upon first meeting, request that he be tested again prior to inseminating with his sperm. Most women prefer self-insemination, using a plain syringe or a diaphragmlike cup that sits at the opening of the cervix (see chapter 6) before undergoing more invasive insemination procedures that involve sperm washing and doctor-assisted insemination, such as IUI. If one partner is having difficulty getting pregnant, the other partner may wish to try before graduating to a more invasive workup. Also review chapters 4 and 5 for information on the menstrual cycle and lifestyle habits that can impair fertility.

Finding open doctors

In order to avoid homophobic experiences as expectant lesbian parents, screen for bias when you interview your doctors. The best places to find doctors who are open to lesbian parents is to ask other lesbians for information, or to find a lesbian or gay doctor through the gay/lesbian community. Many lesbian couples can go the midwife/doula route, too, but this depends on how low-risk and uncomplicated the pregnancy is. You may still need to have a doctor waiting in the wings. (Consult my book *The Pregnancy Sourcebook* for more information on finding obstetrical care.)

Finally, if you are experiencing infertility as a lesbian couple, all your questions should be answered in previous chapters.

How Two Daddies Can Meet Mommies

The popularity of coparenting arrangements can be ideal for a gay couple to father children. In this case the following scenarios can take place:

1. Gay couple may initially approach the lesbian couple as before, but the result is still two mommies and two daddies.
2. Gay couple approaches a single lesbian to be a surrogate for one partner's offspring. (See surrogacy section in previous chapter.) After the birth of the child, the legal parents would be the mother who carried the child and the father, while the other gay partner would adopt the child. In this case, the child would have one mother and two fathers.
3. Gay couple approaches a heterosexual woman or lesbian to be a surrogate mother; the surrogate is simply paid for her services and then gives up her legal connection to the child, resulting in simply two fathers.
4. If the gay couple desires a child that has both partner's genetic traits, the female sibling or cousin of one partner could donate her egg, have it fertilized with the other partner's sperm via IVF, and then have the embryo implanted into a surrogate mother. (See IVF and surrogacy section in chapter 9). Or, the female relative (sibling or cousin) of one gay partner could be approached to be inseminated with the sperm of the other partner, get pregnant, and carry the child to term.

Who Should Father the Child?

Siring offspring is certainly not the same as going through childbirth. The only factors that would physically prevent one partner from siring over the other would be HIV status or low sperm count. Factors to consider is who will be staying home with the infant, and therefore doing the primary nurturing, who has a more demanding job, and so on. Most of the factors involved with this decision are personal issues, not medical. The partners could also take turns siring children with the same or different surrogates, although surrogacy arrangements are far trickier to negotiate than donor sperm arrangements.

Adoption

No matter how genetically related both partners are to the child, one partner will always have to adopt the child as a legal parent. In a coparenting arrangement, the partners who are not biologically connected to the child must legally adopt the child if they want to be the other father or mother. It is easier for same-sex couples to adopt their coparented children than it is to adopt in the traditional way.

Only thirteen states in the United States allow lesbians or gay men to adopt children, while a recent poll found that 47 percent oppose gay and lesbian adoption.

But even if society were more tolerant, the demand for children to adopt by heterosexual couples is so great, same-sex couples are often not at the top of the "list." The only route for most same-sex couples is international adoption (see chapter 12). In many Eastern European countries, for example, nobody cares if you're single or married, which makes it accessible for lesbian and gay couples alike. Even in the states that allow same-sex couples to adopt, only one parent is the parent of record, leaving the other partner out in the cold, although some states allow the partner to adopt as a second parent in a "traditional" adoption.

Whether you're adopting your partner's biological child or want to adopt in the traditional way, find a family law practitioner who specializes in same-sex family law issues. Friends who have been through the process are the best sources for names of lawyers, or contact your gay/lesbian community centers and organizations for referrals.

Legal Stuff

Coparenting arrangements usually involve contracts, which will outline the following:

- *Legal surnames.* This may be a combination of the birth mother's and father's names; the birth mother and her partner's or the birth father and his partner's; or a new name that has components of everyone's surname. In cases where surnames can double as first names (as in Lester, David, Irwin, James, and so on), one surname can serve as a middle name.

- *Child support.* Common arrangements are for the father to pay monthly child support, but all kinds of arrangements can be made that depend entirely on how much contact the coparent wants with the child. Often the male biological parent has no financial or legal obligation.
- *Visitation rights.* Often the child with two mommies spends weekends with his daddy or daddies. But again, arrangements are entirely individual. In cases where a coparent is really more of a donor or surrogate, no visitation rights may be the preferred arrangement.
- *Parenting rights in case you break up.* In this case, you need to work out, in advance, who will retain custody of the child, who will pay child support, and so on.

There are a host of other issues involved, which you can access by contacting the National Center for Lesbian Rights at www.nclrights.org.

Where to Live

One of the last decisions to be made by a same-sex couple who is planning a family is deciding where to live. The translation: The safest places to live. Large urban centers, preferably with major universities such as Boston or Chicago, are good choices. Cities with large gay populations such as Los Angeles and San Francisco are also popular. In Canada, Toronto and Vancouver are good choices. What you want to avoid is a situation where same-sex families are not tolerated, which could lead to harassment and violence.

Diverse neighborhoods, where families are biracial may also be places to consider, so that your children will be just another kind of family, instead of the only family that seems different.

Same-sex couples are not immune to pregnancy loss. Even in routine, uncomplicated pregnancies, one in six pregnancies ends in miscarriage. The risks are higher with IVF-like procedures. All the information you need to know about pregnancy loss is next, while chapter 12 discusses the myriad of alternative families and lifestyles. Same-sex families, however, may lead the way for all kinds of families to be more open about how they came to be.

11

Pregnancy Loss

I wish I didn't need to write this chapter but, unfortunately, many couples who have struggled with fertility have a higher risk of losing the pregnancy. Repeated pregnancy loss is considered to be another form of infertility, even though initial conception may not have been a problem.

This chapter discusses the types of problems that can occur during the first trimester and early second trimester of a pregnancy that can lead to pregnancy loss. Issues surrounding *repeated miscarriage*, which refers to having three or more miscarriages in a row (that is, consecutive miscarriages) before twenty weeks are discussed in a separate section. Under these circumstances, it's important that both partners undergo a full workup to eliminate problems that may be contributing to the pregnancy loss.

While factors leading to pregnancy loss can occur later in a pregnancy, resulting in premature birth in the third trimester or even in a stillbirth at term, this chapter will *not* discuss pregnancy loss issues beyond the early second trimester. You see, the risk of pregnancy complications dramatically *drops* as the pregnancy progresses. For couples who conceived through an ART procedure (see chapter 9) or with fertility drugs (see chapter 8), the risk of pregnancy loss beyond the early second trimester is no greater than that of the general pregnant population. (At that point, you can graduate to my book *The Pregnancy Sourcebook*, which will discuss everything you need to know throughout the entire course of pregnancy and the postpartum phases.)

Finally, this chapter also includes information on a unique pregnancy loss issue known as vanishing twin syndrome. This is essentially the loss of one twin while the other develops normally. Many women who have had fertility drugs may be susceptible to this problem, which has been largely ignored by the medical community until the last decade or so.

What Are the Odds?

If you haven't had any ART procedures and are pregnant solely as a result of fertility drugs, such as clomiphene citrate or human menopausal gonadotropin (see chapter 8), you have a greater risk of having a multiple pregnancy, but your risk of miscarriage is not any higher than that faced by the general population: one in six. If you've already had more than two miscarriages in a row, please review the section entitled "Repeated Miscarriage." You should not attempt conception again before a complete workup is done.

What you *will* need to do is to make sure your levels of human chorionic gonadotropin (hCG) are checked regularly in the first two months of pregnancy (high levels are signs of multiple pregnancy). You should also request an alphafetoprotein (AFP) screening and an ultrasound as early on as you can, which can also confirm or rule out a multiple pregnancy. If you're pregnant as a result of fertility drugs such as bromocriptine or gonadotropin-releasing hormone (GnRH) (see chapter 8), your risk of a multiple pregnancy or a miscarriage is no greater than that faced by the general population.

If you've had any kind of tubal repair surgery, your risk of an ectopic pregnancy is greater than that of the general population because your tubes may have scarred as a result of the repair procedure. You'll need to review the symptoms of ectopic pregnancy discussed in this chapter. Seek medical attention if you notice any of them.

If you're pregnant as a result of artificial insemination, your pregnancy is no more risky than a routine pregnancy (except for the multiple pregnancy issue if you had fertility drugs). If your pregnancy resulted from in vitro fertilization (IVF), gamete intrafallopian transfer (GIFT), intrauterine insemination (IUI), or any similar procedure (including microinjection), you not only have a higher risk of miscarrying but you also have the multiple pregnancy issue to rule out. Anything transferred directly into your fallopian tubes will make you more susceptible to an ectopic pregnancy. However, if your ART procedure involved transfer of gametes or embryos directly into your uterus, your risk of ectopic pregnancy is nil. You should definitely be seeing an obstetrician trained in reproductive endocrinology once your pregnancy is established, however, regardless of which ART you had.

Problems in the First Trimester

When something goes wrong at this stage, it has to do with the pregnancy not "taking." This usually means two things: a miscarriage (bleeding and cramping are the main symptoms) or an ectopic pregnancy (sharp, abdominal cramping or searing pain on one side—it depends on the tube). Often, women don't even *realize* they're pregnant until they experience a first-trimester problem like this. But these problems are common even in the general pregnant population.

Ectopic pregnancies were considered a less common occurrence until about five years ago, when the results of STDs, pelvic inflammatory disease (PID), and assisted reproductive technology started to factor into the childbearing population. If you've had PID (and well over one million North American women do), you are at a higher risk of suffering an ectopic pregnancy. If you're walking around with chlamydia or gonorrhea, you're also at risk. *Studies estimate that as many as 50 percent of all women between the ages of eighteen and thirty have chlamydia and don't know it.* This is why it's important to be screened for STDs prior to conception.

As for miscarriage, one in six pregnancies in the general population ends in miscarriage, *and 75 percent of these miscarriages occur before twelve weeks.* The risk of a miscarriage also increases with age. If you're over thirty-five and pregnant as a result of an IVF-like procedure, your risk of miscarrying is quite high.

Bleeding

Bleeding during pregnancy isn't normal, but it's not *unusual* either. Nor does it mean that a miscarriage is imminent. Some women may continue to have scant periods during this trimester. In fact, in the general population, some women don't realize they're pregnant until about three months into the pregnancy because of this. Although menstrual cycle changes usually won't be noticed until about weeks four and five, you can spot as early as seven days after conception. This is known as *implantation bleeding* and is a normal vaginal spotting caused by the formation of new blood vessels, but it's rarely experienced.

It's crucial to note whether any *pain* accompanies your staining or bleeding. Staining or bleeding with no pain is better news than staining or bleeding with cramps. Nevertheless, bleeding or spotting of *any* kind during this stage should be reported immediately to avoid any risk.

The most dangerous kind of bleeding at this point is heavy bleeding. The definition of heavy bleeding means that you need to change your pads about every hour. Other danger signs to watch out for are *additional symptoms* accompanying the bleeding, such as cramps, pain in the abdomen, fever, weakness, and vomiting. If the blood has clumps of tissue in it, this is also a bad sign. If this is the case, save your pad. Just stick your whole pad, clumps and all, in a baggie and save it for the doctor to look at. Put the baggie in the refrigerator until you take it to the doctor. If this isn't done (particularly if left overnight), the tissue degenerates and smells, and a pathology exam cannot be done. The clumps may be important clues to what's going on. You may also notice an unusual odor accompanying the bleeding. If light bleeding or spotting continues for more than three days, this is another, less obvious danger sign.

Does your bleeding *always* mean that you're losing the pregnancy? No. Vaginal bleeding can occur if you have an infection of some kind, lesions, a polyp, or a fibroid.

Regardless of why you're bleeding, you'll need to follow the emergency procedures outlined in this chapter. You'll then need to undergo an internal pelvic exam, a blood test to see if your level of hCG is normal, and an ultrasound.

Miscarriage

There are several reasons why a miscarriage occurs. Some studies indicate that about 60 percent of all first-time, first-trimester miscarriages occur because of genetic abnormalities. It's your body's way of doing its own "genetic engineering," expelling malformed fetuses. More than 90 percent of women who miscarry once will go on to have successful pregnancies.

Symptoms

Heavy bleeding and cramping anywhere between the end of the second month to the end of the third month are classic signs that you're in the process of miscarrying. Cramps without any bleeding are also a danger sign that you're miscarrying. The bleeding can be heavy enough to soak several pads in an hour, or may be "manageable" and more like a heavy period. You may also be experiencing *unbearable* cramping that renders you incapacitated. Sometimes you can pass clots, which are dark red clumps that look like small pieces of raw beef liver. Sometimes you may pass grayish or pink tissue. A miscarriage can also be taking place if you have persistent, light bleeding and more mild cramping at this stage.

If you suspect a miscarriage . . .

In the United States, if you're under the care of a private physician, you will usually have a chance to consult with your doctor about your symptoms over the phone (most of them are on twenty-four-hour pagers). Depending on your situation, your doctor may be able to evaluate what's going on just by what you're describing over the phone, ask you to come into his or her office for an ultrasound, which can determine the status of the pregnancy, or ask you to meet him or her at the hospital. If you *are* miscarrying, sometimes a dilation and currettage (D & C) procedure can be scheduled at a convenient time for you, rather than as an "emergency" procedure. In fact, many doctors in private practice can actually do a better job of evaluating the problem in their offices than in a hospital emergency room.

For American women in less exclusive health care plans, as well as Canadian women (whose physicians do not have appropriate ultrasound equipment in their offices), you will need to inform your doctors' offices of your symptoms and *go directly to the hospital (or your birthing facility)*. Ask your doctor(s) to meet you there. Someone will take care of you when you get to the hospital or birthing facility.

Once you're in the hospital, your doctor will be able to tell whether you're indeed miscarrying and what stage the miscarriage is in. He or she will do a gentle pelvic exam and/or ultrasound. You might be sent home with a list of instructions and told to wait it out, which is often the only thing to do. Sometimes it takes several hours for a miscarriage to run its course. Or, depending on what's going on, you might need to stay and have an emergency D & C procedure.

When you miscarry before twenty weeks, it's actually called a *spontaneous abortion*. However, there are several kinds of spontaneous abortions. Staying in the hospital or going home will depend on what kind of miscarriage you're experiencing, what stage it's in, and so on.

- *Threatened abortion*. Your cervix is still closed and holding everything in securely, but you're having cramps, bleeding, or staining. Your doctor will examine you and check the fetal heartbeat. You may also need an ultrasound. Then you'll be ordered to bed. In some cases, the bleeding will stop and the pregnancy will continue normally. Sometimes you might miscarry anyway because of unsalvageable problems, such as severe genetic deformities.
- *Inevitable abortion*. In this case, nature has already taken its course, and the process of miscarriage has started. Bleeding is heavy, cramps increase, and the cervix begins to dilate. You may wind up expelling everything while it's still intact: the fetus, amniotic sac, and placenta, accompanied by a lot of blood. This is the most traumatic kind of first-trimester miscarriage because you'll need to *save* what you've just expelled. Sometimes you'll have to retrieve these things from the toilet. If you're going through this, try not to be alone. Call a friend or make sure your partner is with you. If your doctor suspects an inevitable abortion, abnormal bleeding is usually heavy enough to warrant a D & C before any tissue passes out on its own. However, if a D & C is not done, the pregnancy tissue would come out on its own eventually. You'll need to save what you expelled in case your doctor wants to perform tests. But in general, it's difficult to determine the cause of an abortion by examining or testing expelled tissue.
- *Incomplete abortion*. This is when you're not naturally expelling all of the uterine contents. Some, but not all, pregnancy tissue has been spontaneously expelled. Usually what remains are fragments of the placenta. This needs to be

corrected with a D & C procedure, which will clean out the uterus and help it to heal. You'll still need to save part of what comes out, but it will just look like clumpy pieces of blood. You may be sent home from emergency only to have to go back into the hospital a couple of days later for the D & C.

- *Complete abortion.* This is when all pregnancy tissue is passed spontaneously. You will be sent home and will *slowly* expel everything by steadily bleeding. This will feel like a miserable period, but everything will come out in time. You still may need a D & C anyway just to clean out little bits of tissue left behind, but this usually isn't necessary. The bleeding can actually go on for days until you're finally done. In this case, save anything that looks like pregnancy tissue and show it to your doctor.

- *Missed abortion.* The fetus dies in the uterus but doesn't come out. You may not have symptoms for quite some time. This is when you just lightly spot and can mistake it for the "good bleeding." In this situation, all your pregnancy symptoms will gradually disappear, and you obviously won't progress at all. This condition is frequently diagnosed during a routine exam, and the fetal heartbeat can no longer be heard. Treatment depends on the duration of the pregnancy.

Will it happen to me?

Again, the risk of miscarriage increases with age. The risk is about 10 percent for women in their twenties and skyrockets to 50 percent for women in their mid-forties. This means that a significant portion of thirty-something pregnancies will end this way. There are all kinds of reasons why you might be miscarrying, but most women who miscarry either once or twice do go on to have normal pregnancies and deliveries. The odds of having a miscarriage tend to increase exponentially with each *recurrent* miscarriage. In general, with no past history of miscarriage, your odds of having one are about 12 percent. After one miscarriage, the odds remain at about 12 percent. After two miscarriages in a row, the odds of having another are 27 percent; after three in a row, the odds jump to 36 percent; and after four miscarriages in a row, the odds skyrocket to 60 percent. Because of this, it's important to *stop* trying after two consecutive miscarriages to be evaluated for factors causing pregnancy loss.

After one miscarriage, the expelled contents will be examined for any clear signs of why the miscarriage happened. Usually, a fetus is "self-terminating" because it wasn't developing properly. If this is the case, then there usually isn't a known cause for your miscarriage. You'll need to wait anywhere from three to six months after a miscarriage before you can try again, or resume fertility treatments. Choose an appropriate barrier method to prevent conception during this period.

One cause cited for miscarriage is an *incompetent cervix*. Some women are just born with an incompetent cervix, but it can be weakened by a previous miscarriage or therapeutic abortion. Other causes are chromosomal abnormalities, infections, hypertension or diabetes, and progesterone deficiency. Possible causes of miscarriage at this stage involve hormonal deficiencies that interfere with fetal development, uterine structural problems, genetic error, and blood incompatibility.

It's helpful to seek out other women who have gone through pregnancy loss as well. There are several support groups for women who have miscarried once or twice. Some women may have more severe reactions to pregnancy loss than others. These reactions may include sleep disturbances, psychosomatic illness, worsening of a previous illness (such as asthma), irritability, and avoiding social contact (particularly friends with children or friends who are pregnant). A good therapist can help you work through some of these feelings, which are valid and common under these circumstances.

Ectopic Pregnancy

An ectopic pregnancy, also known as a tubal pregnancy, occurs when the embryo never makes it to the uterus and starts to develop in the fallopian tube. Sometimes the embryo can even develop on the ovary or in the abdomen; in this case, it's known as an *abdominal pregnancy*, which *has* been known to go to term (but that's *Guinness Book* material). If an ectopic pregnancy goes undetected, it strains the tube, which isn't designed to expand like the uterus. Then, six to eight weeks after conception, the embryo will cause severe abdominal pain and possible vaginal bleeding. If the pain is more pronounced on one side, this is a textbook symptom of ectopic pregnancy.

Ectopic pregnancies are very dangerous. If your tube ruptures, you could suffer severe internal bleeding, which is a life-threatening situation. Common symptoms of ectopic pregnancy are sharp abdominal cramps or pains on one side. The pains may start out as a dull ache that gets more severe with time. Neck pains and shoulder pains are also common. You may also have a menstrual type of bleeding along with the pain, but the pain is the most *obvious* sign.

The problem with ectopic pregnancies in the general population is that often women don't realize they're pregnant until they have one. If you've been seeking fertility treatment, you'll typically have a pregnancy test before the start of each new cycle. There are also other high-risk groups for ectopic pregnancies that will help to alert you to the possibility.

- Women who wore intrauterine devices (IUDs).
- Women with a history of PID.

- Women with a history of pelvic surgery (scarring may block the tube and prevent the egg from leaving).
- Women with a history of ectopic pregnancy.
- Women pregnant as a result of assisted conception techniques, where gametes or embryos have been injected into their fallopian tubes.
- Women with endometriosis (see chapter 7).

If you have symptoms of ectopic pregnancy or suspect it, follow the instructions outlined in the emergency procedures section following. Your doctor will check your hCG levels (a pregnancy test), and an ultrasound will be done to see the condition of the uterus and fallopian tubes. Once the ectopic pregnancy is confirmed, you will need *emergency surgery and a skilled surgeon*. The surgery involves removing the embryo from your fallopian tube. This is delicate surgery, and you'll want someone who is capable of saving your fallopian tube if possible. Sometimes this isn't possible, and your fallopian tube will need to be removed (known as *salpingectomy*). Depending on the progression of the pregnancy, you may need one ovary removed as well (known as an *oophorectomy*). You'll then need to recuperate from surgery for at least a week. After surgery, you'll need to repeat some blood tests to make sure no embryonic tissue is left. Usually, women go on to have normal pregnancies afterward. You'll need to have at least two natural periods before you try to conceive again. If you have only one fallopian tube or one ovary, the remaining tube or ovary will "pick up the slack" and you'll ovulate regularly.

Although the incidence of ectopic pregnancy has increased, the fatalities from it have *decreased*. This is largely due to major innovations in *laparoscopy*. Many surgeons can safely remove the embryo, preserving the tube, through laparoscopy (operating with a thin telescopic instrument with the aid of a video camera), instead of doing more invasive abdominal surgery. In addition, some ectopic pregnancies can be diagnosed *before* there are any symptoms simply by checking levels of progesterone and hCG. Transvaginal ultrasound and uterine curettage are also helpful diagnostic tools.

How common is it?

Since 1995, ectopic pregnancies, once a fairly rare occurrence, are considered fairly common. Between 1970 and 1987, the incidence of ectopic pregnancies rose from 18,000 to 88,000, a *huge* increase, now accounting for 1.5 percent of all pregnancies in the United States alone. The consequences of an ectopic pregnancy may be upsetting. In women who aren't fortunate enough to have the ectopic diagnosed early, over half will not conceive again. Meanwhile, 10 to 15 percent of all ectopic sufferers will have a repeat episode.

What researchers *do* know is that many of the lifestyle habits discussed in chapter 3 seem to play a large role in ectopic pregnancy risk. Women who smoke less than ten cigarettes a day have been found in some studies to have a 40 percent greater risk of ectopic pregnancy. Women who smoke more than thirty cigarettes a day are *five times* more likely to have an ectopic pregnancy. Nicotine affects the mobility of the fallopian tubes. This may delay implantation because the tube contractions (which move the embryo along into the uterus) are affected by estrogen levels, which smoking seems to reduce. In addition, smokers can't fight off infections as effectively as nonsmokers, which puts them more at risk for certain STDs, which can lead to PID. Again, the increase in chlamydia and PID directly corresponds to the rise in ectopic pregnancies. One British study revealed that 76 percent of women who had ectopic pregnancies were also found to have antibodies for chlamydia.

Emergency Procedures

What's the definition of an *emergency* at this stage? Heavy bleeding, severe pain (cramps or abdominal), sudden, severe vomiting that doesn't seem to be related to your morning sickness, loss of consciousness, and, in later trimesters, symptoms of early labor. If you're taken by surprise by the symptoms discussed in the two sections above and feel that they are severe, immediately call your fertility specialist, gynecologist, or primary care physician's office. If it's during business hours, ask the receptionist or answering service at which hospital your doctor practices (they all will be affiliated with a hospital). Have the receptionist inform the doctor that you will meet him or her there and that you're leaving *now*! *Then, get yourself to the emergency unit of that hospital as soon as possible.* If you can't drive yourself or can't find someone to take you, by all means *call 911 and request an ambulance.* If it's after hours, there should be a recorded message at your doctor's office that gives out an *emergency number* and the *address* of the hospital he or she is affiliated with. If you're well enough to go on your own, have someone (friend, mother, spouse, neighbor) call that emergency number and arrange for the doctor to meet you at the hospital. If you're going by ambulance, the ambulance staff will call for you.

If for some reason you can't get a hold of any doctor, and he or she does not have pre-recorded emergency instructions, get yourself to the emergency unit of *any* hospital as soon as possible, either on your own or by ambulance. Once you're there and being looked after, the hospital will sort everything out and find the doctor and appropriate hospital for you. Never wait for the doctor to call you back. Also review the section "If you suspect a miscarriage" above.

Problems in the Second Trimester

The risk of ectopic pregnancy is almost nil beyond the twelfth week of pregnancy, while the risk of miscarriage really dramatically drops by this stage. Yet those women in a high-risk category will continue to worry about the pregnancy beyond the first trimester. Because of this, I've provided information on the kinds of problems to look out for beyond twelve weeks, even though your "danger time" technically has most likely passed.

When something goes wrong in the pregnancy at this point, it usually has to do with either *your* health—be it infection, structural problem, or injury—that might trigger a miscarriage or premature labor, or a problem with the *placenta*, which may trigger the same things.

Bleeding

This time, light or spotty bleeding is often caused by an increasingly sensitive cervix, which may be irritated in an internal exam or Pap smear (if you need one for any reason) or sexual intercourse. Notify your doctor immediately about the bleeding. Heavier bleeding at this stage can also be caused by either a low-lying placenta (*placenta previa*) or the premature separation of the placenta (*abruptio placenta*), but these problems are more commonly found in the third trimester. Bleeding can also be a sign, once again, that you're losing the pregnancy or that you're experiencing premature labor.

Late Miscarriage

Between the third month and twentieth week of pregnancy, a spontaneous abortion is known as a late miscarriage. The symptoms are similar to the first trimester miscarriage variations. In many cases, a condition known as an incompetent cervix is responsible. This is when the cervix dilates prematurely and cannot "hold in" the fetus. This condition is also known as a weak cervix. For the most part, the causes of an incompetent cervix are unknown, but trauma to the cervix as a result of infection, for example, can trigger premature dilation.

Incompetent cervices are also more common if you're a DES daughter due to a possible malformation of the cervix. See chapter 2 for more information on DES daughters. If an incompetent cervix is caught early enough, as may be the case if you've had repeated miscarriages at this stage, the cervix can be stitched up and the pregnancy can be resumed. Then, at around thirty-eight weeks or prior to labor, the stitches can be removed and a normal vaginal birth can take place. Some stitching techniques are permanent, however, and a cesarean section is necessary.

If the miscarriage is inevitable and can't be prevented, a D & C can be performed up until the twentieth week. A miscarriage after twenty weeks is no longer a miscarriage and graduates to either a premature birth or, in unfortunate cases, a stillbirth. Under these circumstances, you'll need to follow the steps outlined above under "Emergency Procedures."

Premature Labor

Premature labor is characterized by contractions accompanied by vaginal bleeding, vaginal discharge, or even a vaginal pressure anywhere from the twentieth week to the thirty-seventh week. Premature rupture of the membranes (the amniotic sac) occurs in 20 to 30 percent of all premature deliveries and is a sign that something is wrong as well. Other symptoms of premature labor are menstrual-like cramps with possible diarrhea, nausea or indigestion, lower back pain, and all the other symptoms of labor.

Between 5 and 8 percent of all deliveries are premature. The health of the premature newborn depends greatly on how premature the delivery is, what kind of neonatal care is available, the weight of the newborn, and how developed the newborn is. Babies born before twenty-five weeks (weighing slightly more than 2 pounds) have about a 50 percent chance of surviving, *assuming* that they're receiving appropriate treatment in a neonatal unit. When the newborn weighs 3 pounds or more, his or her survival jumps to about 95 percent.

What causes premature labor at this stage?

The causes of premature labor at this stage are unknown, but there *are* some factors that can trigger it:

- Poor general health: cigarette smoking and inadequate nutrition can increase your risk of premature labor.
- Diabetes and/or thyroid problems that have not been treated appropriately.
- Cocaine use.
- Syphilis (review chapter 2 on STD screening).
- Placental problems.
- Physical trauma, such as a car accident or a bad fall.

What should you do?

This is an *emergency situation* and can be treated with medications to postpone the labor. As soon as you begin contractions, contact your doctor immediately. You'll need to go directly to your birthing facility or the emergency room at the nearest hospital. Follow the "Emergency Procedures" outlined above. If you're successful in halting the contractions with medication, you may be put on strict bed rest for the duration of the pregnancy.

Depending on how severe the situation is, your doctor may decide to proceed with delivery. If your membranes have ruptured or you're having vaginal bleeding, there is no way you can stop the labor; you'll need to go ahead and deliver. If, however, you have ruptured your membranes but are experiencing *neither* contractions *nor* any vaginal bleeding, the pregnancy may be "saved" with medications and continue to term. This happens in about 25 percent of the cases. In the worst-case scenario, the baby is delivered prematurely and treated in a neonatal unit. Premature labor is more commonly a third-trimester problem, however.

A word about the premature labor "device"

A common drug used to delay the onset of labor is called terbutaline, administered via intravenous. This drug is normally used in asthma, but has shown to work in preventing the onset of labor, although the FDA has never actually approved terbutaline for premature labor.

The popularity of this drug has led to a "terbutaline pump," an at-home device designed to continuously pump terbutaline into women at risk of premature labor. Women are usually sent home with this pump armed with a very powerful medication. The FDA doesn't think it's a very good idea for women in delicate conditions to be alone and unmonitored with this very potent medicine. Some women are expected to use this medication for days or even weeks, even though there is no evidence that the pump is effective and is "potentially dangerous" according to the FDA. After it received numerous complaints by the National Women's Health Network, the FDA issued a warning to doctors against prescribing the terbutaline pump.

As of this writing, one pregnant woman has died as a result of the terbutaline pump. Other women have experienced a range of the drug's side effects, such as chest pain, irregular heartbeat, shortness of breath, or fluid in the lungs.

If you've been prescribed this pump, question your doctor about the risks before you use it. If you're using it now, call your doctor immediately and ask if you can stop using it.

Vanishing Twin Syndrome

Vanishing twin syndrome used to be considered more rare than it is now thought to be. Again, with the popularity of fertility drugs and assisted conception techniques, multiple pregnancies are on the rise. As many as 80 percent of all twin pregnancies will experience this phenomenon, in which the pregnancy starts out as a multiple pregnancy, but only one fetus actually develops.

Symptoms of vanishing twin syndrome are actually similar to symptoms of miscarriage: vaginal bleeding, cramps, or decreased hormone levels, but then a healthy fetus may be discovered during the ultrasound. More often though, there are no symptoms and the second twin is reabsorbed by the body, while remnants of the placenta and membrane may be delivered at the birth of the surviving twin. In some cases, remnants of a second placenta during delivery may be the only clue that a twin has "vanished."

This syndrome probably would not even have been discovered if it weren't for ultra-sound technology. With ultrasound, two fetuses may be detected as early as the first trimester, and then, in the second trimester, you may be told that one has "vanished." This can be traumatic for many women and is an experience that is not well documented or openly discussed. As ultrasound technology improves and more twin pregnancies are diagnosed in the first trimester, perhaps we will learn more about the reasons behind this phenomenon.

As a result of some of the risks associated with carrying multiple fetuses, some couples in very high-risk situations are opting for a procedure known as "selective reduction." Here, one or more fetuses is aborted to save the life of one or more fetuses in utero. This is a situation reserved for women who are in danger of losing all their fetuses preterm. Usually, this situation arises after an assisted reproductive technology procedure where multiple embryos are transplanted into a woman's uterus. In some cases, this situation arises in women with a history of difficult pregnancies and pregnancy loss. If you feel that you are a candidate for selective reduction, you'll need to discuss all the risks involved with your obstetrician.

Repeated Miscarriage

If you've miscarried more than twice in a row prior to twenty weeks, you're prone to what's known in lay terminology as "repeated miscarriages." (Clinical terms for this are *habitual abortion* or *recurrent fetal loss*.) This is considered a form of infertility, but in my opinion, labeling "repeated miscarriage" as "infertility"—meaning inability to conceive—is inaccurate! Repeated miscarriages have to do with an inability to complete the pregnancy. This is truly a different kind of problem than not *becoming* pregnant to begin with. Nevertheless, women who suffer from repeated miscarriages will need to undergo a battery of tests under the care of an "infertility specialist"—a reproductive endocrinologist/gynecologist.

If you have no history of full-term pregnancies, then you suffer from *primary repeated miscarriage*. If you've had one child or even a stillbirth at term, you have *secondary repeated miscarriage*. Tests include an *endometrial biopsy* (see chapter 6) and a *hysterosalpingogram* (where a dye is injected into your fallopian tubes, checking *not* for blockages, as discussed in chapter 6, but for uterine abnormalities). In most cases of repeated miscarriage, the cause is found; in a few cases, nothing is ever discovered as the definitive cause. Women who have suffered as many as six or seven miscarriages, however, can go on to have a successful pregnancy.

One cause of miscarriage has to do with untreated bacterial infections, such as mycoplasma. As discussed in chapter 2, if left untreated, mycoplasma can lead to an inflamed endometrium (endometritis), which can interfere with the embryo implanting. Another cause of some miscarriages is the effect of certain toxins, discussed in chapter 3, that include anesthetic gases (that's why the consent form for a surgical procedure tells you about a risk of miscarriage). Exposure to lead and mercury are also causes, but usually these toxins are discovered before a *second* miscarriage.

Other causes cited for repeated miscarriage include genetic problems, structural problems involving the uterus or cervix (such as an incompetent cervix, discussed before), luteal phase defects (discussed next), diabetes, and thyroid disease (if it's not treated promptly).

Luteal Phase Defects

Some doctors believe that a significant number of repeated first-trimester miscarriages are caused by a progesterone deficiency; others don't subscribe to this theory at all, even though there is strong evidence to support it.

Once your ovary spits out a follicle, the empty shell turns into a corpus luteum. If you imagine a single pea pod, the pea is the follicle, which will become the egg, while the pod is what will turn into a corpus luteum, which should produce progesterone once the embryo implants. Human chorionic gonadotropin (hCG), secreted from the developing placenta, stimulates the corpus luteum to make progesterone. As the placenta matures at about seven weeks, it takes over progesterone production. However, if the corpus luteum is not functioning properly and is therefore not making adequate amounts of progesterone, you will miscarry. Hormonal tests that include an endometrial biopsy will confirm whether you have this type of luteal phase defect.

The treatment is simple, involving daily dosages of natural progesterone in vaginal suppository form during the luteal phase of the menstrual cycle. Then, if conception occurs, progesterone suppositories are prescribed daily for the first twelve weeks of pregnancy. The average dosage is 50 milligrams of progesterone twice a day, but some women will be given a stronger prescription of 100 milligrams of progesterone taken two or even three times a day. Some doctors will also prescribe clomiphene citrate prior to conception, which will increase the amount of progesterone throughout the early stages of pregnancy. The progesterone suppositories are given once the pregnancy is established. Clomiphene citrate is also associated with lower incidences of miscarriage. Progesterone supplements are successful about 80 percent of the time in averting another miscarriage.

Repeated miscarriages can be caused by a scrambled LH (luteinizing hormone) surge. Normally, the LH surge occurs just prior to ovulation, but in some women, the surge can take place at the beginning of the cycle—common in women suffering from polycystic ovarian syndrome (PCO). The treatment is to be placed on a urofollitropin (pure FSH) or a GnRH analogue (see chapter 8 for details). This is still in the experimental stages, but studies show that this treatment is promising.

Immunological Factors

Between 20 and 25 percent of all repeated miscarriages are due to immunological problems. The woman's immune system causes her body to reject the fetus as foreign tissue for the same reason transplant patients reject organs. In this case, the mother's body is rejecting the father's antigens (also known as paternal antigens) that make up the developing fetus. This problem can often be solved through either passive immunization (injecting the mother with the father's antibodies prior to conception) or active immunization (injecting white blood cells from both the mother and father into the mother's body before conception). In either case, the point of this treatment is for the mother's body to get used to the father's cells so that they recognize the fetus later on as friendly. Some clinics report about a 70 percent success rate using this method. Usually, giving the mother only paternal white blood cells yields the best results.

Phospholipid antibodies and recurrent miscarriage

About 15 percent of immunological causes involve women who produce antibodies that indirectly cause clotting in blood vessels that lead to the developing fetus. The fetus is deprived of nutrients and dies in utero, which triggers a miscarriage. The good news is that there is now treatment for this condition, with the aid of aspirin, heparin (an anticoagulant), and corticosteroids.

If your doctor recommends daily aspirin therapy, you can start with a very low dose of baby aspirin (78 to 81 milligrams per day). There are very few side effects with this dosage. Women who take adult aspirin or high dosages of aspirin have complained of side effects such as nausea, heartburn, upset stomach, decreased appetite, and even microscopic amounts of blood in their stools. (Blood in the stools could be caused by hemorrhoids or may be evidence that you are having bleeding from your gastrointestinal tract.)

Experts also recommend that you avoid the following foods when you're taking daily low-dose aspirin: curry powder, paprika, licorice, prunes, raisins, gherkins, tea, and other than the occasional use of nonabsorbable antacids (Maalox, Rolaids). All of these are foods that can irritate your gastrointestinal tract.

Heparin is an anticoagulant often prescribed to prevent blood clotting problems. It's administered by subcutaneous (under the skin) injection (see Table 8.1, "Getting to Know Your Fertility Drugs" on page 173). Since some women have allergic reactions to it, a trial dose of 1,000 IU of heparin should first be done as a skin test. You should discuss all the short- and long-term risks associated with heparin use during pregnancy; it is not free from side effects and has also been associated with osteoporosis (bone loss). Because of this, many doctors will prescribe a calcium supplement along with heparin during pregnancy. You should also ask what conditions may prevent you from taking heparin.

Make sure you notify all your doctors if you're taking heparin (you should carry an ID card stating so in case of an emergency or accident). You should also stay alert to warning symptoms, such as:

- nose bleeds
- blood in the toilet, your urine, or stool
- uncontrolled or excessive bleeding lasting longer than fifteen minutes
- unusual bruising not at the injection site

Less Common Causes

About 15 percent of all repeated miscarriages are caused by a uterine structural problem, where tissue interferes with fetal development. This is usually correctable with surgery, depending on the severity of the defect. About 3 percent of repeated miscarriages are caused by an "incompetent cervix." This problem leads to second-trimester miscarriages and can be prevented by stitching up the cervix. While about 5 percent of repeated miscarriages (as opposed to single episodes) are caused by chromosomal abnormalities, this is not a "correctable" problem, but a "luck of the draw" cause. It is also the cause of most first-time miscarriages, which occur once in six normal pregnancies. In this case, couples need to keep trying until they strike a good mix of chromosomes.

How Many Miscarriages in a Row Should We Endure?

After two miscarriages, you should stop trying and go for diagnostic tests to see *why* you're miscarrying. Often, the reasons are unknown and you'll go on to have a successful third pregnancy. Even after two miscarriages, there's a 70 percent chance that your third pregnancy will be fine. But if a reason does turn up, it may be easy to fix, and finding the cause at this point will prevent further trauma to you. Keep in mind, though, that one or two miscarriages do not make you infertile and are generally *not* precursors to future problems.

When Should You Cut Your Losses?

There is no right answer to this question. For some couples, one miscarriage or ectopic pregnancy is enough for them to seek alternatives to natural conception. For other couples, natural conception is still a goal even after seven or eight miscarriages. The point is not how many pregnancy losses you *should* endure, but how many you *can* endure. Of course, it's always important to find out, if possible, what the cause of your pregnancy loss was. There are often logical explanations behind the loss, and they *can* be treated.

While no one can prevent you from trying to conceive as many times as you like, the following is a list of guidelines to help you decide what "enough" means to you, personally. This list was compiled with the help of several couples who have been through pregnancy loss.

How Do You Define "Enough"?

1. *What was the nature of your loss: miscarriage or ectopic pregnancy?* Repeat ectopic pregnancies are rare if you're clear of STDs and had your tube salvaged or removed. A second miscarriage in a row is statistically less common than a successful pregnancy following a second miscarriage.

2. *How many miscarriages have you had?* Again, if no cause for your second miscarriage was found, you're statistically more likely to have a successful pregnancy on your third try than a third miscarriage. And with every idiopathic (that is, no cause found) miscarriage, no matter how many in a row, the odds of having a successful pregnancy on the next try are greater than another miscarriage.

3. *If a cause was cited, is it treatable?* If a cause has been found for your pregnancy loss or losses, but there's no way of treating it, trying again will not make the problem go away. In fact, it will put you at risk for another loss. On the other hand, if there is treatment available and your doctor feels that your chances of carrying to term on the next try are better than half, you may regret not trying again.

4. *How old are you?* The risk of miscarriage increases with age, while the risk of Down's syndrome increases as well. You will need an amniocentesis procedure if you're over thirty-five, which carries a risk (albeit small) of miscarriage. Can you handle all these statistics? Can you handle the risk of Down's syndrome if you opt not to have an amniocentesis?

5. *How much technological intervention is involved with each conception?* If you're conceiving spontaneously with no fertility drugs and no ART procedures, obviously each conception attempt will involve less financial and emotional strain. You'll also need to take the above guidelines into consideration.

6. *How has the loss affected your relationship with your partner?* If the stress of your pregnancy loss or losses is straining your relationship, can it survive another loss? Or even the *risk* of a loss?

7. *How are you?* Are you a basket case at work? Are you having repeated nightmares? Are you sleeping? Are you depressed? Are you consumed with the loss/losses? Are you still in mourning? You shouldn't try again unless you're in good, emotional health, which leads us to the next guideline.
8. *Have you sought out counseling of some kind?* No one is emotionally "fine" after even a single episode of pregnancy loss. You need to seek out other couples who've gone through the experience and to air your feelings to a knowlegeable, qualified counselor. Again, you shouldn't attempt another pregnancy unless you're both in solid emotional shape.

Some of you may take the above guidelines, as well as those provided in chapter 9, and move on to the final chapter, "All the Alternatives." Some of you may have stopped reading this book long ago and are into your second or third trimester of a normal pregnancy (a fate I wish for all of you). Nevertheless, for many couples dealing with unsalvageable fertility problems (see also chapters 5, 6, and 7), the next chapter is one not to miss. Alternatives mean *options*, not failure.

12

All the Alternatives

THROUGHOUT THIS BOOK, each of you will have radically different fertility journeys and different outcomes to those journeys. Some of you may have solved your fertility barrier by simply adjusting your lifestyle habits. Some of you may have found a specific problem that was easily remedied through medical treatment. Some of you may have required more aggressive treatments involving fertility drugs or surgery, while some of you may have opted for one of the many assisted reproductive technology (ART) methods. Some of you may have conceived but have experienced one or more episodes of pregnancy loss. And, hopefully, many of you are well on your way to successful pregnancies.

Yet happy endings to infertility are usually not that simple. Somewhere along the way, when biological conception isn't happening, many of your different journeys will converge on one word: *alternatives*. Yes, there are alternate, fulfilling lifestyle choices that do not involve biological parenting. There are also alternative healing systems you can turn to, which may offer hope for infertile couples. This chapter will discuss all the alternatives you can consider, but since many of the topics covered here can become books themselves, please look on this chapter as an introduction to alternatives, not as a detailed treatise on the subject.

In addition to covering topics such as alternative medicine, alternative coping strategies, alternative parenting, and childfree living, there are some issues you need to deal with first: refusal of treatment and stopping treatment. These are decisions you need to make *before* you consider other options.

Refusal of Treatment

Although many people look upon infertility as an "illness" that requires treatment, there are few causes of infertility that are life-threatening. In other words, many conditions that cause infertility are compatible with a full life expectancy. Obviously, conditions such as cancer, infections, or abscesses would need immediate attention. But many hormonal imbalances, genetic or anatomical anomalies, or diseases such as mild endometriosis do not technically require treatment. Limited time and financial resources are very real considerations when you contemplate treatment. For some, treatments can take place only with great financial sacrifice: second mortgages, bank loans, loans from family members or friends, sales of cars and personal possessions, lost income from time off work. Sometimes, lost *jobs* due to poor performance or *too* much time off can be the consequence of treatment.

Refusal of treatment also has a social stigma attached to it. Other couples—both fertile and infertile—may view your decision as selfish and say things like, "You obviously don't want a child badly enough to make the *necessary* sacrifices." Parents may view your decision as a personal affront to deny them grandchildren. Refusal of treatment is a highly individual choice. There is no right or wrong candidate for this decision. I've provided guidelines that will help you decipher whether this very personal choice is a valid decision for *you*. This list was compiled through a variety of sources, including couples who have chosen not to seek treatment.

Guidelines for Making Your Choice

1. *Have you had a workup?* I suspect many of you reading this chapter haven't even *seen* a doctor yet! At least find out what the cause of your infertility is before you decide to "refuse." What if you have chlamydia or prostatitis? These infections could lead to other health problems that antibiotics can avert.

2. *Is your problem easily treated?* There's a big difference between taking antibiotics for an infection and having reconstructive surgery. Does your treatment involve a few urine samples (for retrograde ejaculation) or undergoing a vasovasostomy? Does the treatment involve some lifestyle adjustments or fertility drugs? In other words, is treatment invasive or noninvasive? Time-consuming or incredibly involved? Refusing a simple treatment may lead to regrets down the road.

3. *Is the treatment expensive?* Everyone has a different definition of "expensive," but if the cost of your treatment will interfere with your mortgage payments and other essential bills, you probably can't afford it without financial aid. (Don't be coerced by friends who may taunt you with: "It's *just* another thousand a month.

We spend that on eating out alone!" Or comments like: "That's *nothing* for what you're getting in return!")

4. *What financial aid is available?* Have you looked into this? If you're in good financial shape (that is, a low-risk borrower from a bank's perspective), a low-interest loan or refinancing a previous loan or mortgage may make your treatment affordable. On the other hand, if you're already in debt up to your eyeballs, the stress of treatment and paying for it might break you. Finally, if you have a poor credit history and no bank will give you a loan, this will also factor into your decision.

5. *What are the health risks of your treatment?* Chapter 8 describes all the risks involved with some fertility drugs, which may be enough to turn off any woman. Some people have severe reactions to anesthetics; others have chronic conditions that may cause adverse reaction to recommended treatments. If you don't want to risk future or short-term health problems from various drugs, this is a valid reason for not going ahead.

6. *What are your spiritual beliefs?* Some people truly feel that if they are meant to have children, it will happen naturally. This is absolutely valid.

7. *What are your moral beliefs?* Do you have a problem with the "playing God" overtones involved with fertility drugs and many ART procedures? If you do, this is a perfectly valid reason to refuse treatment.

8. *How does your partner feel about treatment?* This is a decision you need to make together. Some of the factors you'll need to look at are: Who has the problem? Whose body will require treatment and/or drugs? If you can't agree, you'll need to sort this out before you come to a final decision about treatment. Sometimes compromising and trying a single cycle of treatment (as opposed to the usual three to six months) solves the dilemma.

Stopping Treatment

Many people find that they can't stop treatment. Fertility treatment can become an addiction. Each new cycle offers new "hope" and that can be a "rush" that's hard to let go of. Being in treatment also occupies your time and distracts you that much longer from the reality that you don't have, and may never have, a biological child. There is also the issue of new treatments. There will always be something around the corner that has "promising" or better success rates. Coming to terms with stopping treatment may require the expertise of a counselor. Refer to "Addicted to Hope" on page 227 in chapter 9, which provides some information on stop signs you should watch for. There comes a point for every fertility patient when enough is enough.

Coping strategies when you're "in between"

Once you've opted for an alternative to "being in treatment," life can be filled with awkward moments that can catch you off guard. There will always be those family gatherings where someone is pregnant or announcing a pregnancy, or breast-feeding Junior at the table (which, as a breast-feeding advocate, I fully support, but recognize that it can be painful to watch). Here are some strategies to help avoid unwanted surprises and difficult experiences:

- Make an announcement of your own to family members, either privately (and they will spread the word) or in one fell swoop at a gathering. Something akin to this: "As many of you know/have guessed, John/Joan and I have been trying to have a baby. But things just aren't working out as we have planned, and we hope that you'll all support us in this difficult period. We have decided not to pursue/continue fertility treatments and are in the middle of exploring alternatives. All we ask is that you respect our decisions and be sensitive to our pain." The subtext to such an announcement is a warning to family members that you will not take kindly to the "just relax" or "I read that X or Y works" comments; nor will you appreciate sudden announcements of a sibling or sibling-in-law's pregnancy; or the hiding of such a pregnancy followed by the awkward "discovery." Fawning over (versus enjoying) babies in your presence would not be polite, either.
- If you'd rather not make an announcement about your infertility, you can discreetly make it known to certain family members you suspect may be trying to conceive that you'd like to be informed of any pregnancy announcements in private rather than in public.
- Have a few good rehearsed responses to "Do you have children?" or "When are you two going to announce?" When asked these questions, I always say: "It just wasn't in the cards, I'm afraid. But we tried." (Of course, a few clods have then said, "You know, they have treatments for that now," to which I respond, "I know; I wrote the book!")
- If holidays are difficult (Christmas, Jewish holidays, and so on), go away or make yourself unavailable via "unexpected deadlines" or the old standby, "I've already accepted at so and so's." If that's not possible, minimize your time at gatherings, by coming later or leaving earlier, staying at a hotel, and so on. Volunteering at soup kitchens or food banks is also a good way of refocusing your holiday spirit.
- Practice random acts of indulgence. (Comfort foods, good videos, and, especially, weekend getaways with room service at adult-only resorts.)

- Children-filled malls on weekends or during the holidays can easily be avoided, especially with the advent of online shopping and catalogs.
- When you're invited to children's birthday parties, or children-centered parties or gatherings, just say "I'd love to but can't." And don't you dare feel guilty, either.

Alternative Healing Systems

If you find the Western approach to infertility unsatisfactory and are uneasy about fertility drugs and ARTs, there are other systems of healing available to you. Couples who have already undergone some sort of conventional fertility treatment, or who have problems with repeated miscarriage, are often most attracted to alternative therapies.

All ancient, non-Western cultures, be they in native North America, India, China, Japan, or ancient Greece, believed that there were two fundamental aspects to the human body. There was the actual physical shell (clinically called the corporeal body) that makes cells, blood, tissue, and so on, and then there was an energy flow that made the physical body come alive. This was known as the life force or life energy. In fact, it was so central to the view of human function that each non-Western culture has a word for "life force." In China, it is called *qi* (pronounced chee); in India it's called *prana*; in Japan it's called *ki*; and the ancient Greeks called it *pneuma*, which has become a prefix in medicine having to do with breath and lungs.

Today, Western medicine concentrates on the corporeal body and does not recognize that we have a life force. However, in non-Western, ancient healing, it is thought that the life force heals the corporeal body, not the other way around!

Non-Western healers look upon the parts of the body as "windows" or "maps" to the body's health. In China, the ears are a complex map, with each point on the ear representing a different organ and part of the psyche. In reflexology (discussed later), it is the feet (which are "read") that can tell us much about the rest of the body and spirit. In Ayurveda, the tongue is read, while other traditions read the iris of the eyes. Western medicine doesn't really do this. Instead, it looks at every individual part for symptoms of a disease and treats each part individually. To the Chinese healer, the health of the uterus is connected to deeper causes of imbalance in the body. You'll be asked about your personal relationships, your diet, your emotional well-being, and your job. And, the treatment may involve a host of dietary changes, stress-relieving exercises, and herbal remedies. In other words, the body part is not seen as separate from the self.

The following outlines a few of the more popular systems of healing. There are, of course, no guarantees that your infertility will be reversed, but the following therapies can work wonders for your emotional and spiritual self. These therapies aim to ready the body for conception, and people exploring any of these systems are counseled that it can take time for your body to heal itself.

Ayurvedic Medicine

The Ayurveda is an ancient Indian approach to health and wellness that has stood up quite well to the test of time. It's roughly three thousand years old. Essentially, it divides the universe into three basic constitutions or "energies" known as *doshas*. The three doshas are based on wind (vata), fire (pitta), and earth (kapha). These doshas also govern our bodies, personalities, and activities. When our doshas are balanced, all functions well, but when they are not balanced, a state of disease (dis-ease as in "not at ease") can set in. Finding the balance involves changing your diet to suit your predominant dosha (foods are classified as kapha, vata, or pitta, and we eat more or less of whatever we need for balance); doing certain yoga exercises; practicing meditation; and avoiding or incorporating certain lifestyle habits.

Chinese Medicine

About three thousand years old and in the same way that Ayurvedic medicine bases the universe on three constitutions, Chinese medicine bases the entire universe on two: yin and yang. Temperaments, organs, foods, activities, and individual personalities are yin or yang. Yang is considered a male constitution, while yin is female. But in all individuals, both yin and yang coexist. In addition to yin and yang, there are five elements (similar to doshas in Ayurvedic medicine) that are based on fire, earth, wood, metal, and water. Different organs in our bodies correspond to different elements. Similar to Ayurvedic practice, when everything is balanced, all is healthy and the life force (qi) flows uninterrupted; when all is not balanced, qi can be disturbed and disease can set in. So, finding the balance is the goal of Chinese medicine. To restore balance, diet is either adjusted or supplemented with herbs, and pressure points in your body are stimulated through acupuncture (part of Chinese medicine) or massage, while your lifestyle habits may require change as well.

Acupuncture and infertility

This is an ancient Chinese healing art, which aims to restore the smooth flow of life energy or qi in your body, explained above. Acupuncturists believe that your qi can be accessed from various points on your body, such as your ear, for example. (The energy flows along meridians, or pathways.) And each point is also associated with a specific organ. An acupuncturist will use a fine needle on a very specific point to restore qi to various organs.

Each of the roughly two thousand points on your body has a specific therapeutic effect when stimulated. Acupuncture can be used in many ways to treat fertility issues:

- as an anesthetic
- as a pain reliever
- as an aid in controlling hormone levels (it is believed to help normalize hormones in the endocrine system by "opening up the right doors for the body")
- as a means of aiding tubal-factor infertility

Shiatsu and infertility

This is a form of massage that uses systematic stimulation along meridians to help restore the flow of energy throughout the body. If, for example, the ovaries are not functioning properly, a shiatsu therapist would attempt to decrease emotional stress (which is believed to cause upset in the nervous system) in order to regulate the function of the ovaries and the uterus. Shiatsu works with the premise that an imbalance (be it hormonal or emotional) can produce symptoms of infertility and that these symptoms can be improved by regulating overall energy balance in the body.

Herbal Therapy

Herbal therapy accompanies all healing systems but is discussed separately because you don't necessarily need to go toward any one healer to find herbs; they're in abundance in health food stores or nurseries, if you know what you want to grow. And we're flooded with information from numerous books on herbs to newspaper health columns telling us about cumin or garlic.

Every culture in the world has relied on plants and herbs to treat illness. Herbal therapies were taken as early as 4000 B.C. by the Sumerians, one thousand years before Chinese herbs were first used. By 3000 B.C., the Chinese were using over one thousand medicinal herbs.

North America is divided at the U.S. and Canadian border over where to classify herbs. Alternative medicine practitioners argue that pharmaceutical companies won't fund research into herbal therapies because these remedies are natural and, hence, cannot be patented.

The United States has sold over $880 million of herbs and vitamins a year since about 1993. Plant drugs are classified as "food" or "food additives" in the United States, and therefore many herbs are sold in grocery and health food stores or pharmacies. Canada allows the sale of drugs that have received a drug identification number—something which many herbs do not have. Those that cannot be found in pharmacies can be found in health food stores or Chinese herb stores (which large Canadian cities have in abundance). But a few natural products are actually banned in Canada, including melatonin.

Recommended herbs to promote fertility are:

- Black cohosh, blessed thistle, and dong quai are considered uterine tonics, helping to initiate the appropriate buildup of lining and to stimulate the hormone production. These herbs are also thought to stabilize both the adrenal glands and blood sugar levels (see PCO in chapter 7).
- Wild yam extract helps to raise progesterone levels and is considered helpful for treating endometriosis, as well as poor cervical mucus.
- Chase tree and beta carotene are considered helpful for improving luteal phase defects.
- Vitamin E and essential fatty acids are recommended to improve sperm counts.

Holistic Medicine

Holistic medicine was begun as a reaction to the rather narrow, body-focused approach of Western medicine. A holistic doctor will look at the whole person—body, mind, and spirit—and use a variety of Western or non-Western techniques to treat, based on the individual. Essentially, a holistic doctor enters into partnerships with patients, encouraging them to learn how to reduce risks of illness and how to choose therapies that they're comfortable with. It is an approach to health that emphasizes self-care and personal responsibility for wellness.

Homeopathy

This began in the early nineteenth century as a reaction to "heroic measures" commonly used to treat disease at that time, such as bloodletting, induced vomiting, and the application of massive doses of drugs. Pioneered by Dr. Samuel Hahnemann, a German physician who was trained in conventional medicine and chemistry, homeopathy was born out of a disillusionment with conventional approaches to disease.

Homeopathy is based on the theory that "like cures like," or what Hahnemann called the Law of Similars. Essentially, a substance that produces certain symptoms in a healthy person can cure a sick person who shows the same symptoms. He coined the term *homeopathy* from the Greek *homoios* and *pathos* (similar sickness).

To treat disease, a homeopath will use minute doses of substances over large amounts of substances. Hahnemann found that he could preserve the healing properties and eliminate side effects of a medication through a pharmacological process he called "potentization," a process where substances are diluted with distilled water. The more diluted a substance, the more potent it was found to be. As a result of this discovery, Hahnemann discovered the controversial Law of Infinitesimals, which basically means that good things come in small quantities. In fact, to prove the theory, Hahnemann constantly referred to the minute amounts of hormones our bodies produce, which are so potent that they govern our bodies.

Homeopathy was particularly popular in the nineteenth century with treating infectious diseases—particularly epidemics. Homeopathy is often confused with "holistic" medicine, but it's actually a different discipline. Homeopaths call their approach holistic because they believe they're not just treating one organ, but the entire patient. They see symptoms as positive signs that the body is trying to defend itself against an underlying disease. In fact, homeopathic drugs might even aggravate symptoms. A homeopath will say that a worsening of symptoms is really a sign that the body is stimulating its own self-healing mechanism.

Homeopathy involves very long medical-history-taking sessions. There are more than two thousand remedies used by a homeopath, all derived from various plant, mineral, animal, and chemical sources. Some examples include marigold flowers, onions, graphite snake venom, honeybee extract, and other wild concoctions. At first, these treatments may sound dangerous, but since the doses are so diluted, they are widely recognized as, at worst, harmless among the general population.

Naturopathy

Naturopathy encompasses a broad spectrum of natural therapies. In fact, it's now a recognized graduate degree in North America with two colleges in the United States and one in Canada, which grant the degree of naturopathic doctor (N.D.).

Naturopathy is not any one tradition of healing, but instead, an umbrella term that refers to an entire array of healing approaches, all based on the body's intrinsic healing powers. This tends to appeal to people who distrust prescription medications or are interested in preventive therapies.

N.D.s will aim to educate their patients about improper lifestyles, which can lead to more degenerative diseases, such as osteoporosis, for example. In many ways, N.D.s will probably not differ much from the advice of conventional doctors regarding low-fat, high-fiber diets, stress reduction, and so on. What they may do, however, is to treat blocked tubes through nutritional means instead of recommending surgery. They instill the belief that prescription drugs are costly and encourage reliance on natural medicine, including acupuncture, herbs, hydrotherapy, homeopathy, vitamin and mineral supplements, and so on. For example, certain oils can help to stimulate or regulate hormone production, such as evening primrose oil, flaxseed, and vitamin E.

Iridology

No healer believes that the eyes are "windows to the soul" more than an iridologist, who reads the iris. Iridology is not really a therapy but a diagnostic tool used by a wide variety of non-Western healers. Iridology observes changes in texture and color of the iris and correlates them with your physical and mental state of health. An iridologist may not only tell you about an unsuspected thyroid problem but tell you that you have an unhealthy relationship with your spouse. Many people have found the experience very accurate and helpful.

Iridology is also used to identify dietary deficiencies and accumulation of toxic chemicals in the body. In fact, in the same way that a Western doctor may send you for an ultrasound, a natural medicine doctor may send you to an iridologist to expand a diagnosis.

Originally developed in the nineteenth century by Ignatz von Peczely, a Hungarian physician, iridology was adapted for modern practice in the 1950s by Bernard Jensen, an American chiropractor. Jensen based his practice on detailed diagrams of the left and right irises. He then assigned every organ, many body parts, and bodily functions to a specific location on one or both irises.

Iridologists believe that the degrees of light and darkness in the iris give enormous clues to the body's general health. They also examine textures of fibers in the iris. Of course, Ayurvedic or Chinese practitioners will also examine the eyes not just for nearsightedness, but for clues to the body's general health. Iridologists will counsel you about nutrition or lifestyle habits, but for the most part, will send you elsewhere for treatment.

Reflexology

This is a twentieth century version of an ancient healing and relaxation technique that's as old or older than acupuncture. Western reflexology was developed by Dr. William Fitzgerald, an American ear, nose, and throat specialist, who talked about reflexology as "zone therapy." But in fact, reflexology is practiced in several cultures, including Egypt, India, Africa, China, and Japan. In the same way that the ears are a map to the organs, with valuable pressure points that stimulate the life force, here the feet play the same role.

In a nutshell, the "sole is qi to the soul." By applying pressure to certain parts of the feet, reflexologists can ease pain and tension and restore the body's life force.

Reflexologists don't limit themselves to the feet, however. They will also work on hands and ears, although the feet are the most common site. Like most Eastern healing arts, reflexology aims to release the flow of energy through the body along its various pathways. When this energy is trapped for some reason, illness can result. When the energy is released, the body can begin to heal itself.

A reflexologist views the foot as a microcosm of the entire body. Individual reference points or reflex areas on the foot correspond to all major organs, glands, and parts of the body. Applying pressure to a specific area of the foot stimulates the movement of energy to the corresponding body part.

Are There Risks?

Out of the roughly six hundred herbs available in the United States (fewer are available in Canada), less than twelve have been tested in scientifically controlled trials, which is the process that usually determines whether an herb is safe and works better than a placebo. About fifty of these herbs have been tested under more lax conditions.

As of this writing, the American Herbal Products Association, which is a trade group of herbal manufacturers, is compiling a reference manual on six hundred herbal ingredients, including directions for safe use. Some experts suggest comparing most of the herbs sold to coffee when weighing "dosage": Two cups of coffee per day is considered safe; five cups may cause headaches and nervousness; fifteen cups can cause serious side effects.

It's important to keep in mind that when it comes to researching alternative therapies, most Western researchers don't know enough about them to design proper studies. And many of these ancient disciplines just don't lend themselves well to Western-style research, such as double-blind controlled studies.

There are other risks with non-Western medicine that you should be aware of:

1. There is no scientific proof to support most of the treatments you'll be offered, or claims of the therapies.
2. Since there is no advisory board or set of guidelines that govern non-Western practitioners, the alternative "industry" attracts quacks and charlatans, and costs for some therapies are often prohibitive.
3. Academic credentials are all over the map in this industry. Again, beware of humbugs.

4. Certain preparations are boiled down in clay or metal pots, leaving residues of lead, mercury, arsenic, gold, or cadmium. And it's been reported that sometimes Chinese herbal preparations are laced with prescription drugs. You have to be careful and purchase from reputable places.

5. Dosages are all over the map. For example, the active ingredient in many herbs may not be accurately measured. One reason modern medicine moved away from herbal preparations is that drugs were easier to purify and standardize. When you buy ten 50-milligram tablets of a particular drug, that's what you get. But when you buy ten capsules of an herb, the dosages may vary from capsule to capsule.

6. Sometimes you're "blamed" for a treatment's failure. In other words, your body would have responded if your mind was more "open."

Finding Ethical and Qualified Healers

First, do some homework on the type of tradition that attracts you. Use this section as a guide to more thorough sources on the various traditions available. Then, use your "hairdresser" rules to find non-Western healers. Try to go to people recommended by other people with infertility. Keep in mind that depending on where you live, there may not be anyone practicing the kind of medicine you want. You may need to travel to a main urban center for your treatment.

Parenting Without Pregnancy

You can still parent a child without experiencing pregnancy and childbirth. In fact, this is often a satisfying solution to many infertile couples and is preferable to assisted reproduction procedures. Even in a book devoted to infertility issues, it's not possible to cover the range of adoption scenarios that exist, or the range of issues that surround each individual scenario, be it open, private/independent arrangements, or international adoptions. Entire books have been written about just one of the arrangements discussed in this chapter. Therefore, consider this a "get started" section about adoption, and consult the appendix for adoption resources. They can direct you to more detailed books that devote adequate space to the subject.

Creating Spiritual Offspring: Adoption

Adopting after the experience of infertility means that you need to revise your original definitions of parenting. There is considerable stress involved with repeated workups and reversing certain causes of infertility. Many couples will and *should* ask, "Is all this worth it for a biological child?" After reviewing their true motivations for wanting a biological child, many couples will *not* pursue infertility testing and assisted conception and decide to love a child that's already here. This is a logical decision, considering how many unwanted children there are who *need* parents! Unfortunately, there are two societal myths that interfere with a couple's decision to adopt: "Biological parents make *better* parents, and biological children make *better* children." *This just isn't true*!

I liken the decision to adopt to the experience of finding a lifetime partner. When we're in our teens, most of us fantasize about an ideal mate. The fantasy mate is far removed, of course, from *realistic* human relationships. Yet these fantasies are perfectly normal; *everyone* does it! After a while we learn through our own individual processes to let go of our fantasy mate. It is usually around this time that we meet our lifetime partner, who might have been there all along, or who we may seem to suddenly meet (when in fact it's more a case of recognizing qualities you were previously blind to). And, in cases where we *do* meet who we *think* is our fantasy mate, there is a period of "let down" when that person makes a mistake, and we are forced to admit that he or she really *isn't* perfect after all. Ultimately, whether we've met that person on a blind date, through the personals, or because we spilled coffee on him or her, most of us feel as though that person is supposed to be in our lives. If we didn't, we wouldn't make a lifelong commitment.

The process of adopting a child is similar. For all couples, there is a "fantasy child" that doesn't reflect the realistic experience of being a parent at all. Parents who have biological children soon discover that there is far less fantasy involved than hard reality when it comes to the real McCoy. But for an infertile couple, that fantasy child becomes a stronger image, which only reinforces the pain of infertility. The real truth is, having a biological child is *no* guarantee of lifelong happiness! To emphasize this point, an award-winning foreign TV commercial went to hilarious extents. The commercial opens with the line: "Two good reasons to use Brand X Condoms." Then, we are shown two sets of proud parents, circa 1900, fawning over their newborns. Their names flash across the screen: "Mr. and Mrs. Hitler" and "Mr. and Mrs. Mussolini."

The point is that couples who choose adoption need to let go of their fantasy child and accept that the child they're supposed to be with is not biological offspring, but *spiritual* offspring.

A Brief History of Adoption

Until the 1970s, adoptions in North America were handled by public or private agencies that had more babies up for adoption than couples who were willing to parent them. Yet because of greater sophistication regarding birth control, the legalization of abortion, and the destigmatization of parenting a child outside of marriage, there are more couples seeking to adopt a baby than there are available babies. Today more than half of *all* North American adoptions are *independent adoptions* (also known as *private adoption*). This is when birth parents are actively involved in finding an adoptive family. Although public and private agency adoption is still alive and well, the process usually takes longer and many of these agencies still allow no contact between the birth parents and adoptive parents.

It's crucial to note, though, that if you're willing to adopt an older child, a child who is a visible minority (even if you are, too), or a special needs child, you can expect a child from a public or private agency almost immediately. The average wait in these same agencies for a Caucasian infant is *four to eight years*. The wait is much less through independent/private adoption, translating into roughly six to nine months.

Today, many couples need to go outside their countries to adopt an infant or toddler, which is known as international adoption. I'll discuss some of the issues you need to be aware of if you're going the international route.

Getting Started

The maze of decisions, bureaucracy, and paperwork can be extremely overwhelming once you make your decision to adopt. The following are guidelines I've compiled from a number of sources to help you take your own baby steps into the adoption process.

General steps

1. *Contact local adoption and infertility support groups.* Your best source of information regarding adopting are from people who live in your community who have gone through the process successfully. Pick as many brains as you can. Infertility groups are also tremendous sources of information. Many people who join these support groups already have one or more adopted children.
2. *Search for government programs.* Whether these programs are at the local/municipal, state/provincial, or the federal level, find out *what* programs exist that can help you adopt a child in your own country or internationally.
3. *Read everything you can on the subject.* Before you decide what kind of adoption process is right for you, educate yourself about what's involved with each route: costs, time/wait, available children, necessary paperwork, and so on.
4. *Lawyer-shop.* Don't hire anyone yet. Just shop around and ask people you know and trust. (Use some of the strategies outlined in chapter 2.) Ask people you've met through the support group venue. To avoid the average $350 consultation fee, ask if the lawyer can send you information on his or her practice or give you names of satisfied clients. Ask if you can take the lawyer out to lunch for an hour or so just to meet. (Once you discuss your case, the lawyer may charge

you.) Or, as a last resort, ask for a ten-minute meeting. This will give you a chance to check out the office, the feel, the lawyer's initial persona, and so on.

5. *Beware of adoption "facilitator" services.* These usually translate into high fees with few leads.

6. *Hire a lawyer who specializes in adoption.* Do this before you tell anyone about your decision to adopt. That way, if you get an immediate lead, you'll have your lawyer there to negotiate the details. (If you're going the international route, see the separate section below.)

7. *Tell everyone and his or her dog that you want to adopt.* Even if you're planning on adopting internationally, the more people who know about your situation, the more likely you are of finding a child.

Independent Adoption

In independent adoption, also known as private adoption, the adoptive parents take an active role in searching for an infant to adopt. A lawyer represents the adoptive parents and makes all the legal arrangements for the adoption. The birth parents consent to placing the child directly with the adoptive parents, rather than using an agency as the middleperson. Usually, the birth mother is found during the later stages of pregnancy, and the baby goes directly from the hospital into the adoptive parents' home.

There are no set rules to adopting independently, but the best method is to find a family law practitioner who specializes in adoption. First, lawyers who specialize in adoption have a network of contacts that may lead to a child sooner. Second, it's crucial to have someone who can expertly negotiate a clear, contractual arrangement with the birth parents to avoid future legal battles over the child. Make sure that you and your lawyer sign a contract or agreement that clearly states costs in various scenarios, and outlines fees under more complex circumstances (such as adopting twins or siblings, waiting longer than expected, and so on). Your lawyer should also make sure that any money that's exchanged between you and the birth parents is confidential (that is, disbursing all money through an escrow account).

Announce your decision to everyone you can think of. Ask people to put out feelers for available children, and you may just get the call you've been waiting for: "The woman my aunt's cousin's sister works with is pregnant and unmarried and looking for a home for her child."

The next step is conducting a campaign, just as you would if you were starting a small business. Set up an unlisted toll-free number. Then create a print advertisement to be placed in various newspapers and specialty magazines. The headline may go something like: "Forty-something Couple Looking to Adopt." The body copy may read something like: "We're very eager to share our love with a child and form a family. Sadly, we cannot have children of our own, but we want to offer our love, values, and sense of family to a child who needs a home. For more information, call us at 1-800 555-5555." You may also want to consider a radio ad and even a television ad (on cheaper, cable-access stations) if your media budget permits. Some couples have even gone as far as using billboards to advertise their message.

Then, you'll need to conduct a *direct-mail* campaign. Compile the names and addresses of obstetricians, hospitals, clergy, family doctors, other family law practitioners, abortion counselors, high school counselors, student health services, women's health clinics, and other adoption services. (There are companies that have mailing lists you can purchase.) A good number to work with is about one thousand. Then, write a one- to two-page form letter to these people stating who you are, why you want to adopt, where you live, what your income is, what your cultural/religious beliefs are, what your professions are, and how you can be contacted at all times (business and home numbers, and numbers of friends or family in case you're away). You should also include your toll-free number and a business card. Photos of yourselves (one picture with two of you in an embrace), your home, other family members, and pets are also helpful. Attach letters of recommendation from colleagues or friends, as well as your professional résumés, so your work experience and education are crystal clear. Send out this package and see if you get a response.

Once you find your lead, you and your lawyer will work out financial details that may involve paying for the birth mother's medical and counseling expenses, some living expenses that pertain to the health of the child while the birth mother is pregnant, and, of course, all prenatal and neonatal medical expenses. You should not be expected to pay enormous sums of money for the child (a fee of, say, $20,000, over and above all reasonable expenses). Keep in mind that some sort of fee to the birth mother may be expected as a way of compensation, but this usually isn't done. (Compensation fees for the birth mother are legal in some places and illegal in others.)

There are agencies that claim to be independent adoption facilitators, but there are numerous horror stories about many of these services, which require an up-front nonrefundable fee and eventually yield no leads. Be careful. Ask to see a list of satisfied clients and check out the credentials of the people running the agency first.

If all goes well and you've found a birth mother who consents to place her child with you, you'll need to cough up your birth certificates, marriage certificates, medical records, notarized current financial statements, income tax returns, and employer letters verifying your position and salary. You'll also need to have what's known as a "home study" done. This is where a social worker (either independent, or as part of an agency) comes into your home and asks you invasive questions about your private life, assesses your home and neighborhood, assesses your personal qualities and values, and so on. A report is prepared for the birth parents prior to their consent. This same social worker may conduct follow-up visits during the first six months you have the child.

Again, independent/private adoptions are the most popular form of adoption in North America. (Often, many couples will move on to international adoption if they're unsuccessful in adopting independently.)

The independent steps

The following is a summary of the general steps involved with independent/private adoptions:

1. Self-educate (read, network with other adoptive parents, and so on).
2. Hire your lawyer. (See above for more details.)
3. Assemble your paperwork (birth/marriage certificates, letters of recommendation).
4. Contact a certified social worker to do your home study. (This may also be a later step once you find the birth parents.)
5. Install an unlisted toll-free number and plan your ad and direct-mail campaign.

Steps when you get a response . . .

1. Put together a list of interested birth parents and screen out the "undesirables" (you'll have your own criteria for this).
2. Make a short list of birth parent candidates and ask to meet them *with your lawyer present*. Keep in mind that it's a birth parent's market, though. They may not want to do this and may wish to meet with you privately without disclosing any identifying information, or they may not want to meet until the child is transferred to you.
3. Have your lawyer do all the necessary checking regarding background, medical records, test results for HIV, alcohol, or drugs. Your lawyer will also help the birth parents find legal representation.
4. Contact your pediatrician and let him or her know that information about the child might be forwarded in the near future.
5. Wait for the birth of the child.

Open or shut?

Independent adoptions may be open, semi-open, or closed. In an open adoption, you meet the birth parents in person and share full identifying information. You may also have ongoing contact over the years, either in person or through correspondence. The birth parents may visit the child as frequently as you and they are comfortable with, and may even become extended family members. This is a new and healthy approach to adoption, but it only works if *all* parties involved are mature individuals.

In a semi-open adoption, you meet the birth parents but they don't give you any identifying information about themselves. In turn, you agree to send them pictures and updates on the child for a limited period of time, to be negotiated by your lawyer.

In a closed adoption, you never meet the birth parents and have everything done through your lawyer. You essentially have no direct contact with the birth parents, and you don't send them any pictures or updates on the child.

Public and Private Agencies

Private adoption shouldn't be confused with private *agency* adoption. There's a huge difference. Official adoption agencies are state- or provincially regulated private or public agencies that "project manage" the adoption from beginning to end. While the wait can be longer, these adoptions are considered safer in that there's less risk of the birth parents changing their minds; the birth parents have relinquished their legal rights to the children, placing them in the agency's care. However, as long as you have a lawyer handling your independent adoption, this perception of more safety is a bit of a myth.

The usual process involves contacting the agency, being informally screened, and discussing the agency's fees and rules. The agency will then screen you for acceptability before they put you on a waiting list. They'll also conduct a home study (in fact, the home studies now required for independent adoptions were borrowed from these agencies). Then the wait begins. When a child is placed with you, there is a three to twelve month adjustment period you'll have to live through until the child is legally yours. If there are adjustment problems, a social worker will try to resolve the problem rather than take away the child.

The only steps involved in this process are educating yourself about the types of adoptions possible *before* choosing this one, and then shopping around for the agency you think will best serve you. Try to use an agency that someone has referred you to. You should also have a lawyer representing you who can negotiate any documents or contracts you need to sign and find anything potentially fishy about a contract you sign.

International Adoption

If you're willing to spring for airfare and a long list of other costs, you might consider this option. Outside of North America, there is a very high orphan population. You'll need an immigration lawyer and possibly a family law practitioner to help you, but the exact process involved in an independent adoption really depends on the *country* you want to adopt from. Every country has its own rules and required documentation. Throughout North America, there are consultant agencies set up to act as a liaison between your own country and the child's country. *You cannot get anywhere without a liaison.* These liaisons locate foreign child-placing sources on your behalf. They'll make contact with the foreign source and will assist you in compiling your documents.

International adoption is a huge topic that I cannot possibly do justice to in one section. However, I've outlined some of the requirements involved for the most popular regions. For all regions, it's important that the adoptive parents try to visit the country prior to adopting. In many cases, one parent can visit the country and bring the child back to North America within a couple of weeks. There are lists of international adoption agencies and liaison services through local adoption networks, infertility networks, and departments of immigration.

Europe

Any married couple of any age, regardless of divorce history or number of previous children, may adopt here. Europe is also open to single parents. Each country in Europe monitors adoption through local courts of the country of the adoptive parents and of the child. These children are of Byelorussian, Ukrainian, Russian, Slovakian, and other European origins. Most of these children are either in orphanages or hospitals, where they were abandoned by their unmarried mothers at birth. There is often no reliable information about their histories. Many of the children are malnourished and therefore have slightly stunted physical growth that resumes normally once they're fed and clothed properly. There are many babies that are newborn or older that are immediately available.

Immigration requirements for the United States and Canada involve filing various documents and fees with local and federal immigration services so that your child can receive a visa to travel back to North America. This process, including application fees, registration fees, and dossier fees, can cost roughly $10,000 or more. This does not include transportation costs or legal fees. The entire process costs $40,000 (a conservative estimate).

China

Married couples thirty-five years or older without children may adopt, while single adults are not given priority. If you're younger than thirty-five or already have children, some exceptions may be made, but don't count on it. Look for another country. You must be willing to adopt girls, because generally the only children available are girls ranging from newborn to two years old. Infants from Hunan and Jiangsu provinces are available, and some will have correctable handicaps. You're looking at roughly the same costs as a European adoption, once you factor in legal fees and plane fares.

Latin America (Central and South America and Mexico)

Couples over twenty-five years of age who are childless will be given preference to couples who already have one or more children. The countries most popular include Bolivia, Brazil, Chile, Colombia, Ecuador, Guatemala, Honduras, Panama, and Peru. Paraguay and Mexico are also popular areas. The children are mostly of Hispanic or Indian heritage, and in one or two countries, children of African heritage are available. The costs involved are roughly the same as a European adoption.

Documentation requirements

1. Certified birth certificates for each adoptive parent and family member
2. Certified marriage license and/or divorce decrees
3. Financial statement
4. Medical examination for each adoptive parent and each family member
5. Police clearance forms by local police, stating that each adoptive parent has no criminal record
6. Advanced approval through either the Immigration and Naturalization Service (advance processing approval document I 171-H) in the United States, or Immigration Canada (Undertaking of Assistance document, issued by Immigration Canada and accompanied by the Letter of No-Involvement, issued by MCSS Adoption Desk for immigration purposes)
7. Approved home study by licensed agency
8. Employment letter for each adoptive parent
9. Letters of reference
10. Photo of home and adoptive parents
11. Intention to adopt form (prepared by your liaison agency)
12. Power of attorney (prepared by your liaison agency)
13. Passport
14. Photocopy of your most recent tax form

Two sets of your documents need to be supplied: one set in English, for North American proceedings, and one set in the language of the country you're adopting from, for the adoption proceedings in that country.

Adoption Myths

"So-and-so adopted and then got pregnant. If you start the process, you'll probably get pregnant, too!" This is one of those stories *every* infertile couple hears from a reliable source, who *swears* it really happened. Well, it *rarely* happens, and unfortunately, it's the kind of myth that's really not helpful for anyone looking to adopt. All you can do is reply with something like, "If I wanted to get pregnant, I'd (still) be in treatment."

Myth number two: "Well, you *know*, these kids might have learning disabilities and other problems . . ." *This is the exception, not the rule.* Although it's true that many older children who are put up for adoption may have been born to drug-abusing mothers or raised for a time in an abusive home, no agency in the 1990s will withhold this information from you. A child's medical records and history will be *made absolutely clear to you*! If the child you want to adopt is dysfunctional emotionally, this will surface during your adjustment period, before the adoption is legal. The child may take longer to trust you or may need extra therapy, but these problems are usually workable. In more extreme cases, the agency will categorize that child as a "special needs" child from the outset, so any emotional problems will come as no surprise, and you'll *choose* whether you want to take them on.

In an international adoption, children's medical histories are less straightforward. You can have the child checked out by a qualified pediatrician before you agree to take him or her back to North America. If you suspect an abusive background, appropriate therapy and your influence as a loving parent can help that child overcome it.

However, more adoptions now go the independent route anyway, which means that you'll meet the birth parents (or at least the birth mother) and you will have complete access to the parents' and child's medical histories. These stipulations can be negotiated in your contract!

As for the learning disability issue and psychological adjustment problems, this is a societal bias. All children, whether biological or adopted, may experience periods of emotional turmoil. It's all part of the precarious nature of life on earth. This can be caused by an unstable home environment, by an experience that traumatizes the child (witnessing something frightening, getting lost, and so on), or by external factors, such as school adjustment problems. How well your child adjusts to life in general has more to do with who *you* are as a parent. If you're a psychologically stable, loving, and mature person, this will have an impact on how well your child adjusts to the emotional challenges (including finding out about the adoption) he or she will confront. Remember, *nobody* is immune to trauma and adversity.

Childfree Living

Every family has that one kindly aunt and uncle who "never had any children." And, until you *yourself* have struggled with infertility, you probably never wondered *why* they had no children; you just accepted it. Well, if that aunt and uncle of yours are now seniors, in their day they could have adopted from a wide assortment of newborns. *But they didn't.* Today, they probably live comfortably in a small condo somewhere, travel a great deal, are enjoying their retirement, and dote on a large selection of nieces and nephews. When they pass on, they'll probably leave their money to their "favorite" niece or nephew and will always be fondly remembered.

Now, compare *that* lifestyle to the "other" aunt and uncle who have three miserable sons who "eat their hearts out." Everyone in the family knows that these sons scammed their own parents out of their life savings. One son is a stingy businessman who nobody in the family likes, the other is a cocaine addict who sold his father's collector's edition car to buy more coke, while the third son is a bum and has never worked an honest day in his life!

I exaggerate these two lifestyles to point out that there is no guarantee of happiness either way. Some couples with children wish they'd never had them; couples with no children may regret it. The decision *itself* is not as important as how *comfortable* you are with your choice.

In the past, a childfree lifestyle was often a *political* decision for many couples. During the 1950s and 1960s, many couples chose this because they feared a nuclear holocaust. By the 1970s, the issue of overpopulation became the motivating factor for the choice. For example, research at Cornell University recently concluded that the world's population must be reduced from its estimated six billion to roughly two billion by the year 2100. However, population predictions for that year, given current fertility trends, are for roughly fifteen billion. Once we factor in available natural resources, energy reserves, and arable land, a world population of that size would throw the majority of individuals living at that time into "absolute misery, poverty, disease, and starvation" (according to the Cornell paper). Overpopulation is also a major factor in gender inequity, according to many sources. Where there's high birth rates and high poverty rates, the economic value of female children goes down. Yet by the 1980s, childfree living became a symbol of infertility and failure, a symbol that has prevailed into the 1990s. This is a pity, considering what a liberating lifestyle option it can be. Obviously, you'll need to review your original reasons for wanting children before you make this choice. You'll also need to research the decision: Interview other couples who are living childfree and investigate *their* lifestyle. Interview couples with children and find out how much of their own lives are sacrificed.

Some fertile couples are choosing childfree living because of environmental and financial concerns. Many truly feel that the world is an environmental disaster area and they do not wish to raise children in a world of questionable health hazards. Other couples find that they can barely meet their bills as it is, and opt not to add more stress to an already badly strained budget. Remember, parenting is a selfless, largely self-sacrificing job. Choosing a childfree lifestyle may be an appealing option in an economically turbulent and difficult world.

Some of the traditional reasons for having children were *purely* economic. Children, many people thought, guaranteed financial security in old age. Today, with so many college-educated adults living at home because they cannot get jobs, the economic benefits of progeny are no longer visible. And you'll find that most senior-age parents of financially successful children today do not want to be a financial burden and will choose to be independent as long as they can. Another traditional reason for having children was fear of loneliness in one's old age. Twenty years from now, the majority of the population will be over age sixty-five. You won't be lonely.

The Benefit Package

1. *Freedom.* You may have the time and extra money down the road for all the things you dreamed of: going back to school for that second degree, buying a vacation home, traveling, early retirement, or whatever you want.
2. *Control of your life.* When you have children, you lose a certain amount of control over your own life. Children can have lots of problems. They may have difficulty at school, they get sick, they have accidents, they get in trouble, they get pregnant, and so on. You never stop being a parent.
3. *Self-expansion.* You'll have the time to explore parts of yourself that you never knew existed, because you'll have time to *yourself*. Insights about your life, your gifts, your talents, your desires, your interests can be explored. Here are two images to keep in mind: Katharine Hepburn at age seventy, and any other seventy-year-old whose life was ruined because of his or her children. I'll take Katharine Hepburn's life any day.

At any rate, whatever your reasons are for living childfree, the decision is, of course, *reversible* anytime you wish.

Social Parenting

This is what you get when you cross adoption with childfree living. You can become involved with the children in your life: nieces, nephews, godchildren, or friends' children. One woman I interviewed has a toy chest and children's book library that is the envy of all her friends. She spends precious quality time with many of her friends' children of all ages. The children love her, the parents love it because they get a break from their kids, and she benefits enormously. She has become that one special grown-up the children can confide in, yet she can also influence their developing values and skills. She shares in their successes and trials of childhood. "I've never met a child who doesn't have room to love one more person," she tells me.

If you're like me, this may be the first section you've turned to in this book. Whether you're heterosexual or gay/lesbian, just in the planning stages of conception, going through a conception struggle or workup, experiencing repeated miscarriages, undergoing treatment, or experiencing secondary infertility, you haven't been left out of this fertility book. You'll find many of the answers to your questions here, as well as information regarding several difficult issues that may be concerning you. You'll learn how lifestyle or work habits affect your fertility, how to find a fertility specialist, how to gauge your menstrual cycle, the many causes of and treatments for infertility, and all the alternatives to biological parenting. Take this book to the doctor with you, read it, and share it with your friends. Good luck and good health.

Appendix

Links from sarahealth.com

For more information about disease prevention and wellness, visit me online at www.sarahealth.com, where you will find over 300 links—including these fertility links—related to your good health and wellness.

American Society for Reproductive Medicine: www.asrm.com

Center for Endometriosis Care (CEC): information on diagnosis, education, and treatment. Free newsletter. www.centerforendo.com

The Cradle: professional resources and tips about adoption and post-adoption services. www.cradle.org

Fertilitext: information and news on those pursuing fertility treatment. www.fertilitext.com

Infertility at About.com: http://infertility.about.com/health/infertility/mbody.htm

Infertility Center at Women's Health Interactive: assessments, evaluations, tests, and treatment. www.womens-health.com

Infertility Resources: information about IVF, GIFT, ICSI, infertility clinics, donor egg and surrogacy services, sperm banks, adoptions, and so on. www.ihr.com/infertility

International Council on Infertility Information Dissemination (INCIID—pronounced "inside"). Great information on all aspects of infertility and many useful links. www.inciid.org/

IVF.com: home of the Atlanta Reproductive Health Center online. Interesting information, with chat and useful links. Articles on pollution and infertility, and so on. www.ivf.com

Male Infertility: assessment, physiology, clinical findings, pretesticular causes, and diagnosis. www.mindspring.com

Mothers of Supertwins (MOST): information, resources, empathy, and humor for moms of triplets or more. www.mostonline.org

National Adoption Information Clearinghouse: adoption online publications and database with inter-country and special needs information. www.calib.com/naic

Natural Methods: family planning and natural product information. www.3.sympatico.ca/mikeboni/nm/babycomp.html

North American Council on Adoptable Children: www. members.aol.com/nacoc

OBGYN.net: physician-reviewed services for medical professionals and female consumers. Publications, fact sheets, and global interactive resources. www.obgyn.net

Organization for Parents Through Surrogacy: www.opts.addr.com

Parents' Place: information on contraception, conception, infertility, and secondary infertility. Chats. http://parentsplace.com/fertility

Poly-Cystic Ovarian Syndrome Association Inc: www.pcosupport.org

RESOLVE: advocacy, support, and education. www.resolve.org

State Infertility Insurance Laws (from the American Society for Reproductive Medicine): www.asm.org/patient/insur.html

Surrogate Mothers Inc: alternatives to infertility and current trends in surrogacy. www.surrogatemothers.com

Turner's Syndrome Society of the United States. www.turner-syndrome-us.org

Glossary

AH. Assisted hatching; a technique used to dissolve the outer coating of the embryo so that it can properly implant.

AI. Artificial insemination; where sperm is inserted into the vagina or uterus through artificial/assisted or unnatural means.

AIDS. Acquired immune deficiency syndrome; caused by the human immunodeficiency virus. Someone with AIDS has a compromised immune system and is vulnerable to a host of infections.

Amenorrhea. No menstrual cycle.

ART. Assisted reproductive technology; once known as artificial reproductive technology, a range of techniques used to assist couples or single women with conceiving.

Asthenospermia. Poor sperm motility (movement).

Azoospermia. No sperm.

BBT. Basal body thermometer; a special thermometer that measures optimal body temperature for conception.

Candidiasis. Vaginal yeast.

Chlamydia. One of the most common STDs in North America right now, chlamydia is usually asymptomatic, but can lead to complications during pregnancy or childbirth.

Cryopreservation. Freezing of gametes or embryos and other reproductive materials.

Cystitis. Inflammation of the bladder.

Cytomegalovirus (CMV). A virus that is only a danger to pregnant women, or those with a lowered immune system.

D & C (dilation and curettage). A procedure used to scrape out the contents of the uterus, often done after a miscarriage.

D & E (dilation and evacuation). A procedure used to terminate a pregnancy in the second trimester. It involves a synthetic dilation of the cervix and a subsequent suctioning out of the contents of the uterus with a vacuum pump.

DES. Diethylstilbestrol; a synthetic estrogen used between 1941 and 1971 in the United States.

DES daughter. Any woman born to a mother who took diethylstilbestrol (DES) runs a higher than normal risk for reproductive organ abnormalities, cervical and vaginal cell changes, and cancer.

DI. Donor insemination; a procedure that uses donated sperm. Pregnancy is achieved using artificial insemination (AI) or another assisted reproductive technology (ART) procedure.

Dysmenorrhea. Painful menstruation.

Egg retrieval. An ultrasound-guided needle aspiration procedure where eggs are retrieved from the ovary.

Embryo. A fertilized egg after it divides.

Embryo biopsy. A procedure where cells are taken from the embryo to screen for genetic anomalies or sex selection.

Embryo transfer. The process of transferring the embryo from the petri dish into a woman's uterus.

Endometriosis. A condition where pieces of the uterine lining grow outside the uterus, which can block the fallopian tubes and cause infertility.

Endometritis. Not to be confused with endometriosis, this is an inflammation of the endometrium.

Endometrium. The uterine lining.

Epididymovasostomy. A procedure where blockages in the epididymus (see next) are repaired through microsurgery.

Epididymus. A coiled, tubular organ attached to the testes where mature sperm learn to "swim" and fine-tune their capacity to move.

Fecundity. The capacity to reproduce.

FSH. Follicle-stimulating hormone; the sex hormone that stimulates a woman's ovaries to produce follicles, which become eggs.

Gestational diabetes. Diabetes during pregnancy.

GIFT. Gamete intrafallopian transfer; an outdated procedure where eggs and sperm are transferred directly into the fallopian tubes. Some clinics are still offering this as a cheaper alternative.

GnRH. Gonadotropin-releasing hormone; the hormone that both sexes secrete to kick-start the other sex hormones.

Gonorrhea. Another fairly common STD that is more damaging to women than it is to men.

Group B streptococcal (GBS) disease. Group B streptococcus is bacteria that normally lives in your vagina, rectum, or throat but is the leading cause of infections in newborns.

hCG. Human chorionic gonadotropin; a hormone that is produced by the developing placenta in pregnancy, which is what a pregnancy test detects.

Hepatitis B. A virus that causes inflammation of the liver. This is a serious STD that is transmitted through contaminated needles or blood.

hMG. Human menopausal gonadotropin, once made from the urine of menopausal women. This is a powerful fertility drug that stimulates the ovaries to produce eggs. It is a potent form of follicle-stimulating hormone (FSH).

HPV. Human papillomavirus; a sexually transmitted disease that causes genital warts. It is also the virus believed to cause cervical cancer. Safe sex can prevent HPV.

HSV. Herpes simplex virus; a sexually transmitted disease that causes periodic and painful sores and/or blisters above and below the waist. Safe sex can prevent HSV.

Hyperthyroid. Too much thyroid hormone, as in Grave's disease.

Hypothyroid. Too little thyroid hormone, as in Hashimoto's disease.

ICI. Intracervical insemination; where semen is artificially placed directly into the cervical canal via catheter.

ICSI. Pronounced "ixy," intracytoplasmic sperm injection is a procedure where a single sperm is injected into the egg to create fertilization artificially.

Incomplete abortion. When some, but not all, pregnancy tissue has been spontaneously expelled.

Inevitable abortion. When the process of miscarriage has started. Bleeding is heavy, and you may wind up expelling everything while it's still intact.

IUI. Intrauterine insemination; where semen is artificially placed directly into the uterus via a catheter.

IVF. In vitro fertilization; where egg and sperm are placed in a dish and fertilized. The resulting embryo is then transferred back into the uterus for implantation.

Laparoscopy. A surgical procedure that uses a thin telescopic instrument with the aid of a video camera.

LH. Leutinizing hormone; a sex hormone that stimulates the ovary to "spit out" the follicle or egg, known as the "LH surge" in a woman's cycle.

Menarche. A woman's first period.

Menopause. A woman's last period, technically.

Menorrhagia. Heavy bleeding during menstruation.

MESA. Microsurgical epididymal sperm aspiration; a procedure where sperm can be extracted directly from the epididymus (where mature sperm gather) in males who cannot ejaculate due to obstruction rather than sperm production.

Missed abortion. When the fetus dies in the uterus but doesn't come out. Treatment depends on the duration of the pregnancy.

Mycoplasma or ureaplasma urealyticum. An asymptomatic bacterial infection that is more often than not a sexually transmitted disease (STD).

NRTs. New reproductive technologies; a term sometimes used instead of assisted reproductive technology (ART).

OHSS. Ovarian hyperstimulation syndrome; a dangerous condition where the ovaries enlarge due to overstimulation from fertility drugs.

Oligospermia. Low sperm count.

Oocyte. Egg.

Oocyte donation. Egg donation. (A younger woman is stimulated with fertility drugs to produce numerous follicles or eggs, which are then retrieved and used to achieve pregnancy in an older woman or a woman who cannot produce eggs.)

Oophorectomy. Removal of the ovary(ies).

Oophoropexy. Where the ovaries are surgically moved aside to allow for radiation therapy to the abdominal region.

Ooplasm. A liquid material in the oocyte that enables it to mature.

PCO. Polycystic ovarian syndrome; a condition characterized by small cysts on the ovaries that interfere with normal ovulation.

Pyospermia. High white blood cell count in a semen analysis, indicating possible infection.

Repeated miscarriage. Clinically called *habitual abortion* or *recurrent fetal loss*, this term is reserved for women who have miscarried more than twice in a row prior to twenty weeks.

Rh incompatibility. Occurs when your partner is Rh positive, you are Rh negative, and your baby's blood type does not match yours. Can be a problem during delivery or even during a miscarriage or therapeutic abortion.

ROSNI. Round spermatid nuclear injection; where immotile or immature sperm can be obtained directly from the testicle.

Rubella. Also called *German measles*, this condition can damage the fetus in early pregnancy.

Salpingectomy. Removal of the fallopian tube.

Secondary infertility. Infertility after giving birth to one or more children. Age and/or endometriosis are usual causes.

Selective reduction. Where one or more fetuses is aborted in order to save the life of one or more fetuses in utero.

Spontaneous abortion. Miscarriage before twenty weeks.

STDs. Sexually transmitted disease, which replaces the outdated term venereal disease (VD).

Syphilis. Once a very serious, incurable sexually transmitted disease (STD) of which "madness" was sometimes the result; syphilis is now easily treated with antibiotics.

Teratospermia. Poor sperm morphology (shape).

Therapeutic abortion (TA). Deliberate termination of pregnancy for medical or social reasons.

Threatened abortion. When your cervix is still closed and holding everything in securely, but you're having cramps and bleeding or staining. In some cases, the bleeding will stop and the pregnancy will continue normally. In other cases, you might miscarry anyway because of unsalvageable problems, such as severe genetic deformities.

Urinary tract infections (UTIs). Very common bacterial infections that afflict about 10 percent of pregnant women.

Viscosity (of semen). The consistency of semen (thickening is abnormal).

Volume (of semen). The amount of semen (about 1 teaspoon is normal).

ZIFT. Zygote intrafallopian transfer; where the fertilized, but undivided sperm and egg are artificially placed directly into the fallopian tubes. An outdated procedure, which some clinics still may be offering.

Zona pellucida. The "shell" of the embryo, which must dissolve before it can implant.

Zygote. A fertilized egg before it has undergone cell division.

Bibliography

Chapter 1

"Advocates Cite Cancer Rates in Calling for Pesticide Curbs." *The New York Times*, 18 February 1994: 6.

"Body of Evidence: The Effects of Chlorine on Human Health." Greenpeace, 1994.

Castleman, Michael. "Down for the Count." *Mother Jones*, February 1996.

"The Childless Outcasts of Africa." *Globe and Mail*, 12 August 1995.

Colborn, Theo, John Peterson Myers, and Dianne Dumanoski. *Our Stolen Future*. New York: Dutton, 1996.

Cotton, Paul. "Environmental Estrogenic Agents Area of Concern." *The Journal of the American Medical Association* 271 (9 February 1994): 414, 416.

"Counts Rising Since 70s." *The Journal of Urology* 157 (1997): 840–843.

Davis, D. L., et al. "Medical Hypothesis: Xenoestrogens As Preventable Causes of Breast Cancer." *Environmental Health Perspectives* 101, no. 5 (1993): 372–377.

"Decline in Danish Sperm Counts." *Fertility and Sterility* 68 (1997): 1059–1064.

"Decline in Sperm." *Reuter Information Service*, 2 January 1997.

DeMarco, Carolyn. "Military Research: Endometriosis and Environmental Toxins Linked?" *Wellness MD* 4, no. 2 (March/April 1994): 23.

Eighth Biennial Report on Great Lakes Water Quality, Under the Great Lakes Water Quality Agreement of 1978, to the Governments of the United States and Canada and the State and Provincial Governments of the Great Lakes Basin. Washington D.C.: International Joint Commission, 1996.

Emanuel, E. J., and Emanuel, L. L. "Four Models of the Physician-Patient Relationship." *Journal of the American Medical Association* 267, no. 16 (1992): 2221–2226.

"EPA to Study Safety of an Insecticide." *The New York Times*, 24 October 1993: 10.

Epstein, Samuel S. "Pesticides Pose a Lifelong Threat." *The New York Times*, 29 August 1994: 14.

"Estrogens Influence Male Fertility." *Nature* 390 (1997): 449–450, 509–512.

"Evidence for Estrogen." *The Medical Post*, 9 April 1996: 75–76.

"Families Are Shrinking." *Globe and Mail*, 8 July 1995.

Findlay, Deborah A., and Leslie J. Miller. "Medical Power and Women's Bodies." In *Women, Medicine and Health*, edited by B. S. Bolaria and R. Bolaria. Halifax: Fernwood, 1994.

Fox, Maggie. "Expert: Sperm Counts Falling Around the World." *Reuters*, 24 November 1997.

Gillis, Anna Maria. "Wildlife Indicators Worrying." *Bioscience* 44 (May 1994): 296–298.

———. "Research Update: From the Washington, D.C. Meeting on Estrogens in the Environment: Global Health Implications." *Bioscience* 44, no. 5: 296–298.

Highfield, Roger. "Gender-bending Chemicals 'May Cause Cancers.'" *Daily Telegraph*, London, 26 July 1995: 4.

Hodges, John. "Sperm—Down for the Count?" *Wellness MD* 3, no. 4 (July/August 1993): 10.

Immen, Walter. "B.C. Study Quantifies Risk of Delaying Childbirth." *Globe and Mail*, 28 October 1997.

Johnson, Jeff. "Will Our Stolen Future Be Another Silent Spring?" *Environmental Science & Technology News* 30, no. 4 (1996): 168–170.

Kelsey, Jennifer L., and Esther M. John. "Lactation and the Risk of Breast Cancer." *New England Journal of Medicine* 330, no. 2 (13 January 1994): 136–137.

Khatamee, Masood A., M.D. "Infertility: A Preventable Epidemic?" *International Journal of Fertility* 33, no. 4 (1988): 246–51.

———. "Putting Infertility Prevention Before Treatment—A Physician's Plea." *The Journal of Clinical Practice in Sexuality* 7, no. 3. (1988): 11–18.

LeBlanc, Gerald A. "Are Environmental Sentinels Signaling?" *Environmental Health Perspectives* 103, no. 10 (October 1995).

"Male Infertility on the Rise." *Infertility Helper* (March 1996).

Mastroianni, Anna C., Ruth Faden, and Daniel Federman, eds. *Women and Health Research: Ethical and Legal Issues of Including Women in Clinical Studies,* vol. 1. Washington: National Academy Press, 1994.

Occupational Exposures May Affect Sperm Counts. Retrieved November 15, 2001 from http://www.medem.com/medlb/artcle_detaillb.cfm?article_ID=ZZZJ9D9TMGC& sub_cat=624

Ontario Task Force on the Primary Prevention of Cancer. *Recommendations for the Primary Prevention of Cancer: Report of the Ontario Task Force on the Primary Prevention of Cancer to the Ontario Ministry of Health*. March 1995.

Raloff, J. A. "Plastics May Shed Chemical Estrogens." *Science News* 144 (3 July 1993): 12.

Raloff, Janet. "Ecocancers." *Science News* 144 (3 July 1993): 10–13.

Rather, John. "L.I. is Pressuring Albany to Check Perils of Pesticides." *The New York Times*, 27 February 1994: 1.

Reaney, Patricia, "Report Probes Chemical Link to Disappearing Sperm." *Reuter's News Service*, London, 25 July 1995.

Sex, Teens, and Public Schools. PBS, October 1995.

Sex Under Siege. Canadian Broadcasting Corporation, 1994.

Sherwin, Susan. *Patient No Longer: Feminist Ethics and Health Care*. Philadelphia: Temple University Press, 1984.

Shore, Laurence S., Michael Gurevitz, and Mordechai Shemesh. "Estrogen as an Environmental Pollutant." *Bulletin of Environmental Contamination and Toxicology* 51 (September 1993): 361–366.

Soto, Ana M., Honorata Justicia, Jonathan W. Wray, and Carlos Sonnenschein. "p-Nonyl-Phenol: An Estrogenic Xenobiotic Released from 'Modified' Polystyrene." *Environmental Health Perspectives* 92 (1991): 167–173.

Soto, Ana M., Kerrie L. Chung, and Carlos Sonnenschein. "The Pesticides Endosulfan, Toxaphene, and Dieldrin Have Estrogenic Effects on Human Estrogen-Sensitive Cells." *Environmental Health Perspectives* 102 (February 1994).

Steingraber, Sandra. *Living Downstream: An Ecologist Looks at Cancer and the Environment*. New York: Addison-Wesley, 1997.

Stevens, William K. "Pesticides May Leave Legacy of Hormonal Chaos." *The New York Times*, 23 August 1994: C1.

Thornton, Joe. "Chlorine, Human Health and the Environment: The Breast Cancer Warning." Greenpeace, 1993.

"Toxics that Tamper with Hormones." *Eagle's Eye: World Wildlife Fund Canada Newsletter*, Summer 1995.

Winnett, Richard A., Abby C. King, and David Altman. *Health Psychology and Public Health: An Integrated Approach*. New York: Pergamon Press, 1989.

Worzel, Richard. *Facing the Future*. Toronto: Key Porter, 1992.

Wright, Lawrence. "Silent Sperm." *New Yorker*, 15 January 1996.

Chapter 2

Auger, Jacques, M.D., Ph.D., et al. "Decline in Semen Quality Among Fertile Men in Paris During the Past 20 Years." *The New England Journal of Medicine* 332, no. 5 (2 February 1995).

Cain, Joanna M., M.D., and Albert R. Jonsen. "Specialists and Generalists in Obstetrics and Gynecology: Conflicts of Interest in Referral and an Ethical Alternative." *The Jacobs Institute of Women's Health* 2, no. 3 (Fall 1992).

Centers for Disease Control and Prevention, National Center for Infectious Diseases and the U.S. Department of Health and Human Services. "Group B Steptococcal Infections." Brochure. Washington, D.C.: August 1997.

Chez, Ronald A., M.D., and Franklin J. Apfel, M.D. "Women's Health Care: Rights and Responsibilities." *The Jacobs Institute of Women's Health* 2, no. 3 (Fall 1992).

Dewitt, Don, M.D. "Family Physicians, Pap Smears, and Colposcopy." *American Family Physician*, January 1992.

Howards, Stuart S., M.D. "Treatment of Male Infertility." *The New England Journal of Medicine* 332, no. 5 (2 February 1995).

Infertility: Your Role on the Medical Team. Utica, N.Y.: Ferre Institute, Inc., 1994.

Jones, Howard W., Jr., M.D., and James P. Toner, M.D., Ph.D. "The Infertile Couple: Current Concepts." *The New England Journal of Medicine* 329, no. 23 (2 December 1993).

Malesky, Gale, and Charles B. Inlander. "Book Extra: What You Should Know About Pap Tests." *People's Medical Society Newsletter* 10 (April 1991).

————. *Take This Book to the Gynecologist with You: A Consumer's Guide to Women's Health.* New York: Addison-Wesley, 1991.

Maurer, Janet, M.D. *How to Talk to Your Doctor.* New York: Simon & Schuster, 1986.

Morales, Karla, and Charles B. Inlander. *Take This Book to the Obstetrician with You.* New York: Addison-Wesley, 1991.

"Patient's Bill of Rights." Ottawa: Infertility Awareness Association of Canada patient information, 1994.

Rees, Susan. "Doubting Our Doctors." *Weight Watchers*, May 1993.

Rosenthal, M. Sara. *The Gynecological Sourcebook.* Los Angeles: Lowell House, 1994.

————. *The Pregnancy Sourcebook.* Los Angeles: Lowell House, 1994.

————. *The Thyroid Sourcebook.* Los Angeles: Lowell House, 1993.

Chapter 3

"Chemicals, VDTs Affect Fertility." *Journal of Occupational and Environmental Medicine* 39, no. 2 (1997): 138–146.

Howards, Stuart S., M.D. "Treatment of Male Infertility." *The New England Journal of Medicine* 332, no. 5 (2 February 1995).

"Infant Health Effects Noted at Landfill." *Environmental Health Perspectives* 105, no. 8 (1997): 856–861.

Miller Chernier, Nancy. *Reproductive Hazards at Work: Men, Women, and the Fertility Gamble*. Ottawa: Canadian Advisory Council on the Status of Women, 1982.

"Parental Age Gap Determines Sex of First Child." *Reuters*, 24 September 1997.

Petrenko, Alexa. "Creating Fertile Ground: Safe and Natural Approaches to Overcoming Infertility." *Vitality*, November 1992.

Rowland, Andrew S. "Reduced Fertility Among Women Employed As Dental Assistants Exposed to High Levels of Nitrous Oxide." *New England Journal of Medicine*, 1 October 1992.

"Shampoo Chemicals Linked to Sperm Quality." *The Canadian Press*, 28 September 1995.

"Sperm-density Study Surprising." *Globe and Mail*, 10 June 1994.

Chapter 4

"Basal Body Temperature Charts." Mississauga, Ontario: Serono Canada, Inc. patient information, 1994.

Garner, Catherine H., and Grant W. Patton, M.D. *Pathways to Parenthood*. Mississauga, Ontario: Serono Canada, Inc., 1994.

"Getting Pregnant Naturally Depends on Your Combined Fertility." Toronto: Justisse Group client information, 1994.

"Justisse Method for Fertility Management." Toronto: Justisse Group client information, 1994.

Rosenthal, M. Sara. *The Gynecological Sourcebook*. Los Angeles: Lowell House, 1994.

"Saliva Shows Fertile Period." *Globe and Mail*, 24 January 1996.

"Saliva Test Aids Conception." *Reuters*, 27 February 1997.

"Temperature Record." Ottawa: Infertility Awareness Association of Canada client information, 1994.

Chapter 5

Adler, Alexis. "The Importance of Semen Analysis in Assessing Male Factor Infertility." Ottawa: Infertility Awareness Association of Canada client information, 1994.

Blank, William, M.D. "Electroejaculation and Vibratory Stimulation for Sperm Retrieval in Men with Ejaculatory Disturbances." Ottawa: Infertility Awarness Association of Canada client information, 1994.

Braverman, Andrea Mechanick. "The Psychosocial Issues in Male Infertility." Ottawa: Infertility Awareness Association of Canada client information, 1994.

Gagnon, Claude, Ph.D. "The Study of Male Infertility." *Journal of the Infertility Awareness Association of Canada* 3 (October 1996).

"Getting Pregnant Naturally Depends on Your Combined Fertility." Toronto: Justisse Group client information, 1994.

Greendale, Gail, et al. "The Relationship of Chlamydia Trachomatis Infection in Male Infertility." *The American Journal of Public Health*, July 1993.

Howards, Stuart S., M.D. "Treatment of Male Infertility." *The New England Journal of Medicine* 332, no. 5 (2 February 1995).

"Infertile Men May Have Missing DNA." *The New England Journal of Medicine* 336 (1997): 534–539, 576–577.

The Infertility Workup: What to Expect. Utica, N.Y.: Ferre Institute, Inc.

Jackson, Ted. "Male Infertility: Breaking the Silence." Ottawa: The Infertility Awareness Association of Canada client information, 1994.

Jarvi, Keith, M.D., FRCS. "Options for Management of Male Infertility." *Journal of the Infertility Awareness Association of Canada* 3 (October 1996).

———. Interview with author. Mt. Sinai Hospital, Toronto, Ontario, 1994.

Karpen, Maxine. "Varicocele Linked to Ongoing Decline in Fertility." Ottawa: Infertility Awareness Association of Canada client information, 1994.

Lipshultz, M.D. *Male Infertility*. Serono Symposia, USA, 1993.

Meistrich, M. L., et al. "Increase of Cyclophosphamide on Long-term Reduction in Sperm Count in Men Treated with Combination Chemotherapy for Ewing and Soft-tissue Sarcomas." *Cancer Weekly*, 14 December 1992.

Mercer, Todd. "Lost in the Male Factor Maze." *Journal of the Infertility Awareness Association of Canada* 3 (October 1996).

Myers, Michael, M.D. "Male Gender-related Issues in Reproductive Technology." *Psychiatric Aspects of Reproductive Technology*. Washington, D.C.: American Psychiatric Press, 1990.

Shlagman, Roy. "Infertility: A Male Perspective." Somerville, Mass.: Resolve client information, 1994.

Takefman, Janet, Ph.D. "Psychological Issues in Male Factor Infertility." *Journal of the Infertility Awareness Association of Canada* 3 (October 1996).

Zoldbrod, Aline P. "Decisionmaking in Male Fertility." Patient information handout, November 1987.

———. "Men's Reaction to Infertility: Their Feelings Are Concealed." Infertility Awareness Association of Canada's *Insights into Infertility*, Summer 1991.

Chapter 6

Batista, Marcelo, et al. "Comparative Analysis of Progesterone and Placental Protein Measurements in the Evaluation of Luteal Function." *American Journal of Obstetrics and Gynecology*, May 1993.

Doherty, Carolyn M. "Transvaginal Ultrasonography and the Assessment of Luteal Phase Endometrium." *American Journal of Obstetrics and Gynecology*, June 1993.

Domar, Alice D., et al. "The Prevalence and Predictability of Depression in Infertile Women." *Fertility and Sterility* 58, no. 6 (December 1992).

Fritz, Mark, Ronald Holmes, and Edward Keenan. "Effect of Clomiphene Citrate Treatment on Endometrial Estrogen and Progesterone Receptor Induction in Women." *American Journal of Obstetrics and Gynecology*, July 1991.

"General Guideline for Treatment of Infertility." Ottawa: Infertility Awareness Association of Canada client information.

The Infertility Workup: What to Expect. Utica, N.Y.: Ferre Institute, Inc.

Jones, Howard W., Jr., M.D., and James P. Toner, M.D., Ph.D. "The Infertile Couple: Current Concepts." *The New England Journal of Medicine* 329, no. 23 (2 December 1993).

Miller, Kathleen D. "Hodgkin's Disease: Impact on Childbearing." *The Journal of Perinatal and Neonatal Nursing*, March 1994.

Polycystic Ovarian Disease: A Guide for Patients. Birmingham, Ala.: American Fertility Society, 1994.

Rosenthal, M. Sara. *The Gynecological Sourcebook.* Los Angeles: Lowell House, 1994.

The Turner's Syndrome Society. Concord, Ontario: Turner's Syndrome Society of Canada patient information, 1994.

Chapter 7

Braverman, Andrea Mechanick. "The Psychosocial Issues in Male Infertility." Ottawa: Infertility Awareness Association of Canada client information.

"Eggs Could Be Frozen 20 Years." *Guardian Weekly*, 6 August 1995.

Gonzales, Frank, Denise Hatala, and Leon Speroff. "Adrenal and Ovarian Steroid Hormone Responses to Gonadotropin-releasing Hormone Agonist Treatment in Polycystic Ovarian Syndrome." *American Journal of Obstetrics and Gynecology*, September 1991.

Jarvi, Keith, M.D. Interview with author. Mt. Sinai Hospital, Toronto, Ontario, 1994.

Jones, Howard W., Jr., M.D., and James P. Toner, M.D., Ph.D. "The Infertile Couple: Current Concepts." *The New England Journal of Medicine* 329, no. 23 (2 December 1993).

Lipshultz, M.D. Male Infertility. Norwell, Mass.: Serono Symposia, USA, 1993.

Polycystic Ovarian Disease: A Guide for Patients. Birmingham, Ala.: American Fertility Society patient information, 1994.

Rosenthal, M. Sara. *The Gynecological Sourcebook*. Los Angeles: Lowell House, 1994.

Shlagman, Roy. "Infertility: A Male Perspective." Somerville, Mass.: Resolve client information, 1994.

Utiger, Robert, M.D. "Restoring Fertility in Women with PCOS." *The New England Journal of Medicine* 335, no. 9 (29 August 1996).

Wood, Carl E., Jillian M. Shaw, and Alan O. Trounson. "Potential 'Reproductive Insurance' for Women at Risk of Early Ovarian Failure." *Medical Journal of Australia* 166 (1997): 366–369.

Zoldbrod, Aline P. "Men's Reaction to Infertility: Their Feelings Are Concealed." *Insights Into Infertility*, Summer 1991.

Chapter 8

American Society for Reproductive Medicine. *Laparoscopy and Hysteroscopy: A Guide for Patients*. American Society for Reproductive Medicine, 1997.

American Society for Reproductive Medicine. *Ovulation Drugs: A Guide for Patients*. American Society for Reproductive Medicine, 1995.

"Answers to Common Questions About Clomiphene Therapy." Mississauga, Ontario: Serono Canada Inc. patient information, 1994.

Baraldi, Rosanna. "Ovulation Inductors and DES: Is History Repeating Itself?" *DES Action Newsletter*, Summer 1992.

———. "Evaluation of a Long-term Consequences of Drug Testing . . . Where Is the Progress?" *DES Action Newsletter*, Summer 1992.

Contribution of Assisted Reproductive Technology and Ovulation-Inducing Drugs to Triplet and Higher-Order Multiple Births—United States, 1980–1997. Retrieved November 15, 2001, from http://www.cdc.gov/mmwr/preview/mmwrhtml/mm4924a4.htm

"Clomiphene Citrate Tablets." Jerusalem: Serono Laboratories, Inc. factsheet.

Eberlein, Tamara. "Too many babies?" *Redbook*, August 1996, 88.

Fertility Drugs As a Risk Factor for Ovarian Cancer. Retrieved November 15, 2001, from http://cis.nci.nih.gov/fact/3_6.htm

Fertility Drugs Do Not Raise Breast, Ovarian or Uterine Cancer Risk. Retrieved November 15, 2001 from http://www.agi-usa.org/pubs/journals/3210000.html

"Fertility Drugs May Raise Ovarian Cancer Risk." *Journal of the National Cancer Institute* 85, no. 2 (20 January 1993).

"First Recombinant Fertility Treatment Available in the U.S." P\S\L Consulting Group Inc., 30 September 1997.

Fritz, Mark, Ronald Holmes, and Edward Keenan. "Effects of Clomiphene Citrate Treatment on Endometrial Estrogen and Progesterone Receptor Induction in Women." *American Journal of Obstetrics and Gynecology*, July 1991.

Herman, Robin. "Dying to Conceive." *Mirabella*, July 1994.

Howards, Stuart S., M.D., "Treatment of Male Infertility." *The New England Journal of Medicine* 332, no. 5 (2 February 1995).

Infertility Care with Humegon. Scarborough, Ontario: Organon, Canada.

"Infertility Treatment Using Hormone-based Therapies Is Proven Safe and Effective." Serono, Corporate Communications North America news release.

Jones, Howard W., Jr., M.D., and James P. Toner, M.D., Ph.D. "The Infertile Couple: Current Concepts." *The New England Journal of Medicine* 329, no. 23 (2 December 1993).

Maranto, Gina. "Embryo Overpopulation." *Scientific American*, April 1996: 16.

Marrs, Richard, M.D., and Stuart Hartz. "Comments on the Possible Association Between Ovulation Inducing Agents and Ovarian Cancer." Birmingham, Ala.: The American Fertility Society, January 1993.

"Menotropins (Systemic) Advice for the Patient." *Drug Information in Lay Language*, ed. 14 (1994).

"Metrodin." Aubonne, Switzerland: Serono Laboratories Inc. factsheet, 1994.

Mosgaard, Berit Jul, et al. "The Impact of Parity, Infertility and Treatment with Fertility Drugs on the Risk of Ovarian Cancer." *Scandinavian Journal of Obstetrics Gynecology* 76 (1997).

"New Product Brings Recombinant Technology to the Aid of Infertile Couples." P\S\L Consulting Group Inc., 30 September 1997.

"No Proven Link Between Ovarian Cancer and Infertility Drug Treatment." Serono, Corporate Communications North America news release, 1993.

Organon Canada Ltd. *Infertility Care with Humegon*. Organon Canada Ltd., 1997.

"Ovarian Cancer Risk Assessed in Comprehensive Study." Stanford University Medical Center news release, 13 January 1993.

Ovulation Induction. Cambridge, England: Organon Laboratories, Ltd., 1994.

"Pergonal." Aubonne, Switzerland: Serono Laboratories Inc., factsheet.

Pergonal/Profasi Therapy. Mississauga, Ontario: Serono Canada.

Polycystic Ovarian Disease. Birmingham, Ala.: American Fertility Society, 1994.

"Questions and Answers for the Metrodin Patient." Mississauga, Ontario: Serono Canada Inc. patient information.

"Risks of Ovarian Cancer." Mississauga, Ontario: Serono Canada Inc. factsheet.

Rosenthal, M. Sara. *The Gynecological Sourcebook*. Los Angeles: Lowell House, 1994.

Serono Canada, Inc. *Fertinorm HP*. Serono Canada, Inc., 1995.

Tennant, Deborah. "Importing Drugs is Risky." *Infertility Helper*, September 1996.

Wente, Margaret. "Those Troubling Septs." *The Globe and Mail*, 29 November 1997.

Whittemore, Alice S., Robin Harris, Jacqueline Itnyre, and the Collaborative Ovarian Cancer Group. "Characteristics Relating to Ovarian Cancer Risk: Collaborative Analysis of 12 U.S. Case-Control Studies." *American Journal of Epidemiology* 136, no. 10 (1992).

Willemsen, Wim, et al. "Ovarian Stimulation and Ganulosa-Cell Tumor." *The Lancet*, 17 April 1993.

Women's Health Interactive. Infertility Center Website, 1997.

Chapter 9

Alikani, Mina, and Jacques Cohen. "Advances in Clinical Micromanipulation of Gametes and Embryos: Assisted Fertilization and Hatching." *Archives of Pathology and Laboratory Medicine* 116, no. 4 (April 1992).

American Society for Reproductive Medicine. "The Role of Hatching in IVF: A Review of the Literature." A Practice Committee Report, August 2000.

ART: Assisted Reproductive Technologies. Mississauga, Ontario: Serono Canada, Inc.

A.R.T. & Law: Frozen Embryo Custody. Retrieved November 15, 2001, from http://infertility.about.com/library/weekly/aa041500a.htm

ART Success Rates. Retrieved November 15, 2001, from http://www.rscbayarea.com/success_rates.html

Asch, Ricardo H., M.D., and Serono Symposia, U.S.A. GIFT: *Gamete Intra-Fallopian Transfer*. Norwell, Mass.: Serono Symposia, U.S.A.

Assael, Shaun. "Immaculate Deception." *SmartMoney*, August 1993.

Baker, Robin, Ph.D. *Sperm Wars: The Science of Sex*. New York: HarperCollins Publishing, Inc., 1996.

Begley, Sharon. "Infertility: Has the Hype Outweighed the Hope?" *Newsweek*, 4 September 1995.

Belkin, Lisa, "Pregnancy at 51." *The New York Times Magazine*, 26 October 1997: 36.

Bruni, Frank. "Brave New World." *The New York Times*, 8 July 1997.

Canadian Fertility and Andrology Society. "First Hint of ICSI Risks." *CFAS Communique*, January 1996.

Changing Face of Gamete Donation. Seminar presented by the Infertility Network, 1996.

Charbonneau, Leo. "New Procedure Offers 'Truly Outstanding' Pregnancy Rates." Reprinted by Infertility Awareness Association, Canada, November 1993.

Charting, Acupuncture, Shiatsu. Seminar presented by the Infertility Network, 1996.

Clayton, Christine E., and Gabor T. Kovacs. "AID Offspring: Initial Follow-up Study of 50 Couples." *The Medical Journal of Australia*, 17 April 1982.

Cohen, Jacques, et al. "Controversies and Opinions in Clinical Microsurgical Fertilization." *Journal of Assisted Reproductive and Genetics* 9, no. 2 (1992).

Cummins, J. M. and Anne M. Jequier. "Concerns and Recommendations for Intracytoplasmic Sperm Injection (ICSI) Treatment." *Human Reproduction* 10, supp. (1995): 138–143.

DI: Issues, Disclosure, Doctors. Seminar presented by the Infertility Network, 1996.

Domar, Alice D. "The Mind/Body Program for Infertility: A New Behavioral Treatment Approach for Women with Infertility." *Fertility and Sterility* 53, no. 2 (February 1990).

Domar, Alice D., Patricia C. Zuttermeister, Machelle Seibel, M.D., and Herbert Benson, M.D. "Psychological Improvement in Infertile Women after Behavioral Treatment: A Replication." *Fertility and Sterility* 58, no. 1 (July 1992).

"Donor Egg Fluid Helped Overcome Infertility, Researchers Say." *The Associated Press*, 18 July 1997.

"Donor Insemination: A New Beginning." Oakland, Calif.: The Sperm Bank of California patient information.

"Donor Sperm—A Happy Ending." *Lifetime* newsletter, Toronto East General Hospital and IVF Canada, April 1993.

"Ethics and New Reproductive Technologies." *Infertility Helper*, June 1996.

"Fertility Clinics: What Are the Odds?" *Consumer Reports*, February 1996.

"Fertility Treatment May Pose Risk." *The Toronto Star*, 21 November 1997.

Frontiers of Cloning. *The New York Times*, 27 November 2001.

Gordon, Jon W. "Controversies in Assisted Reproduction: Current Unresolved Controversies in Micromanipulation-Assisted Fertilization." *Journal of Assisted Reproduction and Genetics* 9, no. 3 (June 1992).

Grady, Denise. "How to Coax New Life." *Time*, 15 November 1996: 29.

"Guidelines for Oocyte Donation." *The American Family Society Supplement* 1, no. 2 (February 1993): 59.

Hoffman, Jan. "Egg Donations Meet a Need and Raise Ethical Questions." *The New York Times*, 7 January 1996.

The House of Commons of Canada. Bill C-47, *First Reading*, 14 June 1996.

Howards, Stuart S., M.D. "Treatment of Male Infertility." *The New England Journal of Medicine* 332, no. 5 (2 February 1995).

"How to Choose an In Vitro Fertilization (IVF) Program." Ottawa: Infertility Awareness Association of Canada patient information.

Implementation of the Fertility Clinic Success Rate and Certification Act of 1992: A Model Program for the Certification of Embryo Laboratories Federal Register Notice, 21 July 1999 (vol. 64, no. 139).

Ince, Susan. "What Price Fertility?" *More* (May/June 1999): 149–153.

Infertility Information. Bay Area Fertility & Gynecology Medical Group, 1996.

Infertility Myths and Facts. Retrieved November 15, 2001, from: http://www.resolve.org/mythfact.htm

Jones, Howard W., Jr., M.D., and James P. Toner, M.D. "Current Concepts: The Infertile Couple." *The New England Journal of Medicine*, December 1993.

Kolata, Gina. "Company Says It Produced Human Embryo Clones," *The New York Times*, 26 November 2001.

Kolata, Gina with Andrew Pollack. "A Breakthrough on Cloning? Perhaps, or Perhaps Not Yet. *The New York Times*, 27 November 2001.

Lasker, Judith N., and Susan Borg. *In Search of Parenthood: Coping with Infertility and High-Tech Conception.* Boston: Beacon Press, 1987.

Lee, Felicia R. "The Fertility Market: Support and Solace." *The New York Times*, 9 January 1996.

Lerner, Sharon. "The Price of Eggs: Undercover in the Infertility Industry." *Ms.*, March/April 1996.

Levine, R. J. *Ethics and Regulation of Clinical Research.* New Haven, Conn.: Yale University Press, 1988.

Levine Slover, Sandra. "Third Party Conception: The Ambivalent Solution." *Infertility Awareness* 5, no. 6 (July/August 1989).

"Live-Birth Rates and Multiple-Birth Risk Using In Vitro Fertilization." *Journal of the American Medical Association* 282, no. 19, 17 November 1999.

Marrs, Richard P., M.D., and Serono Symposia, U.S.A. In Vitro Fertilization and Embryo Replacement. Norwell, Mass.: Serono Symposia, U.S.A.

Mattes, Jane. "Should Donor Insemination Information Be More Available?" *Single Mothers by Choice* 44 (March 1993).

Mickleburgh, Rod. "Fertility Programs Attacked in Study: 'Very Alarming' AIDS Risk Cited." *Globe and Mail*, 28 April 1993.

Mullen, Michelle A., MHP, Ph.D. "Informed Consent and Treatment for Male Factor Infertility." *Journal of the Infertility Awareness Association of Canada* 3 (October 1996).

Nagourney, Eric. "A Common Link in Failed Pregnancies." *The New York Times*, 15 June 1999: D10.

"New Applications in Assisted Reproductive Technology: Donor Eggs." The Toronto Hospital.

107th CONGRESS Equity in Fertility Coverage Act of 2001. Retrieved November 15, 2001, from: http://www.inciid.org/HR568-infertility.html

Pedwell, Susan. "Fertile Possibilities." *Canadian Living*, November 1995.

Rosenthal, Elisabeth. "Lives Begun in a Lab Generate Joy, Love, and a New Frontier of Issues." *The New York Times*, 10 January 1996.

Rosenthal, M. Sara. *The Gynecological Sourcebook*. Los Angeles: Lowell House, 1994.

————. *The Pregnancy Sourcebook*. Los Angeles: Lowell House, 1994.

Rutter, Virginia. "Who Stole Fertility?" *Psychology Today*, March/April 1996: 46.

Saltus, Richard. "Postmortem Sperm Donation is Getting More Common." *The Boston Globe*, 28 May 1997.

"Secrecy in DI: The 'Advantages' Are the Disadvantages." Ottawa: Infertility Awareness Association of Canada patient information.

"Senate to Vote on Two Bills." *The New York Times*, 30 November 2001.

"The Sexual Legacy of Infertility: The Separation of Procreation and Recreation." *The Canadian Journal of Human Sexuality* 2, no. 3 (Fall 1993).

Skelly, Andrew. "New Methods Help Mens' Fertilization Chances." *The Medical Post* 31, no. 20 (23 May 1995).

————. "For the Infertile, a High-tech Treadmill." *The New York Times*, 14 December 1997.

State Infertility Insurance Laws. Retrieved November 15, 2001, from http://www.asrm.org/Patients/insur.html

States That Cover Infertility According to the American Society of Reproductive Medicine. Retrieved November 15, 2001, from http://www.inciid.org/bb9/message9/1134.htm

Stolberg, Sheryl Gay. "Bush Denounces Cloning and Calls for Ban," *The New York Times*, 27 November 2001.

————. "For the Infertile, a High-tech readmill." *The New York Times*, 14 December 1997.

"Technological Services for Reproductive Medicine." Toronto: ReproMed Ltd. client information.

Toledo, Andrew A., et al. "Electroejaculation in Combination with In Vitro Fertilization and Gamete Micromanipulation of Anejaculatory Male Infertility." *American Journal of Obstetrics and Gynecology*, August 1992.

Tucker, Michael J., et al. "Treatment of Male Infertility and Idiopathic Failure to Fertil-ize In Vitro with Under Zona Insemination and Direct Egg Injection." *American Journal of Obstetrics and Gynecology*, August 1993.

University Hospital, London, Ontario. "Intracytoplasmic Sperm Injection: The Newest Advanced Reproductive Technology." *Infertility Support Newsletter*, Spring 1995.

Van Steirteghem, André C., et al. "Higher Success Rate by Intracytoplasmic Sperm Injection Than by Subzonal Insemination. Report of a Second Series of 300 Consecutive Treatment Cycles." *Human Reproduction* 8, no. 7 (1993): 1055–1060.

Zolbrod, Aline. "The Emotional Distress of the Artificial Insemination Patient." *Medical Psychotherapy* 1 (1998): 161–172.

Zuckerman, Lawrence. "Couple Now Has No Savings, More Debt, and Little Hope of Having a Baby." *The New York Times*, 9 January 1996.

Chapter 10

Gray, D. P., et al. "Heterosexism in Nursing Education." *Journal of Nursing Education* 35, no. 5 (May 1996).

Katrowitz, Barbara. "Gay Families Come Out." *Newsweek*, 4 November 1996.

Lehey, Kathleen A. "Alternative Insemination: Facing the Conceivable Options." *Brondside* 8, no. 1 (1986).

Winnow, Jackie. "Lesbians Evolving Health Care: Cancer and AIDS." In *Women with Cancer Comfort and Epidemic*. Pittsburgh: Cleis, 1991.

Chapter 11

Carson, Sandra A., and John E. Buster. "Ectopic Pregnancy." *The New England Journal of Medicine* 329 (14 October 1993).

"Depressive Symptoms after Miscarriage (Tips from Other Journals)." *American Family Physician* 45 (June 1992).

Drife, James Owen. "Tubal Pregnancy: Rising Incidence, Earlier Diagnosis, More Con-servative Treatment." *British Medical Journal* 301 (10 November 1990).

"Early Detection of Ectopic Pregnancy: Use of a Sensitive Urine Pregnancy Test and Transvaginal Ultrasonography." *Journal of the American Medical Association* 266 (13 November 1991).

"FDA Warns Doctors About At-home Device for Premature Labor." *The Associated Press*, 20 November 1997.

Jones, Deborah. "Recurrent Miscarriages: News about Causes and Treatments." *Chate-laine*, November 1993.

Rai, R., et al. "Randomised Controlled Trial of Aspirin and Aspirin Plus Heparin in Pregnant Women with Recurrent Miscarriage Associated with Phospholipid Antibodies." *British Medical Journal* 314 (1997): 253–257.

Rosenfeld, Jo Ann. "Bereavement and Grieving after Spontaneous Abortion." *American Family Physician* 43 (May 1991).

Rosenthal, M. Sara. *The Pregnancy Sourcebook*. Los Angeles: Lowell House, 1994.

"Significance of Bleeding During First Trimester (Tips from Other Journals)." *American Family Physician* 44 (November 1991).

"Tubal Pregnancies: Casualty of the Modern Lifestyle." *The Women's Letter* 4 (February 1991).

"Use of Ultrasonography to Diagnose Ectopic Pregnancy (Tips from Other Journals)." *American Family Physician* 42 (November 1990).

Zidar, Donna, "Selective Reduction: Could You Make the Choice?" *Journal of the Infertility Awareness Association of Canada* 3 (October 1996).

Chapter 12

"Adoption in the People's Republic of China." Ottawa: Infertility Awareness Association of Canada factsheet.

"Are You Interested in Adopting from China, Peru, El Salvador, China, Guatemala, Poland, or Bulgaria?" Ottawa: Infertilty Awareness Association of Canada factsheet.

Bagley, Gordon. "Magic or Medicine: In Praise of the Healing Touch." *Wellness MD* 4, no. 1 (January/February 1994): 31–38.

Chihal, H. Jane, M.D., and Sister Mary Madonna Baudier, M.D. "Polycystic Ovary Syndrome." *American Family Physician*, April 1985.

"Childless and Second Class." Ottawa: Infertility Awareness Association of Canada factsheet, 1994.

Chisholm, Patricia. "Healers or Quacks? The Controversy over Unconventional Treatments." *Maclean's*, 25 September 1995: 34–42.

Cunningham, Laura. "The Chosen One." *Hers*, 17 April 1994.

Family Focus Adoption Services. Little Neck, N.Y.: client information.

The Ferre Institute. "How to Cope with the Holidays." *Infertility Helper*, no. 2 (December 1995).

"Friends in Adoption." Middletown Springs, Vt.: Friends in Adoption, Inc. client information.

Galcso, Angela. Welland, Ontario: International Adoption Facilitator client information.

Griffin, Katherine. "Alternative Care: Finally Some Coverage." *Health Magazine*, 1995: Document ID mk-9095a.

Harvey, Rosin. "To Do No Harm; Healers and Heretics." *The Toronto Star*, 27 January 1996: L1.

Herman, Flory G. "Private Adoption." Williamsville, N.Y.: attorney client information.

Independent Adoption Centres client information.

International Adoption Consultants. Grand Rapids, Mich.: client information.

Long, Patricia, "Herbal Remedies Really Can Fight Off Colds, Headaches and Other Ills—If You Know How to Use Them Safely." *Health Magazine*, 1995.

"Openness in Adoption." Kingston, Ontario: Adoption Resource and Counselling Services.

Radis, David J. Los Angeles: attorney client information.

Raphael, Larry. Chicago: attorney client information.

Weiss, Rick, "The FDA May Soon Concede That Billions of Chinese Were Right All Along: Acupuncture Works." *Health Magazine*, 1995: Document ID mrw 195a.

General Texts

Bequaert Holmes, Helen, and Laura M. Purdy (eds.). *Feminist Perspectives in Medical Ethics*. Bloomington, Ind.: Indiana University Press, 1992.

DeMarco, Carolyn. *Take Charge of Your Body: A Woman's Guide to Health*. Winlaw, B.C.: The Last Laugh, 1990.

Duster, Troy. *Backdoor to Eugenics*. New York, N.Y.: Routledge, Chapman, and Hall, 1990.

Etchells, E., et al. "Disclosure." *Canadian Medical Association Journal* 155 (1996): 1083–1086.

———. "Voluntariness." *Canadian Medical Association Journal* 155 (1996): 1083–1086.

———. "Consent." *Canadian Medical Association Journal*. {TK}

Frontiers of Cloning. *The New York Times*, 27 November 2001.

Glazier, Lynn. "Playing God: Medical Ethics and History's Forgotten Lessons." In *Misconceptions: The Social Construction of Choice and The New Reproductive and Genetic Technologies*. Hull, Quebec: Sean Fordyce, 1993.

Gorman, Christine. "How Old Is Too Old?" *Time*, 30 September 1991.

Harkness, Carla. *The Infertility Book: A Comprehensive Medical and Emotional Guide*. San Francisco: Volcano Press, 1987.

Hey, Valerie, Catherine Itzin, Lesley Saunders, and Mary Anne Speakman, eds. *Hidden Loss: Miscarriage and Ectopic Pregnancy*. London: The Women's Press Ltd., 1989.

The House of Commons of Canada. Bill C-47. First Reading, June 14, 1996.

Implementation of the Fertility Clinic Success Rate and Certification Act of 1992: A Model Program for the Certification of Embryo Laboratories Federal Register Notice, 21 July 1999 (vol. 64, no. 139).

Kenen, Regina. "The Genetic Reproductive Technology Scene." In *Reproductive Technologies*. San Diego: Greenhaven Press, Inc., 1996.

Lippman, Amy. "Worrying—and Worrying about the Geneticizaton of Reproduction and Health.: In *Misconceptions: The Social Construction of Choice and The New Reproductive and Genetic Technologies*, vol. 1. Quebec: Sean Fordyce, Hull, 1993.

Mullens, Anne. *Missed Conceptions: Overcoming Infertility*. New York: McGraw-Hill, 1990.

Pullen, Heather, and Jocelyn Smith. *Making Babies: A Complete Guide to Fertility and Infertility*. New York: Random House, 1990.

Purdy, Laura M. *Reproducing Persons: Issues in Feminist Bioethics*. Ithaca, N.Y.: Cornell University Press, 1996.

Raab, Diana. *Getting Pregnant and Staying Pregnant: A Guide to Infertility and High-Risk Pregnancy*. Montreal: Sirdan Publishing, 1987.

Rosenthal, M. Sara. *The Gynecological Sourcebook*, 3rd ed. Chicago: Contemporary Books, 1999.

———. *Women and Depression*. Chicago: Contemporary Books, 2000.

Royal Commission on New Reproductive Technologies. *Proceed with Care* (Final Report). Ottawa: Minister of Government Services, vol. 1, 1993.

Seibel, Machelle M., M.D. *Infertility*. Norwalk, Conn.: Appleton and Lange, 1990.

Sherwin, Susan. "Feminist and Medical Ethics: Two Different Approaches to Contextual Ethics." In *Feminist Perspectives in Medical Ethics*, edited by Helen Bequaert Holmes and Laura M. Purdy. Bloomington, Ind.: Indiana University Press, 1992.

———. *Patient No Longer: Feminist Ethics and Health Care*. Philadelphia: Temple University Press, 1984.

Trewinnard, Karen. *Fertility and Conception: The Essential Guide to Maximising Fertility and Conceiving a Healthy Baby*. London: Ward Lock, 1999.

Thobani, Sunera. "From Reproduction to Mal(e) Production: Women and Sex Selection Technology." In *Misconceptions: The Social Construction of Choice and The New Reproductive and Genetic Technologies*, vol. 1. Quebec: Sean Fordyce, Hull, 1993.

Vatican, Congregation for the Doctrine of the Faith. *Instruction on Respect for Human Life in Its Origin and on the Dignity of Procreation: Replies to Certain Questions of the Day*. Rome: Vatican City, 1987.

Veatch, R. M. "Abandoning Informed Consent." *HCR* 25, no. 2 (1995): 5–12.

Warren, Virginia, L. "Feminist Directions in Medical Ethics." In *Feminist Perspectives in Medical Ethics*, edited by Helen Bequaert Holmes and Laura M. Purdy. Bloomington, Ind.: Indiana University Press, 1992.

Index